KUNDALINI, EVOLUTION AND ENLIGHTENMENT

OMEGA BOOKS

The OMEGA BOOKS series from Paragon House is dedicated to classic and contemporary works about higher human development and the nature of ultimate reality, encompassing the fields of mysticism and spirituality, psychic research and paranormal phenomena, the evolution of consciousness, and the human potential for self-directed growth in body, mind and spirit.

John White, M.A.T., Series Editor of OMEGA BOOKS, is an internationally known author, editor, and educator in the fields of consciousness research and higher human development.

MORE TITLES IN OMEGA BOOKS

LIFECYCLES: Reincarnation and the Web of Life
Christopher M. Bache

THE RADIANCE OF BEING: Complexity, Chaos and the Evolution of Consciousness
Allan Combs

THE MEETING OF SCIENCE AND SPIRIT: Guidelines for a New Age
John White

WHAT IS ENLIGHTENMENT? Exploring the Goal of the Spiritual Path
Edited by John White

KUNDALINI: EMPOWERING HUMAN EVOLUTION
Selected Writings of Gopi Krishna
Edited by Gene Kieffer

BEYOND THE HUMAN SPECIES: The Life and Work of Sri Aurobindo and the Mother
Georges Van Vrekhem

KUNDALINI, EVOLUTION AND ENLIGHTENMENT

Edited by John White

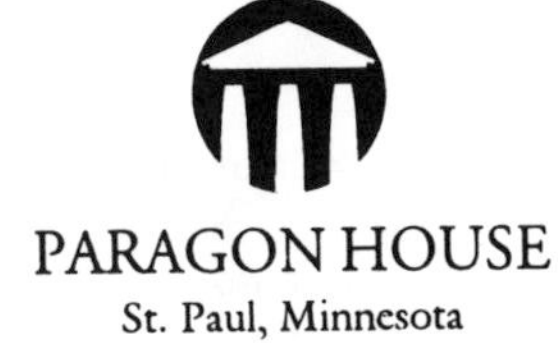

PARAGON HOUSE
St. Paul, Minnesota

First Paragon House edition, 1990

Published in the United States by

Paragon House
2700 University Avenue West
St. Paul, Minnesota 55114

Originally published by Anchor Books, 1979

The Omega Books series from Paragon House is dedicated to classic and contemporary works about human development and the nature of ultimate reality.

Library of Congress Catalog-in-Publication Data

Kundalini, evolution, and enlightenment / edited by John White.—1st Paragon House ed.
p. cm.— (An Omega book)
Reprint. Originally published: Garden City, N.Y.: Anchor Press, 1979.
Includes bibliographical references.
ISBN 1-55778-303-9
I. Kundalini. I. White, John Warren, 1939- . II. Series: Omega book
BL 1238.56.K86K855 1990 89-48894
CIP

Manufactured in the United States of America

The Paper used in this publication meets the minimum requirements of American National Standard for Information Sciences—Permanence of Paper for Printed Library Materials, ANSI Z39.48-1984.

ACKNOWLEDGMENTS

''The Awakening of Kundalini'' is an original article written especially for this book and is printed by permission of the author.

''Kundalini: An Overview'' is abridged from *Kundalini: An Overview* by Swami Sivananda Radha and is reprinted by permission of the author. Copyright © 1977 by Swami Sivananda Radha and published by Timeless Books, Suite 1215, Washington Mutual Building, Spokane, Washington 99201.

''The Psychophysiology of Kundalini'' is excerpted from *Philosophy of Meditation* by Haridas Chaudhuri, © 1974 by Haridas Chaudhuri and published by the Cultural Integration Fellowship, San Francisco, California. Reprinted by permission of Bina Chaudhuri.

''Kundalini Yoga Through Shaktipat'' is an unpublished article and is printed by permission of the author.

''Sri Aurobindo, the Tantra and Kundalini'' is an original article written especially for this book and is printed by permission of the author.

''Signs of an Awakened Kundalini'' is excerpted from *Devatma Shakti* by Swami Vishnu Tirtha, © 1962 by Swami Vishnu Tirtha and published by S. M. Patel, Bombay, India.

''Kundalini and the Tantric Tradition'' is an original article written especially for this book and is printed by permission of the author.

''Is Kundalini Real?'' is Chapter Three of *Nuclear Evolution* by Christopher Hills and is excerpted by permission of the author. Copyright © 1977 by University of the Trees Press, Boulder Creek, California.

''Are the Chakras Real?'' is an original article written especially for this book and is printed by permission of the author.

''Exploring the Myths and Misconceptions of Kundalini'' originally appeared in *Beads of Truth*, 1976, and is reprinted by permission of the magazine and the 3HO Foundation, Los Angeles, California.

''So this Is Kundalini'' is excerpted from ''Simple, Dumb Boring Truths and a Course in Miracles,'' which appeared in *New Realities*, January–February 1977. Copyright © 1977 by Brian Van der Horst.

''Sensual Excitement'' is excerpted from *Play of Consciousness* by Swami Muktananda, © 1974 SYDA Foundation, Oakland, California. All rights reserved. Reprinted by permission.

''Shaktipat'' is a privately published article reprinted by permission of the author.

''Instant Cosmic Consciousness?'' is reprinted by permission from *Fate* magazine, July 1975. Copyright © 1975.

''A Psychic Healer Experiences Kundalini'' is reprinted from *Human Dimensions*, Fall 1975 by permission of the author.

''The Sudden Awakening of Kundalini'' is reprinted by special arrangement with Shambhala Publications, Inc., 1123 Spruce Street, Boulder, Colorado 80302. From *Kundalini, the Evolutionary Energy in Man* by Gopi Krishna, © 1971.

"The Phenomenon of Kundalini" is extracted from a paper by Gopi Krishna presented to the All-India Institute of Medical Sciences at its first seminar on Kundalini research in March 1975. The appended remarks were delivered in June 1975 at a seminar on Kundalini research. Printed by permission of the Kundalini Research Foundation, New York City.

"Kundalini Energy" is reprinted from *Kundalini Quarterly*, Fall 1976, by permission of the Kundalini Research Institute, Pomona, California. All rights reserved.

"The Biological Basis of Kundalini" originally appeared in *Kundalini and Spiritual India*, Vol. 1, No. 1, 1977, and is reprinted by permission of the author.

"Neurochemistry and the Awakening of Kundalini" is reprinted from *Human Dimensions*, Fall 1976, by permission of the author. It is extracted from *Consciousness and the Ergotrophic and Trophotropic Systems of Arousal*, privately published in 1975 by the author.

"Kindling and Kundalini Effects" originally appeared in *Brain/Mind Bulletin*, Vol. 2, No. 7, February 21, 1977, and is reprinted by permission of Interface Press, P.O. Box 42211, Los Angeles, California 90042. Copyright © 1977 Interface Press.

"A Research Note on Kundalini Energy" is excerpted from *American Meditation* by Robert L. Peck, privately published in 1976, and is reprinted by permission of the author.

"Kundalini as Prevention and Therapy for Drug Abuse" is excerpted from "Yoga as Prevention and Therapy for Drug Abuse," which appeared in *Yoga Journal*, Vol. 2, No. 1, March–April 1976. Copyright © 1976 *Yoga Journal*, Berkeley, California. Reprinted by permission of the journal.

"Kundalini: Classical and Clinical" is excerpted from *Kundalini: Psychosis or Transcendence?* by Lee Sannella. Copyright © 1976 by Lee Sannella. Reprinted by permission.

"Micromotion of the Body as a Factor in the Development of the Nervous System" by Itzhak Bentov originally appeared in *Kundalini: Psychosis or Transcendence?* by Lee Sannella and is reprinted by permission of the author.

"Symbolic Expressions of Kundalini Through the Unconscious" originally appeared in *Spiritual India and Kundalini*, Vol. 1, No. 1, 1977, and is reprinted by permission of the author.

"Some Possibilities for Further Kundalini Research" is an original article written especially for this book.

"Stigmata and Kundalini" is an original article written especially for this book and is printed by permission of the author.

"UFOs and Kundalini," by Gene Kieffer, is from *Gods of Aquarius*, copyright © 1976 by Brad Steiger. Reprinted by permission of Harcourt Brace Jovanovich, Inc.

"The Divine Fire: Tumo and Kundalini" is an original article written especially for this book.

''Cults of the Shadow'' is excerpted from *Cults of the Shadow* by Kenneth Grant. Copyright © 1975 by Kenneth Grant and reprinted by permission of the publisher, Samuel Weiser, Inc., New York.

''Christian Mysticism and Kundalini'' is an original article written especially for this book and is printed by permission of the author.

''The Restored New Testament'' is excerpted from *The Restored New Testament* by J. M. Pryse, first published in 1907.

''The Danger of Arousing Kundalini'' is reprinted from *A Treatise on Cosmic Fire* by Alice A. Bailey, by permission of the Lucis Trust, which holds the copyright. No portion of these extracts may be reproduced without permission from the Lucis Trust.

''Kundalini Is Not the Sole Truth'' is abridged and modified from an editorial in *World Union*, March 1976, by permission of the editor.

''The Two Paths to Kundalini'' is extracted from *Kundalini: The Mother-Power* by Sri Chinmoy, © 1974 by the Sri Chinmoy Lighthouse Publishing Co., Jamaica, New York. Reprinted by permission of the publisher.

''Ordered Meditation and Loving Service'' is reprinted from *The Externalization of the Hierarchy* by Alice A. Bailey, by permission of the Lucis Trust, which holds copyright. No portion of these extracts may be reproduced without permission from the Lucis Trust.

''The High Purpose of Kundalini'' is excerpted from *Kundalini: An Occult Experience* by G. S. Arundale. Copyright © 1905 by the Theosophical Publishing House, Adyar, Madras, India, and reprinted by permission.

''Kundalini in Action'' is extracted from *Darshan: The Vision of Light* by Roy Eugene Davis, published by CSA Press, Lakemont, Georgia. Copyright © 1971 by Roy Eugene Davis and reprinted by permission of the author.

To the higher humanity, *Homo noeticus*

And to those sages and seers, ancient and modern, whose selfless service has prepared the birthplace.

Contents

II. A HANDFUL OF PERSONAL ACCOUNTS

III. EXPLORATIONS IN KUNDALINI RESEARCH

IV. KUNDALINI AND THE OCCULT

V. SAGE ADVICE TO THE SEEKER

Introduction

There is a great irony in modern society. At the very moment when science and technology are achieving unprecedented feats in the manipulation of matter, large numbers of people are turning away from them with sadness, even dismay, because these feats have failed to satisfy human aspirations and psychological needs. The ancient dream of peace on earth, world brotherhood, and freedom from the perennial ills of life has not been realized, despite our glittering machines. The dream evades us, and science, for all its genuine benefits, spawns new ills to plague us. It is small wonder that people should look elsewhere for satisfaction and fulfillment.

Call it a Great Awakening, a Rebirth of the Spirit, a Consciousness Revolution, the Coming of the Aquarian Age. Whatever the name, a new and growing phenomenon is making itself felt today throughout society as many people—dissatisfied with a materialistic life-style—seek a higher state of being. These people want to grow spiritually. They want to actualize their inner resources. They want to rise above the old forms that limited freedom and understanding, above the old values that brought about unacceptable conditions. They want to experience the transcendent dimensions of their existence.

Opinion poll researcher George Gallup noted in 1977 that there is a "ground swell of interest in religion" and that tens of millions of Americans are being "energized" by this revival movement. He reports that the United States appears to be in "an early stage of a profound religious revival." Two years earlier, sociologist Andrew Greeley reported in a *New York Times Magazine* article that four out of ten adult Americans have had a mystical experience. The enormous popularity of books such as *Life After Life, Angels, Jonathan Livingston Seagull,* and the Castaneda accounts of Don Juan further indicate the widespread search for the release of human potential.

The search is taking many forms: psychic development, meditation, paraphysics, occultism and true magic, mysticism, eastern religions, transpersonal psychology, UFO cults, evangelical Christianity. What is behind this upsurge of interest in spiritual unfoldment, cosmic contact, and knowledge of supersensible worlds? Is there a common denominator among the multitude of paths claiming to lead to higher consciousness?

This book proposes an answer to these questions—an answer that has vast social and scientific ramifications.

The answer is kundalini.

The Sanskrit word kundalini means "coiled up" like a snake or spring. It implies latent power or untapped potential —the possibility within each person of attaining a new and more fulfilling condition of life. This possibility, of course, is precisely what underlies the surging interest in religious and paranormal phenomena.

Kundalini is traditionally symbolized in yogic texts as a sleeping serpent coiled at the base of the human spine. This indicates its close connection with the reproductive organs and life force. In fact, because according to the kundalini concept there is a direct connection between bioenergy and spiritual experience, some modern scholars translate kundalini as meaning "latent reservoir of energy," "power at rest," and "psychosomatic power center." It objectifies Pascal's maxim, "It is dangerous to tell people of their bestial origins unless at the same time you tell them of their divine potential."

Although the word kundalini comes from the yogic tradition, nearly all the world's major religions, spiritual paths, and genuine occult traditions see something akin to the kundalini experience as having significance in "divinizing" a person. The word itself may not appear in the traditions, but the concept is there nevertheless, wearing a different name yet recognizable as a key to attaining godlike stature.

The kundalini experience, then, considered from the viewpoint of individual transformation, is said to be a path to enlightenment. But if a large number of enlightened people were to appear in society at the same time, the result could well transform society itself. So the kundalini experience, in its broadest aspect, is evolutionary—a path for the advancement of the entire human race to a higher state.

Thus kundalini presents a radical idea that goes to the roots of important social trends involving spiritual seeking and religious reawakening. Just as important, it has significance for a number of related aspects of unfolding human mentality: genius, creativity, intellectual and artistic talent, insanity, psychic powers, sociopathic behavior. Last of all, it is a powerful idea for explaining in a unified way many of the mysteries of the biological, physical, and social sciences. The kundalini concept, it would seem, is a simple, logical, and comprehensive theory of man-in-nature that is accessible to empirical testing.

Some thoughtful members of the scientific, scholarly, and religious communities have already been led to just this conclusion and are seeking to examine the concept in terms of both its ancient traditions and its modern manifestations. Kundalini, as experienced and researched, may well be the means for a higher-level resolution to the antagonism existing in popular thought between science and religion, between technological materialism and unfulfilled human aspirations for a new state of being here on earth. This book is intended to stimulate examination of this possibility by presenting a wide selection of voices from the spectrum of those who have spoken and written about kundalini.

Some of the lines of investigation offered here may appear bizarre or even absurd at first because they are contrary to "common sense" and accepted scientific views. However, nothing need be taken on faith. That would be out of keeping with a basic assumption of this book–namely, that the scientific method can be applied to kundalini as a means of determining its validity and usefulness. All that is asked of you is this. First, examine the evidence critically but with an open mind. Second, judge whether the speculations and inferences are logically derived, coherent, and in accord with those data from science and scholarship that bear on them. Third, do not dismiss the entire kundalini concept if any single part should prove false or untenable. Fourth, remember that a new idea usually does not "make sense" until you have sufficient preparation to receive it. Higher-level integrations often require some degree of dismantling previous mental structures. This can evoke ego-based anxiety, denial, fear, and hostility in which the nonconscious purpose is to prevent change necessary to allow the new integration.

Kundalini is an idea whose time has come–such, at least, is another basic assumption of this book. The invitation offered here is to investigate, experience, reflect, and decide whether the kundalini concept is as significant as this book assumes–my third basic premise.

My final premise is that evolution is still going on, and that it is characterized at the human level primarily by the further development of our mentality. If kundalini is the key to unlocking the spectrum of psychological, psychic, occult, and spiritual phenomena, its importance for you and for all the human race will be enormous, for it would offer no less than an answer to the "riddle of life" and a demonstration of the transcendent cosmic intelligence behind creation.

I

What Is Kundalini?

What exactly is kundalini? The answer has many levels, on which various difficulties and controversies will be encountered. This book will explore them through the words of people whose experience and research have given them insight into the phenomenon of kundalini. However, these articles offer guidelines, not gospel. It will quickly become apparent that there are major divergences of opinion among those regarded as authorities on the subject.

In general, the question can be answered briefly like this. Kundalini is the personal aspect of the universal life force named *prana* by the yogic tradition. This primal cosmic energy is akin, if not identical, to *ch'i* (Chinese), *ki* (Japanese), the Holy Spirit, and various other terms from cultures that identify a life force that is the source of all vital activity. Prana has not yet been identified by modern science, but ancient wisdom maintains that it is the means for raising human awareness to a higher form of perception, variously called illumination, enlightenment, cosmic consciousness, *samadhi*. Kundalini, often referred to as the "serpent power" because it is symbolized by a coiled snake, can be concentrated and channeled through the spine into the brain—a process likewise not yet identified by modern science. The systematized process for accomplishing this upward flowing of energy is known as kundalini yoga.

One of the most ancient treatises on yoga, *Hatha Yoga Pradipika,* describes kundalini this way:

> As one opens the door with a key, so the yogi should open the gate to liberation . . . with the kundalini. The great goddess [kundalini] sleeps, closing with her mouth the opening through which one can ascend to the *brahmarandhra* . . . to that place where there is neither pain nor suffering. The kundalini sleeps above the *kanda.* . . . She gives liberation to the yogi and bondage to the fool. He who knows kundalini knows yoga. The kundalini, it is said, is coiled like a serpent. He who can induce her to move [upward] is liberated. [Vss. 105–10]

Swami Vivikananda, who brought Vedanta to the West at the end of the last century, reinterpreted the ancient wisdom with these words:

> When by the power of long internal meditation the vast mass of energy stored up travels along the *sushumna* and strikes the [*chakras*], the reaction is immensely more intense than the reaction of sense-perception. Wherever there was any manifestation of what is ordinarily called supernatural power or wisdom, there a little current of kundalini must have found its way into the sushumna. Only, in the vast majority of cases, people had ignorantly stumbled on some practice which set free a minute portion of the coiled-up kundalini. All worship, consciously or unconsciously, leads to this end. The man who thinks that he is receiving response to his prayers does not know that the fulfillment comes from his own nature, that he has succeeded by the mental attitude of prayer in waking up a bit of this infinite power which is coiled up within himself. What, thus, man ignorantly worships under various names . . . the yogi declares to the world to be the real power coiled up in every being, the mother of eternal happiness, if we but know how to approach her. And yoga is the science of religion, the rationale of all worship, all prayers, forms, ceremonies and miracles.

Terms such as brahmarandhra, kanda, sushumna, and chakra will be explained in the following pages. Note here, however, that this book is not simply about kundalini yoga and will not give instruction in it.* Rather it is concerned with human potential and the hypothesis that kundalini, as it becomes generally understood by science and society, offers the next step in human evolution. That step will not be a physical development but a change in consciousness.

Dr. Karan Singh, formerly the Minister of Health and Family Planning in the government of India, proposed this hypothesis in October 1974 when he gave the welcoming address to twenty-three hundred scientists gathered in New Delhi for the International Congress of Physiological Sciences. In his speech, he raised these fundamental questions about human potential, scientific research, and planetary society:

> Man's predominant faculty is the capacity to be conscious of himself and his surroundings. What is the texture of this consciousness? What are the links between the genetic structure of man and his capacity for conscious awareness? Can manipulating the one influence the other? What are the functions of those areas of the brain that are still unexplored? Is man, in fact, evolving toward a transmutation of consciousness in much the same way as animal consciousness after millions of years on this planet evolved and developed into human consciousness? Is it possible that man is on the threshold of a new evolution? If so, what will be the concomitant changes required in the human body, particularly the brain?

These questions sketch the cosmic dimensions framing the kundalini concept. However, kundalini as a word and as a

* Yoga in its generic sense from the Sanskrit root *yug*, meaning "yoke" or "union," includes any and all spiritual disciplines that aim at attaining oneness with the Supreme Intelligence. In that sense, this book *is* about kundalini yoga—but as a goal, a state of being, rather than a body of techniques and instructions.

concept presents difficulty for those new to the subject. It is a strange term, and brings with it a host of other terms foreign to our language and our way of thinking. Although I defined it in the Introduction as meaning "coiled up"—because that is what the preponderance of opinion holds—it has also been defined by Yogi Bhajan as meaning "curl of the hair of the beloved" and by Christopher Hills as meaning "to burn."

On a conceptual level, too, there are difficulties and differences to be resolved. The foremost is the dualistic thinking so deeply ingrained in Western culture. We are conditioned from infancy to conceive of mind and body as separate entities, so the dynamics of the kundalini concept—which posit an inherent psychophysical potential for self-transformation—pose a great puzzle to materialist-mechanist-reductionist science.

We can, for example, accept Freud's notion of the libido, the sex drive, because it is purely psychological and intrapersonal. But to say that there is a biological basis called prana to the "purely psychological" and to add that it is transpersonal or cosmic in origin is to challenge one of psychology's most deeply ingrained assumptions. If we add that this can be demonstrated in a way that will radically alter the perspectives of physics and biology, the challenge is extended to the rest of science. And if we conclude with the statement that this demonstration will show the intimate relationship between sexuality and mystical experience, proving that the latter is the *fulfillment* of the former, we will have included the religious establishment in the challenge. All of these groups have conceptual barriers to understanding, let alone accepting, the kundalini concept.

Nevertheless, it is being proposed just this way—and, in part, demonstrated through research. One of the advocates of kundalini research (a topic we will examine in Part III) is Yogi Bhajan. In his recent book *The Teachings of Yogi Bhajan,* he made this statement:

> What is kundalini? The energy of the glandular system combines with the nervous system to become more sensi-

> tive so that the totality of the brain perceives signals and interprets them, so that the effect of the sequence of the cause becomes very clear to the man. In other words, man becomes totally, wholesomely aware. That is why we call it the yoga of awareness. And as the rivers end up in the same ocean, all yoga ends up by raising the kundalini in the man. What is the kundalini? The creative potential of the man.

This integrative view of human nature, transcending the mind-body dualism of Western thought, is articulated by Ken Dychtwald in *Bodymind,* which is concerned with "the evolution to cosmic consciousness":

> Kundalini yoga . . . has recently received a great deal of attention here in the United States. From this particular branch of yoga comes a highly structured method of self-development through careful exercises and meditations, as well as a fascinating way of viewing body/mind relationships. My own interest in kundalini yoga began when I first realized that the kundalini perspective on psychosomatic structure and process is in some ways remarkably similar to several of the popular Western approaches, such as bioenergetics, Rolfing and the Feldenkrais method. Underlying each of these approaches to human development is a strong emphasis on identifying specific psychoemotional qualities and levels of human awareness in terms of their relationships to the body.
>
> Yet kundalini yoga differs from these Western processes in that within this ancient system lies a deeply profound statement about human evolution through bodymind development.

The "bodymind" or holistic perspective—already accepted by science in a limited way as psychosomatic medicine—is being recognized more widely, but the linkages themselves are still imperfectly understood. The question will be dealt with more fully in Part III. Here we will simply note that this perspective, in its fullest form, elegantly unites the best of modern science with the ancient wisdom of spiritual and religious tradition. As Yogi Amrit Desai puts it in *God Is Energy* (see Appendix), to the yogi, God is not a remote superhuman being, but the energy—superintelligent and divine—that regulates man's most intimate life processes. Science, seemingly so familiar with the life processes, has from the yogic perspective lost its perception of the cosmic context that generates those processes, and thus has, in a sense, degenerated to mere mechanism, materialism, reductionism—and is devoid of real wisdom.

This section attempts to re-present the ancient wisdom. It offers ten selections, nearly all by well-recognized spiritual teachers. These selections do not agree in all particulars. One must be critical and discriminating. But reasoning and logical analysis alone are not enough. Personal experience is irreplaceable in the acquisition of knowledge. Likewise, an acquaintance with the ancient traditional scriptures and modern empirical findings is also necessary for separating true knowledge from the false and the partly true.

Therefore in order to seek a balanced, integrative understanding of kundalini, we will deal with all these aspects in the various parts of this book. We begin with the traditional view of kundalini.

THE AWAKENING OF KUNDALINI

Swami Rama

The science of kundalini is one of the most advanced and difficult branches of yoga. In this article I hope to set right some misconceptions and abuses of this science and to give a clearer conception of what kundalini yoga is.

Shiva and Shakti

To understand the meaning of this word kundalini we must consider it in its proper context along with the word *shakti*, for the term kundalini modifies and explains this term, shakti. Kundalini comes from the world *kundala*, which means coiled. The image of a serpent coiled up while resting conveys the idea of kundalini. The word shakti comes from the root *shak*, to have power or to be able. Taken together, these two Sanskrit words might be translated as the coiled-up power, or the resting potential.

But what is this power and why is it resting? To understand this, we must go to the very foundation of tantric philosophy. According to this ancient philosophy, the entire universe is a manifestation of pure consciousness. In manifesting the universe, this pure consciousness seems to become divided into two poles or aspects, neither of which can exist without the other. One aspect retains a static quality and remains identified with unmanifest consciousness. In tantra this quality is called *Shiva*, and is conceptualized as masculine. Shiva is depicted as being absorbed in the deepest state of meditation, a state of formless being, consciousness, and bliss. He remains for the most part aloof from and uninterested in manifesting the universe. Shiva has the power to be, but not the power to become or change. He has no power to act or to manifest. He is the power holder, but has no energy in his own right. Nevertheless, consciousness as the power that builds the world is based on and arises out of this consciousness as being.

The other part of this polarity is a dynamic, energetic, or creative aspect that is called Shakti, the great mother of the universe, for it is from her that all form is born. Shakti is the subtlest of created things. She manifests herself as the entire universe including matter, life, and mind.

These two principles are united, but in the manifest world an illusion of separation is created between pure consciousness and its manifestations. Shakti is a projection of consciousness that veils the consciousness from which she was projected, in the innumerable illusory manifestations (*maya*) that she brings forth and that we call the universe. The scriptures say that when karma ripens, Shakti "becomes desirous of creation, and covers Herself with her own maya."[1]

The creation of this illusion is called *involution,* for we find consciousness *involving* or folding over itself. As a result of this involvement it seems to become complex, bipolar, and formed. After aeons of time, when the universe is dissolved, it is drawn or recollected into that shakti that produced it. This latter process is known as *evolution.* It is a further stage of development in which consciousness becomes uninvolved with its manifestation.

We know from physics that energy exists in two forms: (1) dynamic or active and (2) latent or potential, power at rest. Any activity or force must have a static background. When consciousness manifests itself as the creative or dynamic principle (shakti), she in turn polarizes herself into these two forms. In the manifestation of the universe, part of the energy of shakti becomes involved in the manifestation itself, while a still greater part remains dormant. The dynamic aspect is shakti in specific differentiated form. In Indian mythology the primal power that remains after the ongoing creation is symbolized by coiled-up energy in the form of a serpent that supports the universe.

Organization of Energies in the Human Body

According to tantra, the human being is a miniature universe. All that is found in the cosmos can be found within each individual, and the same principles that apply to the universe apply in the case of the individual being. In human beings the surplus of energy that is not being used to maintain the functioning of the organism is also symbolically described as a coiled or resting serpent. This potential energy is said to rest at the base of the spinal cord, at the muladhara (root support) chakra. The potential energy is called kundalini. Kundalini is the static support of the entire body and all of its pranic or energy forces. "Kundalini-Shakti in individual bodies is . . . the *static center* round which every form of existence as moving power revolves."[2] "Kundalini is the Divine Cosmic Energy in bodies."[3]

The dynamic energy that provides the working forces for the body evolves from the active energy of shakti and is called *prana.* Electrical energy is more subtle than mechanical energy. Its properties have come to be recognized and utilized in the past two hundred to three hundred years. Before that the idea of electrical forces was quite foreign to the thinking of most people. This is the situation today with our empirical understanding of prana. Prana is a still more subtle form of energy that is not yet studied or understood in the mainstream of modern science. However, it has been studied in detail in the introspective science of yoga.

Prana is organized and subdivided according to specific functions in the body. It flows like an electric current through an intricate network of subtle nerves (*nadis*), connecting the body and mind and keeping the entire organism in working order. This vital force of shakti in the body is also organized around specific centers. These are not physical centers, although they have physical correspondences in the various plexes of the body. These energy centers, called chakras, are intricate vortices of energy that help organize the physical body, although they cannot be perceived by it. The chakras influence, vitalize, and control corresponding regions of the body. They also determine the quality of consciousness. When the universal consciousness is manifest in the form of each center, the result is a particular frame of reference through which the individual experiences the world. For example, when mind and energy are expressed through the svadhishthana chakra one may be preoccupied with sensual enjoyment, while at another, the anahata chakra, one becomes loving and compassionate, interested in taking care of others. As Table 1 indicates, each of these centers in the indi-

TABLE 1

No.	Psychic Center in the Human Body	Corresponding Physical Center	Loka or Cosmic Plane	Guna or Quality
6	Ajna	Pituitary	Satyaloka	Sattva
5	Vishuddha	Thoraxic plexus	Tapaloka	
4	Anahata	Cardiac plexus	Janoloka	Rajas
3	Manipura	Solar plexus	Maharloka	
2	Svadhisthana	Sacral plexus	Survarloka	Tamas
1	Muladhara	Coccyx	Bhuvarloka	

vidual has its own corresponding loka or cosmic plane of reality. In other words, there are realms (in Western terminology, earthly, celestial, or heavenly spheres) in which the mode of experience corresponds to that of each chakra.

Although there are many energy centers, six are traditionally considered to be most important. These are located along the central axis of the body in conjunction with the spinal cord (see Figure 1). Energy is usually focused in one or more of these centers to the relative exclusion of others. Differences in where energy is focused from person to person

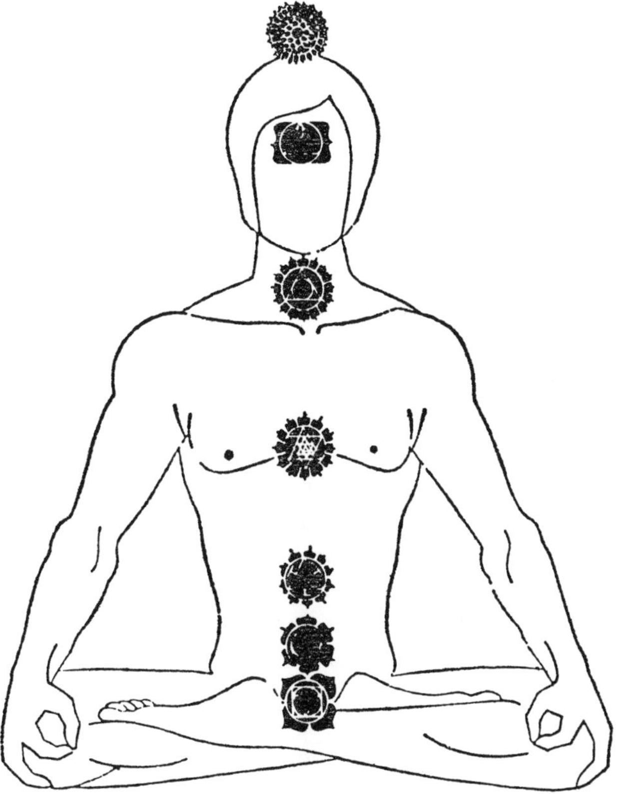

Figure 1. The chakras in traditional symbolic form.

and from time to time help to account for differences in the way the world is experienced from one individual to the next, and from one moment to the next.

The two lowest centers are grouped together because they represent the most primitive expressions of energy, and states of consciousness that are most closely tied to the physical world. They are linked to the basic instincts for individual and species survival. When energy is focused in these centers, pure consciousness is obscured and the individual identifies with the grossest material plane of existence. These chakras have the quality of tamas (inertia or torpor).

The second two chakras, located at the solar and cardiac plexes, represent a turning to more subtle relationships with the world. There is an active involvement in trying to organize and make sense of the world, and to interact on a less physical plane than in the case of the first two chakras. There is a focus on the building up and expansion of one's sense of I-ness. The predominant characteristic is that of rajas (expansion and activity).

The two chakras that correspond to the cervical and pituitary centers in the human body represent a movement away from worldly relationships to a world of pure form. Here one perceives and relates to the underlying forms from which the material universe comes. One who is operating at these levels exhibits creativity, intuition, and wisdom. His manner is predominantly sattvic (serene and devotional).

There is a series of still more subtle chakras above the ajana or pituitary center, culminating in the center of pure consciousness at the crown of the head. This is the abode of shiva, pure transcendent consciousness, in each individual. This center is named sahasrara (the place of luster). Its corresponding cosmic plane is called chandra loka (the world of nectar).

Ordinarily the individual is polarized, with shiva residing at the crown chakra and the latent power of shakti (kundalini) lying dormant at the base of the spine. Only the smallest bit of shakti's energy becomes dynamic and functions in the chakras and nadis (subtle nerve channels) in order to maintain the ordinary functions of the individual. That such an infinite reservoir of energy exists is not even imagined by official science.

It is traditionally thought that shakti contains not only latent energy but also latent memories, both personal and transpersonal. The modern way of understanding this latent power is in terms of the unconscious. Like shakti, the unconscious is conceived of as a vast unknown power. Those individuals who have controlled access to the unconscious experience an abundance of energy, insight, and creativity. So it is with the latent power of shakti. Those who transform this force from its latent to its active form become the dynamic geniuses of every age and culture.

This transformation is called the awakening of kundalini. Usually this is depicted as a sudden, intense, "earthshaking," and transforming experience. But such an experience is rare. It is more usual for tiny bits of this energy to be released through various means. One then experiences breakthroughs, bursts of energy and enthusiasm, peak experiences, a sense of well-being, and similar changes in consciousness. This is analogous to what happens in psychotherapy as bits of the unconscious are brought into one's awareness. Occasionally there are more startling breakthroughs, in which a significant quantity of the latent power is released. This leads to more unusual experiences, which will later be described.

The practice of kundalini yoga involves not only awakening this kundalini shakti but also systematically leading her through each of the chakras to the sahasrara or crown chakra, the abode of shiva. The word *yoga* means union, and this union can be understood as the uniting of kundalini shakti with shiva (pure consciousness). When this is achieved in the individual, he becomes fully conscious. There is no longer an unconscious or latent power–the individual is fully awakened and illumined. When the static shakti becomes dynamic and travels upward, fully energizing each of the centers along the way, the polarization of the body gives way and one attains the highest state of samadhi. Consciousness of the body is withdrawn. Sir John Woodroffe eloquently says:

> When Kundalini Shakti *sleeps* in the Muladhara, man is *awake* to the world; when she *awakes* to unite, and does unite, with the supreme static Consciousness which is Shiva, then consciousness is *asleep* to the world and is one with the Light of all things.[4]

As a static power, kundalini sustains consciousness of the world, but when she unites with shiva she loses consciousness of the world and goes to a state of consciousness without object or form. When she is aroused and moves upward, kundalini withdraws into herself the dynamic forces that maintain the body. This is the reverse of involution, of consciousness involving itself in the universe. It is a process of evolution in which the human being comes to realize his full potential. The final goal of the yogi is to dissolve the universe and abide in that state of pure consciousness.

Outwardly the body may seem no longer to be alive, but it continues to function minimally so that it can again be used as an instrument of the individual who has temporarily left it. The body may even become cold as a corpse. It is said that the union of shiva and shakti generates a nectar that continues to sustain the body in this superconscious state.

This union is the goal of the aspirant, but few achieve it. It is more common, although still rare, for the yogi to awaken kundalini shakti and lead her only part of the way toward her goal.

Means of Awakening Kundalini

A number of methods have been developed in yoga to help the aspirant awaken the sleeping force within him. An appropriate method is chosen by a realized teacher to prepare each student according to his particular inclinations and capacities. Before describing these methods, I would like to warn the student so that he may avoid being misguided by those who claim to be teachers of these practices but do not have the necessary realization to guide their students properly.

Kundalini and tantra yoga are perhaps the most misunderstood and abused of all yoga practices. These sacred, systematic, and extremely advanced traditions for leading the aspirant to the highest state of transcendent consciousness have been caricatured in the West in crude breathing exercises and unfounded claims by a number of teachers that they directly arouse this energy in many of their students through their mere touch or presence. All too often what becomes aroused are the latent hysterical tendencies in the student, who imagines and acts out all sorts of things. The misinterpretation of these ancient, revered teachings has led to self-delusion instead of genuine awakening. Those who offer easy methods for achieving an awakened state of mind are in actuality using suggestion or trickery and are misleading their students. The vast majority of reports of awakened kundalini that we find in the West are merely the expressions of rich imaginations.

It should be no surprise that the study and practice of kundalini shakti should be so abused. Whenever the awakening of power in any form is offered, those who seek to aggrandize themselves flock to those who promise rapid and easy attainment of such power. They are finally duped by their own desire for power. All they catch is the illusion of power, never the real thing. I remember once I asked my master why there are so many false teachers in the world. He said, "They create a fence for those who are genuine. By attracting those students who want to get something for nothing, they free the real teacher to work with a smaller group of sincere aspirants."

To genuinely awaken kundalini, one must first prepare himself. Without long and patient practice in purifying oneself and strengthening one's capacity to tolerate and assimilate such a flood of energy, the awakening of this latent power would deeply disturb, disorient, and confuse the student. Even at the physical level such a charge of energy can threaten the integrity of the body. This has been metaphorically described in terms of the body being a ten-ampere fuse receiving a current of one hundred amperes at a high potential. Only after one has developed considerable self-control can this charge be tolerated without the organism's being strained to the point of danger.

The experience of a "bad trip" after ingesting a powerful psychoactive drug is nothing compared to the release of this force in one who is unprepared. Can you imagine the effect of the sudden and massive release into awareness of what is in your unconscious? This is exactly what happens with the awakening of the kundalini. If through careful training the aspirant has gradually come to recognize and master his unconscious demons—in other words, has purified and strengthened himself—then and only then is he prepared to face the full awakening of all that is latent within him. In Indian iconography shakti

> is painted as riding on a lion as a symbol of strength, courage, magnanimity and majesty. The picture also denotes the fact that when the Kundalini is aroused in a person, She rides the lion of yoga which roars like a hungry lion in the body and begins to devour the weakness (flesh) of the yogi. The Shakti with Her numerous kinds of weapons begins to wage war on the animal passions which . . . hinder spiritual advancement, killing them one by one, till every one of them has been to the last overpowered and killed.[5]

If the aspirant has not purified himself through various spiritual practices, the war that is waged within can be especially intense, even unbearable. Releasing kundalini without preparation is like opening Pandora's box without having cultivated the ability to master what emerges. For this reason the teacher who truly represents a tradition that teaches methods to awaken kundalini will never fully reveal these to an unprepared student, but will do his best to prepare him. Preparation for awakening kundalini is more important than awakening kundalini.

Here is a brief overview of those methods traditionally used to prepare the student and to awaken this latent force.

1. *Physical Means.* The practice of hatha yoga, including purifying exercises, prepares the body to tolerate the heightened energy of kundalini. After considerable preparation, advanced postures, energy locks and seals called mudras and bandhas, and breathing exercises (pranayama) help to rechannel the dynamic energy (prana) and use it to awaken the latent energy (kundalini). Since prana regulates the functioning of body and mind, by acquiring control of this energy the yogi is able to control the mind and body at will. In most people

prana flows outward connecting the mind with the senses, but when this energy is concentrated and channeled upward through the chakras, the mind becomes detached from the senses and the physical body and becomes inwardly absorbed in meditation. A number of related spiritual exercises have the effect of withdrawing energy from two subtle nerve channels (called ida and pingala) that run along the spinal cord, and channeling this energy through a third channel (sushumna), which runs along the center of the spine. A form of prana that normally travels upward (prana vayu) is brought down, while the normally downward-flowing energy (apana vayu) is brought upward so that the two merge. The union of these two pranic currents in the central canal creates intense heat. In the *Upanishads* they are called upper and lower arni. By the friction produced between them, fire is created.

> The position seems to be thus similar to a hollow tube in which a piston is working at both ends without escape of the central air, which thus becomes heated. Then the Serpent Force, Kundalini, aroused by the heat thus generated, is aroused from her potential state.[6]

Kundalini is thereby aroused, and flows upward through a channel at the center of the spine called Brahma nadi.

2. *Concentration and Meditation.* Kundalini can also be awakened by intense concentration and meditation on specific sensory nerves such as the tip of the nose or the root of the tongue, along with concentration and meditation on specific chakras. Such concentration helps to withdraw the consciousness from its absorption in the physical body, and to master the quality of energy associated with a specific chakra. Meditation on a chakra along with the repetition of a particular thought form (mantra) and a visualization (yantra) can awaken energy from kundalini and bring it to that center.

3. *Brahmacharaya* or physical and mental celibacy is still another path that can lead from involution to evolution. Instead of discharging the vital force in the service of procreation, the yogi who follows this path learns to absorb that en-

ergy and direct it upward. The external union between male and female is forsaken; instead an internal union between the male (shiva) and female (shakti) principle takes place.

4. This union is most clearly cultivated in *tantra yoga,* which centers on the worship of Shakti, the mother of the universe. Many people in the West think that tantra means having sexual relations. In some forms of tantra a male-female relationship may be involved, but it is transformed from the physical plane to the sphere of energy and consciousness. The partners relate to one another as embodiments of shiva and shakti rather than as two physical beings. In the more pure form of tantra, Shakti is worshiped through meditation and mantra, so that the aspirant comes into a direct and conscious relationship with the shiva and shakti within himself and unites them. It is considered that the teacher introduces bahiya yag (external worship) to unprepared students. But those who are prepared are introduced to antaryag (inner worship) to make the mind inward and one-pointed. According to the tantra shastras there still exist three great schools, the kaula, mishra, and samaya schools of tantra. While kaula and mishra perform certain rituals and believe in obtaining powers (siddhis), the samaya group does not believe in any external rituals and is considered to be the purest and highest of all.

These are just some of the practices for arousing kundalini. She can also be awakened through intense devotion. And for those who are more intellectual and philosophical, intense study of the scriptures with a competent teacher can also serve this purpose. In fact, any spiritual practice that leads to a genuine awakening and experience of transcendent states of consciousness involves an awakening of this coiled energy.

The word kundalini also means a bowl of fire. In all great mystic traditions of the world there have been similar experiences of kundalini awakening. Moses was moved to take off his shoes before the burning bush; Isaiah in the temple, and Mohammed on the night of power, when the teachings of the Koran were revealed to him, also experienced the awakening of this force. The books of revelation in Judaism and Christianity reveal the signs and symptoms of the awakening of kundalini. Hindu and Buddhist scriptures make up the most extensive literature on the subject. This literature emphasizes that, particularly on this path, a competent teacher is essential.

In most of the spiritual practices, the awakening of this force is not clearly conceptualized or systematically brought under the control of the aspirant. Thus the mystic may have rare, inexplicable, and uncontrolled moments of ecstasy and illumination, but he does not know how to produce these again at will. This is not the case in the systematic practice of yoga under the guidance of a teacher who himself has mastered this latent force. Indeed, it is the awakened master, as the representative of a perennial tradition, who makes it possible through the practice of kundalini yoga, but sincere effort is essential. Under the close supervision of the master and through a series of initiations the student is guided toward his goal. The first initiation on this path is the imparting of a mantra, a "seed" sound to concentrate on, which represents certain aspects of this vital force. Traditionally, mantra meditation is not given as an isolated practice but is considered an early step on the path. It is practiced in conjunction with a number of co-ordinate spiritual exercises and mental and physical disciplines to purify and prepare the student for further steps. If the student is successful in his practice, he is guided through more difficult and intricate forms of meditation in which he becomes sensitive to the forces within and is able to channel them.

These practices may culminate in a higher initiation called shaktipat diksha, in which the master directly transmits his energy to the student to remove the final obstacle, awakening the sleeping serpent and leading her upward. One who is functioning on a higher level may sometimes unconsciously influence those around him in the same way that a magnet influences metal objects in its proximity. But the magnet can only attract a particular metal. As a magnet influences a particular metal, such a teacher influences those who are prepared, though he might inspire many. In shaktipat the influence is conscious and extremely intense. Through a look, touch, or thought the master transmits his own power to the aspirant, who is suddenly transported into a realm of blissful divine consciousness.

This state may last for an hour or a few days. Typically the aspirant is not able to maintain the aroused state and after some period of time kundalini returns to her abode. The awakened energy becomes latent once again. But now the aspirant's faith is strengthened, for he has directly experienced the awakened state. It is not at all like a hypnotic trance or the hysterical outpourings that parody this state. The individual is completely transformed after such an experience. He has glimpsed divinity, and although the experience is not yet completely integrated, it continues to influence him at all levels of his being for the rest of his life. As a result of such an experience, many latent abilities are awakened. The student becomes dynamic, creative, and talented in all aspects of life. He is elevated spiritually, morally, and intellectually. But he must also guard against an inflated ego. He must work systematically, perhaps for many years, to learn how to awaken and guide that energy within and without.

This experience of shaktipat is typically not repeated many times, for it takes considerable time for the student to integrate what he has experienced. If the master does not proceed slowly and cautiously in working with the student, the student could become disoriented and unable to function in the world for a considerable period of time. There is another less widely known practice, called shakti chalana, in which the student is led gradually, and to some extent unconsciously, through transformations in which he becomes more and more able to integrate and handle the awakening shakti.

Fortunately, the master is not working alone when dealing with this powerful force. He has behind him the tradition of sages, which he represents. He is guided by that tradition in determining when and how to release the latent power within his close disciple. I remember my first experience of this sort.

I was still quite young and had recently been initiated by my master after many years of diligent practice under his tutelage. One day he told me that a swami would come the next morning and that I was to touch him on the forehead, thereby initiating him in shaktipat diksha. I protested, saying that I had no such power to arouse the kundalini in another person. But he said to me, "Don't you know, it is not you acting. You are just the instrument of a higher power. Let that power work through you."

I was not reassured. I could not sleep that night. I remained awake thinking, "What if I touch him and nothing happens? He will no doubt be furious with me." I tried touching my finger to various objects to see if there was some vital force passing through me, but I was aware of nothing. When morning came, I met the swami at the appointed time, still not knowing how I would fulfill the task that was given to me. I sat in meditation with him before me, and repeated certain mantras as I was instructed by my guru. Suddenly I found my arm being raised. It was not at all under my control. I touched that swami and he remained in samadhi for several hours. I know this was not hypnosis or my imagination. When I asked my master to explain what happened, he just smiled, knowingly. I find that this power is still not in my control as an individual but is guided by the tradition with which I am linked. There may be someone to whom I wish to impart this experience, but nevertheless I cannot. Yet with a few rare individuals I feel such a strong impulse that I cannot resist.

Signs and Symptoms of Kundalini

There are clear and unmistakable signs when kundalini awakens. Initially there may be involuntary jerks of the body, trembling or shaking, and an intense feeling of pleasure. One of the first and most common occurrences is the experience of intense heat as the energy is passing through a particular center. Here are typical descriptions of the experience of heat:

> I felt a burning sensation in various parts of the body and my whole body was perspiring. I had previously seen flames . . . but they were not so extremely hot as these.
>
> Sometimes it seemed as if a jet of molten copper, mounting up through the spine, dashed against my crown.

As kundalini awakens there is a sensation of something moving along the spine. This has been described as a feeling of frogs jumping, snakes wriggling, or ants creeping in a line from the feet to the head. As the aroused energy passes through the chakras, yoga mudras, bandhas, or breathing exercises, which are usually practiced voluntarily, may occur spontaneously and unintentionally. Kundalini acts as a spiritual guide, governing and leading the individual through various experiences.

The aspirant may have difficulty leading the energy upward. At times it may remain for a while in one of the lower chakras and return again to its resting place. There are three granthis (knots) through which the energy has a difficult time passing. In piercing the abdominal knot, pain or physical disorders may occur. The yogi may have to repeat the process of awakening kundalini a number of times, gradually leading her higher along her path. Specific spiritual exercises are given by the teacher to help the student overcome the obstacles encountered. It is said that bringing kundalini to the anahata chakra at the cardiac plexus is the most difficult task. At this point kundalini is said to pass from an infant state to a mature state.

As the kundalini passes through and energizes each of the chakras, particular visions and sounds are experienced at each center. The disciple passes through the corresponding lokas or cosmic planes. He will typically see a lotuslike flower at each center with its petals hanging downward. When the energy becomes more manifest in that center, the petals turn upward.

The quality or force that exists at each center is seen in the form of a presiding deity. These experiences are consistent and predictable from one individual to another. Here is an example:

> Some days later the navel lotus appeared. It was similar to the lotus of the heart but its petals were slightly different. Many days later the form of Shesasayi (Vishnu sleeping on a snake) appeared. . . . From the navel of Vishnu issued forth a lotus plant and Brahmadeva appeared to be sitting on the flower.

More advanced yogis believe that it is only when the ajana chakra at the pituitary center is reached that anything significant is achieved. Ramakrishna said, "If . . . anybody's mind reaches the spot between the eyebrows . . . he then has direct knowledge of the supreme Self and remains continually in samadhi."[7]

There are a number of lesser-known centers between the ajana chakra and the sahasrara or highest center at the crown of the head.

> When mind rises up to these stages, super-visions of light in various forms such as the moon, the sun, stars . . . etc., appear to the inner vision and sounds of bells, drums, flute, etc., culminating in one resembling thunder, become audible.[8]

St. Teresa of Avila describes the following experience:

> The noises in my head are so loud that I am beginning to wonder what is going on in it. . . . My head sounds just as if it were full of brimming rivers . . . and a host of little birds seem to be whistling, not in the ears, but in the upper part of the head, where the higher part of the soul is said to be; I have held this view for a long time, for the spirit seems to move upward with great velocity.[9]

In the yogic tradition these visions are said to culminate in the union of shiva and shakti at the sahasrara. This is the most transcending and all-encompassing state of consciousness that can be experienced. There is nothing beyond this. The individual consciousness becomes merged with divine consciousness.

If kundalini were to remain at this center, after twenty-one days the body would no longer be maintained. Usually, however, it is not possible to maintain this state of consciousness, and kundalini returns once again to the lower chakras. Gradually, through systematic practice, the yogi learns complete mastery of this energy and is able to direct it at will, maintaining that state of consciousness that is appropriate and useful at a given time.

As far as my own experience goes, I was trained to study body anatomy first, and to have control over the four appetites (food, sleep, sex, and self-preservation). I was told to have a healthy body and to discipline myself in mind, action, and speech. I was asked not to allow my mind to be influenced by anyone's opinion and way of thinking. This took a long time for me to achieve.

It is not possible for an unhealthy body and a disturbed mind to tread this path properly. A healthy body and yogic mind are two necessary instruments to awaken the consciousness and lead it to its source from where the consciousness flows on various degrees and grades. I was trained to have control over bodily functions and internal states, and without them it was not possible for me to think of awakening kundalini and going to the center of consciousness.

I have met others who hallucinate or mistakenly boast of awakening this power, but I was strictly warned not to be guided by my emotions. No doubt emotion is one of the greatest powers, but it needs to be devotionally channeled. Otherwise pleasure and joy on the physical and mental planes can be mistaken for the awakening of kundalini.

I was taught to have perfect control over the unconscious activities of my mind and autonomic and central nervous systems. During my intense sadhana I observed perfect silence with certain dietary rules. Stillness of body and mind were two important signs of my progress. I was instructed not to be guided by any hunch or so-called intuition that comes through an untrained and unpurified mind. After completing my sadhana, which included thoroughly studying all the systems of Indian philosophy, I can assure you that those experiences that ensue from irrationality and from the exhaustion of mental force through pushing, shoving, rolling and tumbling, jumping, shouting, and weeping are not signs and symptoms of kundalini.

I have determined to do research in order to scientifically verify the way this force is brought under systematic control by the yogis. In experiments at the Menninger Foundation we have been showing that the autonomic nervous system can be brought fully under control. In various experiments I have demonstrated the voluntary control of brain waves, heart rate, and skin temperature. But these are only the minor points, the preliminary self-mastery that is necessary to awaken kundalini, which modern science is capable of observing with its instruments and methods. More research, which goes farther and studies the achievement of various higher states of consciousness, can only be conducted when science finds the methods to examine and differentiate these states from one another and from ordinary consciousness.

The awakening of kundalini is a very specialized method of self-realization that can be attained after long, intense practice. Silence and discipline of body and mind through self-effort, as well as sincerity, faithfulness, and truthfulness are necessary requisites in the path of enlightenment. Grace dawns at a certain stage of attainment. It is important to know and awaken the ascending force, kundalini. But it is equally important to be aware of this descending force called kripa (grace). Shaktipat is a form of grace that dawns when sincere, selfless effort is made by the student.

For sincere aspirants it is advisable to study the tantra scriptures in a traditional way, under a competent guide, and then start practicing methods for the awakening of kundalini. Modern students, out of sheer enthusiasm and emotional outbursts, surrender themselves before their emotional ideals and depend completely on their guru for enlightenment. They forget that though the guru is important, he is still a means and not the end. A real guru leads his student on the path of freedom and does not propagate a personality cult. These days many gurus, instead of introducing the subject and instructing the student in the ways and methods, ask students not to do anything except to follow them–least of all to think and to cultivate the mind. Such students may have experiences on the higher levels of consciousness, but the experiences will be temporary and superficial. Direct experience through self-mastery alone enlightens the student and leads him to the final abode. The *Upanishads* declare that without a systematic method of meditation (dhyana yoga) the awakening of kundalini is not possible. The great sages experienced the union of individual consciousness with the cosmic one through meditation. Says *Shvetashvatara Upanishad:*

> The great sages by practicing the method of meditation could awaken the Devatma Shakti.

ते ध्यानयोगानुगता अपश्यन्
देवात्मशक्तिं स्वगुणैर्निगूढाम् ।
यः कारणानि निखिलानि तानि
कालात्मयुक्तान्यधितिष्ठत्येकः ॥ ३ ॥

NOTES

1. *Kulacudamani,* 1:16–24.
2. Sir John Woodroffe, *The Serpent Power* (Madras: Ganesh & Co., 1972), p. 42.
3. Ibid., p. 2.
4. *Sakti and Sakta* (Madras: Ganesh & Co., 1951), p. 446.
5. Swami Vishnu Tirtha, *Devatma Shakti* (Bombay: Sri Sadhan Granthmala Prakashan Samiti, 1962), p. 126.
6. M. P. Pandit, *Kundalini Yoga* (Madras: Ganesh & Co., 1971), p. 56.

7. Swami Savadananda, *Sri Ramakrishna the Great Master* (Mylapore, Madras: Sri Ramakrishna Math, 1952), p. 366.
8. Swami Vishnu Tirtha, op. cit., p. 96.
9. *Interior Castle,* tr. and ed. E. Allison Peers (Garden City, N.Y.: Doubleday & Company, Inc., 1961), pp. 77–78.

KUNDALINI: AN OVERVIEW

Swami Sivananda Radha

Kundalini yoga is a direct path of conscious cooperation with the evolutionary forces inherent in each individual, leading toward higher consciousness. What has come to us from ancient times about kundalini has been preserved in a most interesting picture language. The beautiful symbols represent a very precise path, from the foundation of human life to the heights of an expanded consciousness.

The ancient yogis depicted the evolution of mankind, and the consciousness of the individual in particular, as a progression of seven steps. The seven centers have symbolic locations in the spinal column. These centers are referred to either as chakras or lotuses. Chakra means wheel and symbolizes the process of the movement of life. The lotus, slowly unfolding from a bulb rooted in mud to a full-blown flower above the water, symbolizes the development from a primitive to a highly cultivated and refined being. The chakras are best understood as levels of consciousness.

Each of us, whether aware of it or not, is on the path of evolution of consciousness. The unaware person, through events that are very painful, is often incited to get off the merry-go-round and look for other options. There is more to life than fame, wealth, reaching the top of the social ladder, or—on the other hand—a broken heart, loss of status, the death of a loved one. When these events are given too great an importance, one becomes forgetful of the true purpose of life. Life becomes meaningless sleepwalking. We don't live—we drift. We have lost direction. We have lost sight of our option to stop being sleepwalkers and to begin to consciously cooperate with the forces of evolution that are everywhere at work.

In the beginning of kundalini yoga there is usually much intellectualizing about the meaning of kundalini, the powers, and the new terminology. To learn anything new is a process requiring time and special effort. In many areas of human activity there is a special language that first must be acquired to understand what it is all about. Kundalini is no exception. It has its symbols with specific meanings. Mental acrobatics are necessary to keep the mind flexible. This proves later to be very helpful. Little by little the mind becomes more pliable, learns to accept new ideas, takes greater risks, overcomes old limitations. Gradually old concepts are more easily thrown out. Kundalini, being a state of awareness, is difficult to describe. But then what child can imagine light-years or picture the distance of remote planets? One must study astronomy. Likewise kundalini, by persistent study and practice, will unfold itself.

Because each chakra controls one of the five senses, the practicing yogi takes great care to develop each of the senses to its utmost potential, bringing them all into balance for a smooth interplay of those forces already inherent in them. This gives the yogi a considerable advantage over others who have never paid attention to the senses or considered their development.

The ancient teachings tell us that all human actions originate in the mind. Energy is basically neutral, and each individual forms and shapes it through the expression of thoughts, speech, and action empowered by the undercurrents of strong emotions. Since the chakras are best understood as levels of consciousness, impurities have to be understood, not as a matter of moralizing, but of discrimination. Impurities arise from desires, self-gratification, and self-interest. In the beginning it is hard to let go of cherished beliefs and illusions. Having to accept the hard facts seems unnecessarily cruel. But it is illusion itself that is the source of pain. All pain is caused by ignorance and by staying intentionally blind, when experience has already told us something different. We think that we are victims of circumstances, when actually we have allowed ourselves to remain ignorant. Discrimination and conscious investigation are seldom applied. We are too busy to go into the depth of each experience. We try to escape pain and disappointment by hoping it will go away. If intelligence were used properly there would be discriminating investigation, leading to a proper perception of reality instead of a false one, which causes more pain.

The system of kundalini was designed to assist those who aspire to higher consciousness. It must be emphasized, however, that the release of more energy is not the goal. The first goal is self-development, which is achieved through increasing self-discipline and refinement. This is the only key that can permanently unlock the door to expanded consciousness. In each person there is an interplay of forces and interaction between the chakras. The aim of the yogi is to bring the centers into harmony so that there is a balanced and controlled expression of energy through them.

In many people's minds today there is much confusion about kundalini. One of the difficulties comes from the fact that each person has to begin where he or she is in his own development. There is a tendency for the aspirant to immediately concretize the symbolic expressions of the system. That habit leads one to miss many of the more subtle aspects involved.

It is important for everyone wishing to enter the path of kundalini to follow the progression from the beginning as it has been laid out by the pictorial symbols. Any scientist who is planning to work in a new field will first acquire an understanding of the basics and follow carefully the procedures that have been laid down by other experts in that area. The necessity of this approach is often entirely overlooked when it comes to the investigation of levels of consciousness and awareness.

Unfortunately, there is also a tendency for the reader or listener to exaggerate his or her own stage of development.

The first and last rung of the ladder can be mixed up. Resist this temptation. The yogi seeks to bring all levels into a harmonious balance, and in order to understand what this involved, the new student must begin at the first level. In other words, a firm foundation must be laid and progress made a step at a time.

Because tradition emphasizes the direct teaching from guru to disciple, kundalini has remained mysterious and thereby has created much speculation and confusion. It is unfortunate that today, when there is a great deal of interest and discussion about kundalini energy, it is mainly linked to only one aspect—that of sex. Particularly in the West, it has become a word and a concept that serves as an excuse for many things. Attributing events to kundalini energy and its overwhelming power, men and women throw aside sexual inhibitions and indulge in all sorts of illicit sexual activity. This lack of real understanding of the nature and purpose of kundalini is leading not only to confusion and disaster in human relationships, but also to mental imbalance. This is because the path of kundalini has not been sufficiently understood and the groundwork has not been laid. That emphasis inviting greater freedom and enjoyment of sexual pleasure has been taken out of context from an ancient Eastern culture that was vastly different from that existing now in the West.*

There are two principal schools of thought in kundalini yoga. Both acknowledge the pure energy in the muladhara chakra. One school applies this energy in a concrete way by an emphasis on sex. The other does not concretize the direction of the energy but seeks to transcend all attachments, including sex, through the development of the mental powers. If this difference in the application of the energy is not understood, problems will arise. Even in the case of concrete application, which means the inclusion of the sexual experience, it has to be recognized that all the statements of the ancient texts have been made from a man's point of view. Sex does not burden the male with responsibility for the possible

* The *Kama Sutras,* an Indian sex manual, is not part of the kundalini system but has been confused with it.

offspring because that has traditionally been viewed as the female's responsibility. Neither in the ancient texts nor in the stories is there any clarification of what happens to the female and her offspring when the male aspirant is geared to the attainment of the goal that he has set for himself—that is, using sex for his liberation and to attain higher consciousness. In this case, the woman is taken as an object of practice. Because of the biological result that makes her a mother, she and her child are seen as obstacles to the attainment of his goal. Is that not, in the very end, self-defeating? One cannot help but wonder if a high state of awareness and bliss can be achieved at the cost of the rejection of the mother and child.

If the male and female are indeed complementary to each other and a higher level of bliss can be achieved through sexual union, then the possible result of that bliss, the child, should also be accepted and revered. The West is a throwaway society—one does not mend things—and this is reflected in the relationships between men and women. Without due consideration of the partner involved and without the acceptance of responsibility for the consequences of action, how could a higher state of consciousness be achieved?

In the kundalini symbology, the union of Shiva and Shakti is presented in one body, not two bodies united. Lord Shiva ultimately becomes half man and half woman. The meaning of this symbolism is lost today. True oneness is only achieved in a particular state of mind for which the sex act itself is not essential. The pleasure from the sexual act, which is often misinterpreted as spiritual union, is in fact only the registration of stimulation in the pleasure center of the brain. The experience of union has many levels, beginning with that of the male and female *united in oneself*. This has nothing to do with sex. The final level is union of the individual consciousness with cosmic consciousness. This experience is beyond the ability of language to describe.

We can go a step farther and say that whatever is felt on the physical level is a stimulation and sensation that is interpreted by the mind. In the second chakra, it is stated that the yogi can destroy worlds. These are the worlds of the mind whose creative power has an awesome reach. While the intense practice of kundalini yoga includes a recognition of one's needs, these needs are more often projected into another person, and by so doing the projector does not realize that in reality he sees his needs through the other.

Sexual instinct has almost the power of the gravitational pull. Emotional and sexual dependency are much more than just a hangup created by social upbringing. As long as the emphasis is on the "I" and everything is related to this little word, we have to see behind it a whole chain of construction with the purpose of serving the "I." As the individual progresses in awareness, it becomes clear that the overemphasis or priority given to sex has no place in the other chakras. In the same way, the joy of self-gratification attained through acquiring a lot of material goods and comforts is short-lived, and the list of desires keeps increasing. But at some point in his or her development, the aspirant experiences the joy that has been given to another person echoing back to oneself. This is pure joy.

The other school of thought seeks to transcend the application of the energy in a concrete way by realizing that for thousands of lifetimes human beings have applied and experienced sex, and that at one lifetime it is necessary to loosen all attachments, and the attachment to the sexual experience in particular. The dhyana-yogi wants to preserve energy to pursue the rather arduous path toward liberation. This is really very easy to understand when we consider that in everyday life certain demanding executive jobs are not open to the young person who is still giving too much time and energy to physical interaction with the opposite sex. Only a beginner would assume that by the fulfillment of his desires he can at the same time pursue his development to liberation. When there is attachment to sex, then liberation cannot be achieved.

It must be understood that the kundalini system is for the man and woman who by their own choice have gratified sexual impulses in many lifetimes. Every human being goes through different stages of development. A child plays with colorful toys. A young person has different attractions, and the adult seeks again very different gratification, generally shifting into the pursuit of success and achievements of various kinds. On the spiritual path, and particularly on the path of kundalini, it needs to be understood that kundalini is not for the person for whom life is the continuous seeking of pleasures or the achievements of success in name and fame. All the scriptures point out the same truth.

Each individual makes the decision as to how far he or she wants to go. Kundalini is not necessarily pursued for the sake of its highest goal. For most, this is far in the distance, and there is the need for intermediate goals—goals such as the development of the five senses, greater receptivity, greater acceptance of other people, and bringing more quality into life. Only when a certain development toward one's true potential has been achieved can we truly speak of entering upon the path of kundalini.

In the beginning, the motivation to pursue the path can be compared to the aims of growth workshops: to improve and grow beyond present limitations. But for many this is an ego trip, a desire to be different, to be singled out. Many become not better people but rather more narcissistic. Because one aspires to improve one's self-image, to tell fewer lies, to refrain from always seeking the best place and the most attention, to become a little less critical and judgmental of others does not mean that one will reap spiritual rewards as a fringe benefit. Understanding the true purpose of the spiritual search, and exploring and refining the senses through the different practices come after the basic groundwork of self-control has been achieved.

With all that has been said so far about kundalini, some very significant questions may appear. Why does cosmic intelligence allow a kundalini awakening to occur in an unprepared person? Each individual must first define what is meant by "cosmic intelligence," by "kundalini," and by "awakening."

A comparison from nature may help to clarify this matter. When the branches of a fruit tree are pruned in the spring and placed in a container of water, there is enough energy in the branch to produce flowers with only the addition of water. These flowers, however, will not produce fruit. Manifestations of what is called the kundalini energy can be compared to this process. There is enough energy in the mind and the body to produce certain physical evidence that something is going on—but the fruit of full enlightenment is not produced by the flower of the creative ability of the mind.

By manipulation of the mind through such means as hypnosis people can manifest many unusual actions and much that is startling and bizarre can be achieved. In past years when few lectures or publications about kundalini were available, people would rarely describe circumstances or bodily experiences in the way they do now. The question arises: How much of this is fabrication of the mind? This does not mean in an intentional sense, but simply as a product of what the mind does when it is fed new information.

Another example is that of a woman who is desperate to become a mother and who has convinced herself that she is pregnant. She can then produce all the physical symptoms of pregnancy, and yet when the time comes to deliver the baby, the uterus is empty. The intensity of desire has produced the symptoms but not the genuine fruit. The empty uterus and the lack of the fruit on the branch are comparable to the artificial kundalini experience rather than to the state of true enlightenment.

When the yogis of old gave a mantra to a disciple, they would not disclose the meaning of the mantra so as not to feed the mind of the disciple. The disciple had to find out the meaning of the mantra through personal practice. That was the only way to avoid stimulating the creative powers of the mind to produce results according to the disciple's interpretation of the mantra.

This is not to dispute the fact that there are cases of true kundalini manifestation in "unprepared" individuals. Usually such a person has for many years been filled with a deep longing for a kind of spiritual union, without necessarily being able to express it in the mind in concrete terms. When that experience takes place, the individual is no longer capable of returning to the former way of life. In contrast to this is the individual whose mind has manifested physical changes, also through sincere desire, and yet these are not the true spiritual experience, and enlightenment is not attained. In this case the mental power is there but, because of a lack of underlying spiritual power, the physical changes do not produce the spiritual fruit of enlightenment.

We cannot say therefore that the kundalini energy manifests itself in a totally unprepared person. The energy can be activated in a person who has a deep and sincere spiritual longing. Kundalini can consciously be awakened through numerous spiritual practices and through a change of mental conditioning.

After kundalini is first experienced, the promised powers may not manifest themselves at all for many years because the individual must still build character and lay a firm foundation. The energy will otherwise fizzle out. Just as someone may write only one lovely poem or paint one beautiful work of art in a lifetime, kundalini may be manifested only once, with no further development.

How can a seeker with average knowledge find out about kundalini? It is a matter of finding a teacher, studying texts, doing spiritual practice, cultivating observation, and finally having personal experience little by little.

A major misconception about kundalini is to think that, once it has been raised, kundalini will stay there. Like any spiritual flame in oneself, unless it is nourished and attended to, unless it dominates one's life, kundalini will simply disappear like water in quicksand. As previously mentioned, someone may compose one beautiful melody and never do so again. It was just a temporary flare-up of creative energy. One can only produce according to the skills one has. Therefore if kundalini has been raised inadvertently or unknowingly, one would still have to acquire the skill to handle that energy. There is then, of course, no such question as, "What do you do after kundalini has been raised?" "What do you do after you have developed or cultivated a talent?" Such questions simply do not occur. A true artist always knows that there is something more to be done—something better, finer, more beautiful, more perfect. Nothing is the best, the last, the finished product.

The method a seeker should use to raise the kundalini energy is determined by his or her temperament and inclination and level of development at the time that the desire comes. It could be through worship, through chanting, through raja yoga, through the mystical aspects of hatha yoga (the physical aspects alone being insufficient). Kundalini cannot be achieved or raised by drugs. There can be temporary experiences that are only micromanifestations of kundalini, and only if we consider *all* energy as kundalini. But then if kundalini had been defined in this way, the old texts would never have described the energy as "sleeping" or "latent." So when is the kundalini energy asleep and when is it awake? Awakened kundalini is a level of awareness and consciousness of a very high degree.

A question very often asked by those aspiring to awaken kundalini is, "What really is purification?" A pure mind is a mind that does not scheme to fulfill personal desires. A pure mind does not scheme revenge. A pure mind does not take advantage of the weaknesses or needs of another person. A pure mind will not exploit the emotional dependence of another person. A pure mind will support rather than undermine another's struggles to attain that same purity. A pure mind does not result from simply being a vegetarian. It is not food that makes someone pure. One may be a vegetarian and still take subtle or not so subtle revenge on others.

How can the average person understand and discriminate among the variety of experiences that have been presented as kundalini? A yogi is one who practices yoga, but this does not imply being a fully accomplished master of any yogic path. Anyone who has the genuine experience of kundalini has full control of the latent energy and is comparable in achievement to a person we would call a genius in the West. We simply have to ask: How many geniuses are there in the various fields of art and science? How many Einsteins? Michelangelos? Beethovens? Bachs?

Once again it has to be re-emphasized that the removal of

sexual or emotional inhibitions does not mean that the source of the additional energy to the individual is kundalini. It simply means what it is: inhibitions have been removed.

It takes superhuman strength to renounce the emotional investment in the belief in something that has provided security and gratification so far. The idea of renunciation, a requirement in certain Eastern and Western religious groups, has been seen for centuries as a necessary step toward liberation. Its essential value is not diminished because some individuals do not grasp the idea correctly and have little desire to have their own comfortable beliefs shaken. For most people, the fact that material renunciation has to precede the renunciation of mental-emotional security becomes very clear when certain spiritual experiences begin to take place. These are not proof of kundalini but show that the traveler is on the right road. With proper preparation any fear or anxiety connected with such new experiences is considerably diminished, and the experiencer is free to soar to new heights in joy and jubilation. If one stands on an unusually high tower looking into the distance it takes only a quick glance to realize fearfully how far one can fall. But if one has trained the mind into awareness, fear can be transformed into the ability to stay a little longer with the experience, to remember it and seek to find it again.

Many kundalini experiences that are reported deal with physical and mental manifestations of a rather frightening nature. It stands to reason that here it is rather an experience of powerful emotion that has taken place. States of hypnosis and autosuggestion and strong, powerful emotions have never been considered kundalini energy. The term used in the sacred texts indicates that kundalini energy is "latent." Kundalini has to be awakened. While some people may genuinely believe that they have experienced kundalini symptoms because they have heard or read of their manifestations, others have come to believe this because their descriptions of symptoms have been categorized by someone else as a manifestation of kundalini.

There is certainly today a rising awareness in people of the existence of the kundalini energy. People who have experiences that they erroneously attribute to kundalini arousal or to the "transmission of power from a guru" will find that over time the experience will fade out. Some will return to their normal lives and remember what they experienced as a dream. Others will doubt they experienced anything. And others will have a rude awakening when they see that there was an overstimulation and exploitation of their emotions.

But do not doubt that the true kundalini experience does take place in some people's lives. The measure of the validity of the experience—whether it is a true kundalini increase or not—depends upon what the person does with it. If you have, even for a short time, come "face to face with God," you will never be the same again. A beautiful transformation will take place.

It would be well to emphasize again that the transformations that take place in life after the kundalini experience do not occur suddenly. Neither does the development proceed automatically. Through his touch, Ramakrishna, an Indian prophet of the last century, gave an experience to his disciple, Vivekananda. He told Vivekananda that this was a foretaste but that he must find the key to the door for himself. The kundalini can disappear if you do not clear the channel for higher inspiration. By this is meant building character and seeking self-mastery. It takes time, training, effort, and persistence.

Each aspirant consciously or unconsciously searches for a teacher—that person who will help to guide his or her footsteps on the path of spiritual unfoldment. Be careful and discriminate in your search. Take a little time; listen to and evaluate those who are called gurus. That is your right and responsibility. Be cautious and curtail your vanity in the search. Your search should be done with prayer and meditation on the guidance from within, and with a decision to suspend the old habit of premature criticism. When the aspirant cannot suspend judgment, the time to find a guru has not yet come. Your guru will be one to whom you feel drawn, not emotionally, but by a different attraction: an inner knowing that one can receive. If the inner knowing is not there, the preparation is not yet complete. One has only oneself to blame for becoming involved with the wrong person. We get what we deserve.

The more advanced exercises and lines of thought cannot be written down. For these practices there must be a very close relationship between guru and disciple. The closeness can be and has to be guided by the effort of the seeker, by a prayerful attitude, by requests to the Most High, and by a commitment that allows one to make such a request to the Most High. The commitment to spiritual life by itself is one step. The other is suspension of judgment for the time being, and cultivation of all that which we sum up in the word "I." But above all, have faith that in response to your sincerity and earnest prayer, when the foundation has been properly laid and you are ready, the guru will appear. Blessings on your journey.

THE PSYCHOPHYSIOLOGY OF KUNDALINI

Haridas Chaudhuri

If the meditator keeps advancing on the path of meditation with a sustained depth-exploring thrust, he is in for a spiritual breakthrough. The combined pressure of the breath-libido-ego at the base of the spinal cord brings about the release of a tremendous dormant energy. In yoga psychology this is known as the kundalini, the serpent power, the coiled energy. Tantric yogis believe that it is the nuclear energy of the human psychophysical system. It is comparable to the nuclear energy of the atom. The atomic energy is released through bombardment of the atomic nucleus with high-voltage alpha particles. Likewise, the psychonuclear energy of man is released through high pressure of the concentrated biopsychic energy mobilized by mental focusing. Another pressure brought to bear upon the release is that of the concentrated thought energy resulting from the intensification of consciousness. While the pressure of the biopsychic energy is a tremendous push sideways, the pressure of thought energy is like a magnetic pull from above. The push from below is felt as intense Godward aspiration of the human soul. The pull from above is felt as the irresistible attraction of divine grace or charm. The dynamic interplay of these two forces produces the following results:

1. Transformation of the sexual libido (retas) into the subtler and luminous ego-transcending or transpersonal Being-energy (ojas).
2. Awakening of the psychonuclear energy and its appro-

priation of the newly generated value-energy (ojas) resulting in upward movement along the central canal (sushumna) of the spinal cord.

3. Considerable withdrawal of energy from the vital organs, efferent nerves and externally-oriented musculature.

4. Gradual opening or activation of the various energy centers and associated glands of the body resulting in the exploration of the higher levels of consciousness as the regular practice of meditation continues from day to day, from month to month, from year to year.

5. Gradual change of the body metabolism and brain chemistry facilitating the enhanced functioning of the cerebral hemispheres.

The Psychonuclear or Physionuclear Energy (Kundalini)

The awakened physionuclear energy is invariably experienced by all meditators and yogis as some kind of supernatural or divine energy. The Vedic and Zoroastrian mystics called it the mystic fire. Endless hymns of adoration have been composed in recognition of its ability to carry the human soul to higher realms of consciousness on to the unsurpassable glory of the supreme Godhead. In ancient mythology it is described as the mythical sunbird Garuda which soars up in the sky carrying the serpent in its beak, i.e., transforming the libido energy into passion for the divine.

The more the physionuclear energy rises upward, the more the meditator's energy level rises, and in consequence his consciousness also rises.

In Christian mysticism it is the same physionuclear energy which has been perceived as the Holy Spirit or Ghost. It is the divine spark transmitted to the mortal frame. Since in Christian theology, the body and the spirit, the natural and the supernatural, the impure flesh and the pure divine energy are diametrically opposed substances, it has not occurred to

Western mystics that they might have been made of the same ultimate stuff.

The tantric philosophy of India is in agreement with modern science that there is, in ultimate analysis, only one stuff of all existence, and that is energy. The primordial energy is known as mahashakti. Science analyzes it objectively and declares it to be the matrix of all the infinitely variegated objects of the physical world. Yoga as personal growth process reveals the basic dynamic stuff of the universe as spiritual energy, metaphorically described as the Divine Mother (Jaganmata, Divyashakti). According to Vedanta, the superconscient divine energy is experienced by the meditator at the highest peak of cosmic consciousness. Whereas the primal physical energy of science is the energy as it appears to physical consciousness, the primal superconscient energy of yoga is the same energy as it appears to the eye of illumination or transpersonal superconscient experience of the advanced meditator.

According to some, the kundalini or primal energy is the right vagus nerve[1] that controls the nerve plexes of the autonomic nervous system. When the vagal center in the medulla oblongata is stimulated, the functions of heart, lungs and larynx are inhibited. At the same time the functions of the stomach, intestine and digestive glands are accelerated. By stimulating the afferent nerves of the vagus centered in the solar plexus and forming interconnections with the hypogastric and pelvic plexes, the yogi succeeds in enormously intensifying or expanding his consciousness in both dimensions of the universe. The climax of this process is achieved when, without any interference from the autonomic and unconscious functioning of the sympathetic nervous system, the yogi experiences ecstatic oneness with the cosmic whole.

In the opinion of Sir John Woodroffe the kundalini is the potential energy which stimulates the vagus nerve and therefore is not to be identified with the latter.[2] In this respect, Woodroffe is at one with the most widely accepted traditional view.

The most authoritative interpretation postulates the kundalini as the nuclear energy of the psychophysical system. When awakened, this energy is simultaneously experienced as physical, vital, mental, and spiritual. So in a sense it is immaterial whether it is described as the physionuclear or bionuclear or psychonuclear or somatonuclear energy. It is the nuclear energy of the enormously complicated organized structure of man's existence which we call the psychophysical system.

The kundalini is also referred to as the supraindividual, transpersonal Being-energy (shiva-shakti), or as the all-conquering spiritual or divine energy capable of capturing the kingdom of heaven (the blissful superconscient experience) by storm. It is transpersonal in the sense that it lifts an individual beyond the limits of his circumscribed ego-self, or mind-bound personal existence, or socio-culturally imprisoned self. It is divine in the sense that it is invariably felt as vastly superior to all ego-effort or personal initiative. It has a unique rhythm and law of becoming of its own, an irrepressible spontaneity, a time-scorning, death-defying drive of its own. It may suddenly appear like a thief at unexpected hours, steal your mind and heart with a thrilling touch, devour your sleep, decimate all lethargy and resistance and galvanize your total being into one soaring flame of divine passion. When unchecked in its advance, it is capable of swallowing up the entire ego-self, shattering the bonds of space-time awareness, and annihilating all landmarks of familiar cultural norms. . . .

Can the Body Survive Kundalini Explosion?

If the kundalini or the mystic fire be really the nuclear energy of the human organism, would not its release and explosion entail the disintegration of the entire body?

There are varying degrees of awakening or dynamization of the coiled energy which is the static pole and positive nucleus in relation to the rest of the bodily energies which are dynamic. Whenever a person enters into the condition of immensely intensified consciousness due to his total concentration on an absorbing project, whether scientific, artistic, commercial or political, he feels the thrill and excitement of overflowing energy. What happens is the partial awakening of the coiled energy. His concentrated vital energy (prana), withdrawn from all other affairs of the world, puts pressure at the base of the spinal cord. The coiled energy reacts by rechanneling the mobilized vital energy along the spinal cord toward the brain. This results in the flow of new creative ideas, or exciting new solutions to the problems concentrated on.

In the case of a yogi or advanced meditator the same thing happens in more intensified form. A greater measure of rechanneling of energy from the outer to the upward direction takes place. If and when there comes a time when the coiled energy undergoes total conversion from the static to the dynamic form, the yogi attains what is called bodiless liberation (videha mukti). He leaves the body and becomes one with the vastness of cosmic Being.

But the majority of spiritual seekers wish to attain spiritual liberation while living in the flesh (jivanmukti). After liberation they wish to share with the world some of the joy and perfume, some of the love and glory of their beatific experience. So usually what happens is sufficiently effective dynamization of the coiled energy without its total dislocation from the root center. All that is needed is that such dynamization should be powerful enough to open the highest center of consciousness in the upper cerebrum resulting in enlightenment and liberation.

What is exactly the mechanism involved in the dynamization of the coiled energy?

In the course of yoga practice and concentration, the vital, instinctual, and mental energies are mobilized and marshalled inward. Under the impact of their concentrated attack, the positive nucleus of the psychophysical system (kundalini), the apparently static positive pole of the body's magnetic field, sends forth an emanation or ejection, some kind of "etheric double," as theosophists call it, which shoots up like an electric current along the central canal of the spinal cord.

Regarding the exact nature of this upward-ascending electric current there is room for difference of interpretation. It is possible that the coiled energy of the nuclear power undergoes a partial conversion into its dynamic equivalent. This dynamic equivalent then reacts upon the concentrated psychophysical energy by rechanneling it and converging it along the vertical axis of the spinal cord. Herein lies the basis for the phenomenological experience of the upward-rising kundalini.

Second, the coiled energy may be like unto radium. Its emanations or radiations do not diminish its total store of energy. They perform the task of converging the concentrated dynamic energies along the vertical axis.

There is still another, a third, possible line of interpretation. Under the impact of breath-control and intense concentration, the root center, like an electromagnetic machine, becomes oversaturated. It then produces an inductive action, analogous to electromagnetic action, by which the mobilized dynamic energies operative in the body are converged along the axis. In this case there is no need to postulate the conversion of the static pole into its dynamic equivalent. The root center, like an oversaturated electromagnetic machine, induces in the neighborhood an equivalent and opposite kind of electromagnetism without losing its own stock of energy.[3]

According to an orthodox interpretation, at the highest point of inward concentration in the practice of kundalini yoga, the coiled energy becomes entirely dynamized, leaves its original abode at the base of the spinal cord, shoots up to the top of the cerebrum and becomes blissfully united with the boundless light of transcendental consciousness (paramshiva). Out of this union profusely flows the nectar of spiritual energy and bliss (cerebrospinal fluid) which sustains the body. This bestows complete liberation in the flesh. The body is sustained by the energy-flow of divine bliss until the momentum of the past karma entirely wears out. Then the liberated yogi leaves his mortal coil and becomes one with the absolute Spirit.

Modern interpreters find this orthodox interpretation difficult to accept. It militates against the scientific view of the living organism as a polarized structure of energy. Essential to the aliveness and dynamic functioning of the body is the presence of the static pole, the coiled energy at the base of the spinal cord, without its dislocation or complete depletion of energy.[4]

Higher Levels of Consciousness

The more the psychonuclear energy rises upward richly fueled by the refined oil of sublimated libido, the more the meditator feels celestially high, his total energy level mounts in an ascending scale, and in consequence his level of consciousness also rises in a corresponding measure.

As the fiery sparks emanating from the celestial serpent's mouth reach the cerebral hemispheres, different areas of that marvelous mechanism become more and more stimulated. On the stimulation of the pleasure site the meditator begins to experience intense waves of profound ecstasy, spontaneous joy and ineffable peace. The entire body appears flooded with a downpour of bliss, even the countless blood cells dancing in joy.

When the right hemisphere of the brain is especially stimulated, latent intuitive powers of extrasensory perceptions such as clairvoyance, clairaudience, telepathy, precognition, etc., begin to be unfolded. Consciousness begins to expand and unravel new frontiers and new dimensions of the cosmic whole. The I-consciousness or sense of identity begins to make quantum jumps from larger to larger orbits of cosmic awareness. The increasingly penetrating insight eventually hits the most hidden nontemporal depth dimension of existence. At this stage the sense of time in all its modes, not only the sense of linear time but even the nonlinear now-centered time, is swallowed up in pure timeless consciousness.

NOTES

1. Vasant G. Rele, *The Mysterious Kundalini* (Bombay: D. B. Tarapore Vala Sons, 1970), pp. 50–52.
2. Ibid., p. x.
3. *The Serpent Power,* op. cit., p. 307.
4. Ibid., p. 310.

KUNDALINI YOGA THROUGH SHAKTIPAT

Yogi Amrit Desai

Kundalini yoga is one of the most secret ancient sciences of India, but recently it has been made available to the West. Kundalini can be awakened by several different methods. There is hatha yoga–techniques of asana, pranayama, mudra, and bandha (locks). There is bhakti yoga–the yoga of extreme love, devotion, faith, and mantra chanting. It can also be awakened suddenly and unexpectedly as a result of incomplete sadhana (spiritual discipline) in a past life. In such cases, a person unfamiliar with the subject fails to understand the significance of the experience. If he is not actively searching for the results that this awakening ultimately brings, he will not benefit and progress. Some who experience this awakening without the guidance of a guru become frightened, thinking it to be mental illness, nervousness, or evil spirits.

At such times the grace and guidance of an experienced guru are necessary to sail safely through the varied experiences and attain samadhi (cosmic consciousness). Here it is necessary to point out that anyone who tries to awaken kundalini through forced mechanical techniques without the guidance of an experienced master may encounter dangerous effects. Because shaktipat is like a powerful charge, it is necessary that the nervous system be strong and pure.

Guru's Grace

Many authors describe kundalini yoga as a dangerous approach. Yet the same could be said for learning to drive a car without the supervision of an expert driver. The safest and best method of awakening the kundalini is through the grace of a realized kundalini master. Even if shakti is awakened by other means, the guru's grace is essential on this path.

The guru, when inspired by Divine Will, stirs up the latent kundalini power in the deserving disciple. This process is called shaktipat. The yogi who has control over prana can consciously bring his prana and his whole being to a certain level of vibration where he is able to impart it to others. The charismatic and magnetic influence of such masters can arouse the psychic astral force (shakti) within the disciple. Swami Vishnu Tirtha, in his book *Devatma Shakti,* says, "Such great personalities have their prana and mind on higher potentiality and when approached they tend to raise the prana of others from a lower potentiality to a higher one."

A guru transmits shakti by a pregnant glance, touch, mantra, or simply by thought. Thus he installs his divine energy in his disciple, releasing mental and physiological blocks that had prevented the prana from moving freely within the body. The guru, being in tune with his own master and with God, continues to receive shakti uninterruptedly and abundantly in order to serve the spiritually hungry disciples. When Christians take Holy Communion, they are partaking of the flesh and blood of Christ. This was originally the act of receiving Christ's body into oneself. Similarly, with the shaktipat initiation the disciple unites with his guru and his love and faith increase as he progresses along the path.

Some receive shaktipat by reading the writings of the master or by looking at his picture. This divine energy can be transferred at will or unconsciously. Simply touching any article which belongs to the guru can ignite the spark within the disciple. Christ had this power. A woman who was ill came up behind him and touched his cloak. She was immediately healed, and Jesus, without seeing her, was aware of the occurrence. "Somebody hath touched me for I perceive that the power is gone out of me" (Luke 8:46).

Shaktipat Diksha

During the process of shaktipat diksha (shakti initiation), the astral body of the guru merges with that of the disciple. It establishes karmic ties between the two which last for incarnations. At this time, the master takes on the karma of the initiate, thus speeding up the evolutionary process of his devotee. The same process of karmic ties is expressed in Christianity by the statement that Christ suffered and died for our sins (I Cor. 15:3). Not only did he take on the sins of men but he gave the power to disciples to do the same: "Receive ye the Holy Spirit: Whose soever sins ye remit, they are remitted unto them, and whose soever sins ye retain, they are retained" (John 20:23). The shaktipat initiation creates an astral link between the guru and disciple by which the disciple continues to receive psychic help from his chain of gurus. Unity with the master is accomplished by complete surrender and love for the guru accompanied by a special technique of meditation on the guru.* The link which binds guru and disciple in divine love grows, creating an almost irresistible pull on the aspirant to be near his master. Shaktipat opens an inner door which enables him to experience a tremendous amount of love. This is almost frightening to some who are not used to feeling such unconditional love. They temporarily suffer from typical Christian guilt feelings that they are unworthy of such blessings.

How Shakti Works

Shaktipat kundalini yoga is the yoga of total surrender to God and guru within. This is best accomplished by first surrendering to the external guru and using him as a vantage point.

* Refer to *Guru* by Swami Muktananda.

The phenomenon which occurs during and after shaktipat initiation is the experience of surrender to the God-power (prana or Holy Spirit) within. It is this powerful divine force which becomes the inner protector and guide who is ever loving and forgiving once allowed to be free by the grace of the guru. Through shaktipat and an accompanying longing for freedom and knowledge on the part of the aspirant, the shakti rises through the central canal of the spinal column (sushumna), piercing the six chakras (nerve plexes). This is known as kundalini awakening.

The aroused power of kundalini affects both the autonomic nervous system, which functions by pranic intelligence alone, and the central nervous system, which functions under mental control. Under the effect of the powerful currents traveling through the entire nervous system as a result of shaktipat, the prana assumes its original role as master of the whole being and the central nervous system becomes autonomic for a time. The mind under the influence of the boosted prana becomes a mute spectator of the divine inner intelligence. The prana becomes free from the usual mental tyrannies and functions as a purifying force wherever it is needed within the person. The *Atharva Veda,* one of the oldest Indian scriptures, says, ". . . bowing to the prana, under whose control is all this (universe), who is master of all, by whom everything is supported." So whenever the defenses of the mind are lifted and the prana level is raised, the prana's divine power accomplishes healing, purification and elevating effects in the body, mind, and spirit.

Manifestations

When the empowered prana (shakti) moves through the body, it creates various external and internal movements. On a physiological level one can experience the following: heat, cold, automatic breathing of various kinds, mudras, locks, postures (which are done with perfection even if the aspirant knows no hatha yoga), laughter, tears of joy, utterance of deformed sounds, feelings of fear, the curling back of the tongue, revolving of eyeballs, temporary stopping of breath without effort, an itching or crawling sensation under the skin, and singing with ecstasy and joy.

These cleansing kriyas and exercises may be practiced for many years by those who do not have the fortune to receive shaktipat initiation. Strangely enough, however, the initiate performs them automatically, guided from within, without study of any external source. On a subtle level, one may experience divine harmonies, the sounds of various instruments or mantras, the taste of divine flavors and the smell of sweet fragrances, or divine lights and colors. One may recall past lives, be poetically inspired, feel drunk with the ecstasy of divine bliss, have frightening dreams, or remain completely silent. During all this, the mind remains filled with joy. On an intellectual level, the hidden meaning behind the scriptures and spiritual texts are revealed. Intuition and psychic powers put one in touch with the divine, bringing security, peace, and a feeling of unseen guidance and protection.

Thus, when the automatic kriyas take place and the entire being functions under the control of prana, the nervous and glandular systems are nourished and revitalized. This in turn removes disease and prepares the body and mind for higher states of consciousness. The mind, being still, learns an important lesson, that of remaining as objectively aware as possible, increasing its capacity to maintain objectivity as the disciple progresses along the path.

It is important to understand that the manifestations of shakti, though automatic and involuntary, can be consciously controlled and stopped at any time. The feelings produced and the physical effects are all under objective observation by the mind even during the most intense periods. The mind is subordinate and surrendered as long as the aspirant lets himself go and does not fear. With complete surrender shakti can purify the mind and body very quickly and effectively. Hence, nothing goes wrong because the shakti and the guru psychically protect the disciple. All such manifestations have a cleansing effect, though they may seem terrifying to the outside observer who knows nothing of kundalini yoga.

The physical manifestations which occur with the movement of shakti correspond exactly to the biblical description of the day of the Pentecost: "and suddenly there came a sound from heaven as of a rushing mighty wind, and it filled the house where they were sitting. And there appeared unto them cloven tongues like as of fire and it sat on each of them. And they were all filled with the Holy Spirit and began to speak with other tongues, as the Spirit gave them utterance" (Acts 2:2–4).

Whenever the right conditions are provided, experiences somewhat similar to shaktipat can be observed, as in the Pentecostal Church. Others who experience slight variations of this awakening are those who practice Subud, Quakers (who were originally called that because they quaked), and Holy Rollers. It may also manifest itself on the psychiatrist's couch and in group therapy sessions, or during drug experiences.

However, as soon as the person goes back to his usual living habits, the impurities and distractions return. Most of the systems described above lack the program charted by enlightened masters which leads the aspirant step by step to the highest peaks of spiritual enlightenment. Such experiences, if not properly guided and guarded by the grace of the guru, do not serve their real purpose.

Surrender to Prana

The average person ignores the dictates of the divine prana's inner guidance. This is because modern man has allowed his pranic energies to be dissipated indiscriminately in sense and ego satisfaction. When prana dictates sleep, man will say, "I'd rather go to the movies." Where prana gives the signal for elimination, man will respond after he has finished some work. Thus he ignores and insults God's power that tries to function for his well being. Kundalini awakening reestablishes these natural promptings and hence the higher natural disciplines become a way of life in a most effortless manner. After shaktipat, meditation becomes natural and takes place without strain or striving. Preoccupation with time and/or physical discomfort gives way to joy and ecstasy.

Because man is a creature of habit (the gross karmic effects of samskaras) he receives impulses from the subconsciously suppressed past. As a result, he finds himself performing actions and entertaining thoughts and emotions which obviously destroy his peace and keep him on a merry-go-round of worldly sufferings. His life is sporadically "fun," but each "up" is always accompanied by a "down" leading to an endless pattern of sorrow, depression, fear, and insecurity.

The best way to come out of this self-created, self-imposed compulsive destruction is to truly and sincerely accept the divine force known as Krishna or Christ. When we regard them as savior and say, "My Lord, Thy will be done, not mine," we can be free in the real sense. With the recognition of the divine prana as the basic energy which sustains the entire universe, we may realize its presence within ourselves. At the awakening of this energy within, man is transformed into superman and he assumes his heritage as a true son of God.

SRI AUROBINDO, THE TANTRA AND KUNDALINI

Vasant V. Merchant

Sri Aurobindo (1872–1950) was one of India's–indeed, the world's–foremost mystic seers, philosophers, and poets. Although he came from a background of teaching and political action, he underwent a transformative experience in 1910 that led him to a lifelong calling of service to the world through spiritual endeavor. This included a colossal production of texts–including his masterpiece, *The Life Divine*–and the establishment of an ashram in Pondicherry, India. In 1968, the international City of Dawn called Auroville, which he had envisioned, was established a few miles from the ashram.

Helping him as his spiritual collaborator was Mira Alfassa Richard (1878–1973), born in France, called "The Mother." In Sri Aurobindo's philosophy, "The Mother" refers to the Divine Eternal Forces. In the ashram, "The Mother" is representative of that Supreme Power (Mahashakti), a concrete manifestation in human form of the unfolding energy of consciousness in the universe.

The formation of Sri Aurobindo's vision and the expression of it on the earthly plane in the system called integral yoga is an inspiring story. Too long to recount here, it is nevertheless worthy of investigation and research. Suffice it to say that tantra is of major significance to it. Sri Aurobindo once stated that the tantric system "is in its aspiration one of the greatest attempts yet made to embrace the whole of God manifested and unmanifested in the adoration, self-discipline, and knowledge of a single human soul." He described it elsewhere as "a wide, assured, and many-sided endeavor, unparalleled in its power, insight, amplitude, to provide the race with a basis of generalized psychoreligious experience from which man could rise through knowledge, works of love, or through any other fundamental power of his nature to some established supreme experience and highest absolute status."[1]

Underlying integral yoga is the knowledge of the tantra. Yet integral yoga is nevertheless a genuinely new and unique approach to human transformation. Some of the main principles of tantra enter into integral yoga. The ascent of consciousness, for example, through psychophysical centers (chakras) and other aspects of tantric knowledge are part of Sri Aurobindo's formulation. But for the first time in the history of evolutionary consciousness, he articulated and exemplified the *descent* of consciousness, along with the truth that nothing can be done except through the force of The Mother, the creative as well as the redemptive and executive energy of the universe.

In the integral approach of Sri Aurobindo, there is a full appreciation of the many-sided perspective of tantra on the problems of living. Neither tantra nor integral yoga make a false or radical cleavage between a person's inner and outer life, between the so-called higher and lower. Rather, they embrace the human being in his totality and oneness, and aim to give importance to the whole person in all aspects of life, ennobling and uplifting him to the joy of creation, to the delight of becoming divinized, along with the rest of humanity and the physical world. The destiny of the body is to grow into a divine body, its purpose is to pour out and breathe forth the delight of being and becoming. Thus the body becomes the spirit. Therefore it is not to be neglected, abhorred, or condemned, but understood and transmuted for the higher purpose of consciousness consonant with the integral harmony and balance necessary not only with the physical levels but also with the vital, mental, psychic, and spiritual dimensions and aspects of the being and nature.

Kundalini yoga is one of the most important of the shakta tantras, and it is included in Sri Aurobindo's vision of divinized life, though in a way that is distinctly different from modern forms of kundalini yoga. In Sri Aurobindo's teaching, both the individual and cosmic lives' evolutionary thrusts tend toward divinity. Ultimately, therefore, the goals of the individual and of the collective life of humanity are not at variance, but are both seeking the Supracosmic Transcendent Divinity through the process of the ascent and the descent of consciousness, where the chakras are instrumentalities for both the evolution and involution of consciousness flowing through the energy of prana and the proper awakening of kundalini, as represented in the creative mysteries of the spirit in science, metaphysics, psychology, art, ritual, and life.

In the philosophy of the tantra–especially the shakta tantra–the universe is a manifestation of the two poises or stances of the Supreme Consciousness (Divine Shakti) whose nature is Power. The poise of rest (static aspect) supports the poise of action (dynamic aspect). The interaction of these two poles of Her Being brings out of Herself ananda or pure bliss, the delight of her universal expression, and this becomes the sustaining force of the entire creation. This truth of the macrocosm is reflected and repeated in the microcosm of each individual and entity in the universe at different levels. In the human, too, this divine energy or shakti is operative in keeping one alive and functional in different spheres of life. This power or energy is called the kundalini.

Kundalini shakti is defined in the traditional tantric philosophy as the power that is lying unused in the human body. Tantra aims to tap this reservoir, set in motion by the latent energy, and give full meaning to the individual concentration of power that is man. Kundalini shakti is also described as the thrice-coiled serpent power. It is the treasure house of the life essence, the life force stored at the base of the spine. It is also considered the seat of birth, death, and rebirth.

The Uniqueness of Sri Aurobindo's Yoga

The key to the uniqueness of Sri Aurobindo's yoga lies not only in the ascent of consciousness, but also in the descent of consciousness as the singularly most important feature in the spiritual transformation. This process of the ascent and the descent of consciousness is a reciprocal one, a bipolar process, and hence represents both the evolution and the involution of consciousness. Sri Aurobindo is the first yogi who recognizes, discovers,. develops, realizes, and works with the awakening of the kundalini thus. He acknowledges that there is a tantric knowledge behind the process of transformation, but with this essential difference from other yogas and other tantric practices. In the words of Sri Aurobindo himself:

> The process of the kundalini awakened rising through the centers as also the purification of the centers is a tantric knowledge. In our yoga there is no willed process of the purification and opening of the centers, no raising up of the kundalini by a set process either.[2]

And again:

> In our yoga there is no willed opening of the chakras; they open of themselves by the descent of the Force. In the tantric discipline they open from down upward, the muladhar first; in our yoga, they open from up downward. But the ascent of the force from the muladhar does take place.[3]

The difference between the tantric practices in awakening the kundalini and opening the centers is further explained by Sri Aurobindo as an ascension of the consciousness rising up till it joins the higher consciousness above. This process is repeated and a descent is felt and experienced until all the different centers (physical, vital, mental) and the planes they command and correspond to are opened and the consciousness rises above the body (see Figure 1).

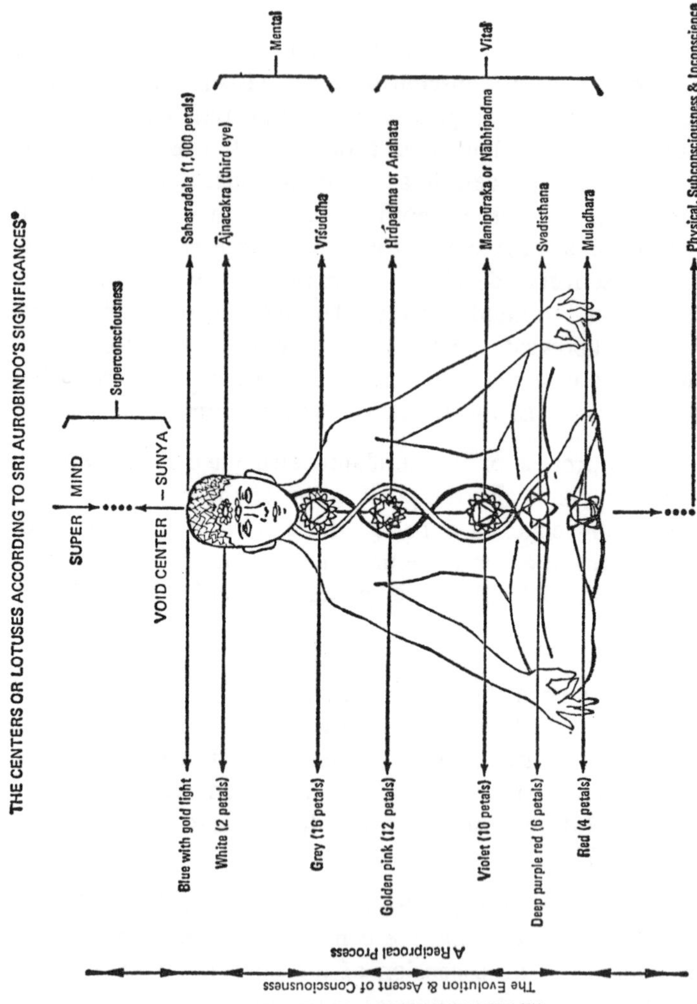
THE CENTERS OR LOTUSES ACCORDING TO SRI AUROBINDO'S SIGNIFICANCES*
SUPER
MIND
Superconsciousness
VOID CENTER
— SUNYA
Blue with gold light
Sahasradala (1,000 petals)
White (2 petals)
Ājnacakra (third eye)
Grey (16 petals)
Viśuddha
Mental
Golden pink (12 petals)
Hrdpadma or Anahata
Violet (10 petals)
Manipūraka or Nābhipadma
Deep purple red (6 petals)
Svadisthana
Red (4 petals)
Muladhara
Vital
Physical, Subconsciousness & Inconscience
The Involution & Descent of Consciousness:
The Evolution & Ascent of Consciousness
A Reciprocal Process
*Traditionally, those who take the centers in the body count only six centers, the *Sahasrara* being excluded because it is above the head center, as also those centers below the feet.

Figure 1.

This consciousness thus can suspend itself, widen itself, and merge into the universal self and cosmic consciousness. This describes a general course, which is subject to a greater rapidity and velocity and the opening above in a sudden, definite, and spontaneous manner.

Another key point of difference between Sri Aurobindo's yoga and the other yogas is that following the enormous and very complicated details and accessories laid down in the tantric books is not necessary. The force of ascent and descent accomplishes itself in this yoga in its own way. Also, the awakening of the kundalini and the consciousness of the openings of the centers do not necessarily occur in chronological order—that is, from center to center or chakra to chakra (although it may or can be so)—but from level to level or plane to plane—that is, from the force descending first to the head, then to the heart, then to the navel, and still below. It is not considered at all imperative to know and become aware of the different deities in the centers according to the descriptions of the tantra, but The Mother's power is felt and experienced in the various centers by the sadhakas (seekers of truth, spiritual practitioners).

Sri Aurobindo in this sense is extremely unorthodox in his integral yoga. He emphasizes in the sadhana (spiritual quest and spiritual practice) no false bondage to the knowledge given in the books, and is totally independent in the sense that his greatest and only allegiance is to the central truth and its pursuit and realization in the unfoldment of the consciousness without any slavery or subjection to the old signs and symbols, or old names and forms. Sri Aurobindo gives a different interpretation, and therefore a new and different value and significance to the centers themselves—whether they are related to psychology, biology, metaphysics, etc. Therefore they are not the same as are given in the tantric books (see Figure 2).

Figure 2.

THE CHAKRAS OR LOTUSES IN

NAME OF CHAKRA	LOCATION/ REGION	GOVERNANCE OF OR CENTER OF
Muladhara	Its apex at end of the spine and projects from there	The seat of physical consciousness proper, commanding the physical consciousness and the subconscient; regulates sex organs and commands sex action.
Svadisthana	Below the navel	The lower vital
Manipura or Nabhipadma	The navel center	The seat of the centralized vital consciousness (dynamic center), which ranges from the heart level (emotional) to the center below the navel (lower vital, sensational-desire center); governs the larger vital.
Hrdpadma or Anahata	The heart center	The seat of the emotional being
Visuddha	The throat center	The physical mind or externalizing mind is in the subtle body in the throat and connected strongly with the speech—but it acts by connection with the brain.

*THIS CHART IS PREPARED FROM THE "CHAKRAS" IN *SRI AUROBINDO ON THE TANTRA*, pp. 19-22.

SRI AUROBINDO'S YOGA*

SPECIAL FUNCTION AND SIGNIFICANCE	COLOR OF THE LOTUS	NO. OF PETALS
The physical center is also the sex-center. The *Muladhara* from which the Kundalini rises is not in the physical body but in the subtle body.	Red	Four
Commands the small movements, the little greeds, lusts, desires, the small sense-movements.	Deep purple red	Six
Commands the larger life-forces and passions and larger desire-movements.	Violet	Ten
Commands the higher emotional being with the psychic deep behind it.	Golden pink	Twelve
Commands expression and all externalization of the mind movements and mental forces; is the center of the physical mind, the center of externalization—in speech, expression, the power to deal mentally with physical mind to the light of the divine consciousness instead of remaining in the outgoing mentality.	Grey	Sixteen

THE CHAKRAS OR LOTUSES IN

NAME OF CHAKRA	LOCATION/ REGION	GOVERNANCE OF OR CENTER OF
Ajnacakra	Forehead center: Between the eyes, but a little bit above	The inner will, the inner vision, the dynamic mind; the third eye (in the center of the forehead).
Sahasradala †	Above head center	The higher consciousness center, *Sahasradala Padma.* (This center is not within the body; it is above the head, above the brain, and acts as a center connecting all that is above the mind with the mind proper, situated in the body.

† USUALLY ONLY SIX CENTERS ARE COUNTED, THE SEVENTH AND THE HIGHEST BEING ABOVE THE HEAD–VIZ, SAHASRARA IS EXCLUDED, AS ALSO THE CENTERS BELOW THE FEET.

SRI AUROBINDO'S YOGA (continued)

SPECIAL FUNCTION AND SIGNIFICANCE	COLOR OF THE LOTUS	NO. OF PETALS
With opening of this center and the force, there is opening of a greater will, power of decision, formation, effectiveness, beyond what the ordinary mind can achieve; bestows inner vision, sees inner forms and images of things and people and understands things and people from within and not only from outside. It is the beginning of the yogic as opposed to ordinary mental consciousness.	White	Two
Commands the higher thinking mind and the illumined mind and opening upwards to the intuition and overmind. It centralizes spiritual mind, higher mind, intuitive mind and acts as a receiving station, a link between individual consciousness and the infinite consciousness around and above; not to be identified with the brain. This center also called the void center, *Sunya,* because it is not in the body but in the apparent void above, entering into the silence of the self or spiritual being.	Blue with light gold around	Thousand-petaled

What then is the true meaning of transformation in integral yoga as opposed to other yogas? How does "transformation" differ from "realization," and what is its relationship to "descent"? Are they the same? Sri Aurobindo's answer to these questions is crystal clear: Transformation in his yoga is not to be equated with sainthood or development of a transcendental body. Rather, transformation means a radical, total, and complete change of consciousness toward the next definite step in spiritual evolutionary growth from the animal-material world to the vital, mental, and psychic. Partial or fragmented or relative realization must not be mistaken for the total transformation to be made in life through integral yoga.

Sri Aurobindo further clarifies that the light of realization is not the same thing as descent. Why? Because a mere realization may only bring an "opening" or heightening or widening of the consciousness at the top so as to realize something in the purusha (static supreme knowledge) part without any radical change in the parts of prakriti (dynamic evolutionary material-energy). Sri Aurobindo continues to emphasize that the light of realization at the spiritual summit of the consciousness may be there, and is necessary, but it is not sufficient in itself, since the areas and aspects below remain the same without any change. In other words, unless there is a descent of the light that enters and permeates not only the mind and mental levels of the being in part, but also becomes an all-powerful ubiquitous force touching and transforming the levels that are physical and below, no real transformation transpires. That light must touch and purify the vital nature and its movements too. Otherwise only a part of the nature is touched, and hence only a portion or fraction is transformed.

Sri Aurobindo declares that even the descent of light is not sufficient. It must be the descent of the whole consciousness—and its manifestations such as peace, power, knowledge, love, ananda (pure bliss). The descent, he concludes, "may be enough to liberate, but not to perfect, or it may be enough to make a great change in the inner being, while the outer remains an imperfect instrument, clumsy, sick, or unexpressive. Finally, transformation effected by the sadhana cannot be complete unless it is a supramentalization of the being. Psychicization is not enough, it is only a beginning; spiritualization and the descent of the higher consciousness is not enough, it is only a middle term; the ultimate achievement needs the action of the Supramental Consciousness and Force."[4]

Another major point of difference in Sri Aurobindo's yoga is that even at its highest, it is to be remembered that the kundalini power of the individual—the shakti embedded in the material or body-consciousness—does not rise beyond the domain of the lower triple creation of the physical, vital, and psychic planes of existence. The divine shakti invoked in the yoga of Sri Aurobindo is the Supreme Power that not only extends itself universally, but also transcends the creation, *para shakti.* It is this *mahashakti* (Supreme Power of the Divine Mother) that is instrumental in becoming the most effective means, and not man's puny will and sense of being the doer in awakening the kundalini, which is described as a "devi" or a goddess. Here, too, not mere personal effort and reliance alone on one's own power is the crux; a total surrender is absolutely essential.

This does not mean that individual effort does not count or assume importance in the earlier or initial stages. Also, aids like mantra, japa, asanas, devotional rituals, etc., are used *only* if necessary and only as long as necessary. But they are not considered indispensable as supports, as in other yogas. The only demands in this yoga on the sadhaka are primarily three: aspiration, rejection, and surrender—aspiration for the highest Light and all its manifestations; rejection of all the wrong movements (at whatever level) of any nature that are an impediment on the way; and surrender of all and everything one is to The Mother or the Divine Power invoked. (A word of caution, however, about the meaning of surrender: This unreserved surrender is not a dull, lifeless surrender. It is the unconditional surrender of a vibrant, living, conscious individual that is *integral*—not the surrender of a robot, an automaton, or a mechanical, unconscious being.)

One other point of distinction in the uniqueness of Sri

Aurobindo's yoga is the concept of the Supermind. It is, in fact, the center, the source, and the crown of Sri Aurobindo's yoga, and manifests itself in all the centers–physical, vital, psychic, and mental. What is the Supermind? How can it be reached, experienced, and retained? To that supreme aim Sri Aurobindo addresses himself thus:

> The Supermind is the vast Truth-Consciousness of which the ancient seers spoke; there have been glimpses of it till now, sometimes an indirect influence or pressure, but it has not been brought down into the consciousness of the earth and fixed there. To so bring it down is the aim of our yoga.
>
> . . . It is not by reasoning but by constant experience, growth of consciousness, and widening into the Light that one can reach those higher levels of consciousness above the intellect from which one can begin to look up to the Divine Gnosis. Those levels are not yet the Supermind, but they can receive something of its knowledge.[5]

In traditional literature, there is no mention of such a center, not even an allusion. This can be explained simply by saying that knowledge of the Supermind is *new* knowledge. No one other than Sri Aurobindo and The Mother, who dedicated their entire lives to their stupendous work on the Supermind, its discovery and manifestation, and the transformation of Earth life through the power of Supramental Truth, have ever been known to have received the living splendor and puissance of the Supermind.

A new light on the philosophical and evolutionary history of consciousness, and its basis, function, and purpose in the cosmic schema, is given in Sri Aurobindo's answer to the question: Did the Vedic rishis ever attain the Supermind?

> The Vedic rishis never attained to the Supermind for the earth or perhaps did not even make the attempt. They tried to rise individually to the supramental plane, but they did not bring it down and make it a permanent part of the earth-consciousness. Even there are verses of

> the Upanishads in which it is hinted that it is impossible to pass through the gates of the Sun (the symbol of the Supermind) and yet retain an earthly body. It was because of this failure that the spiritual effort of India culminated in Mayavada. Our yoga is a double movement of ascent and descent; one rises to higher and higher levels of consciousness, but at the same time one brings down their power not only into mind and life, but in the end even into the body. And the highest of these levels, the one at which it aims, is the Supermind. Only when that can be brought down is a divine transformation possible in the earth-consciousness.[6]

The most important distinction between Sri Aurobindo's integral yoga and other lines of yoga lies in the fact that the lotuses or chakras are set in full activity and the centers opened by Consciousness-Energy that was latent (kundalini shakti) and is now awakened and freed into an expanding and ascending movement. This is not accomplished or pursued by mechanical or similar processes, but rather by an integral spontaneous opening and activating of the centers of consciousness occurring naturally and as a direct result of the Divine Consciousness working in life through will, emotion, action, etc.

Hence, the "left hand" (vama marga) practices of the tantra, akin to the lower aspects of spiritualism and spiritism of the Western kind–revolving around hypnotism, mesmerism, black magic, witchcraft, as well as the uses and abuses of sex and drugs for mind expansion–are *not* to be mistaken for, nor equated with, spirituality or truth of the spirit either in the true emphasis of the tantra, kundalini yoga, or Sri Aurobindo's integral approach.

The paradox of the effortless effort in blossoming of the lotuses in the consciousness is likened by Sri Aurobindo thus to:

> Our hidden centres of celestial force
> Open like flowers to a heavenly atmosphere.
>
> *Savitri,* Book II, Canto 12[7]

In its deep lotus home her being sat
As if on concentration's marble seat
Calling the mighty Mother of the worlds,
To make this earthly tenement her house. . . .

Savitri, Book VII, Canto 5

The Divine Mother responds and an emanation comes down and a reciprocal gigantic movement takes place:

A face, a form came down in her heart. . . .
A mighty movement rocked the inner space—
As if a world were shaken and found its soul. . . .

Savitri, Book VII, Canto 5

It is then that the thrice-coiled kundalini wakes up from its slumber, raises its hood, and stands ready for the tremendous ascent, and the lotus centers are awakened and fragranced by the touch and power of the smiling shakti all through the way in this ascent and evolution of consciousness:

A flaming serpent rose released from sleep.
It rose billowing its coils and stood erect
And climbing mightily stormily on its way
It touched her centers with its flaming mouth:
As if a fiery kiss had broken their sleep,
They bloomed and laughed and surcharged
with light and bliss. . . .

And the mystic serpent

Then at the crown it joined the Eternal's space.

Savitri, Book VII, Canto 5

The supreme power of the Supramental Truth is not confined to any one center, not even to Supermind. But on the experience and the authority of Sri Aurobindo and The Mother, we now know that the center that receives the Supramental Consciousness is *above the head, above the thousand-petaled lotus.* And the power of this Supramental Consciousness extends, sweeps, permeates, pervades, and penetrates, infuses and suffuses all life and consciousness in all the centers, known and unknown.

Integral yoga therefore differs from other traditional yogas, including tantric yoga, not only in its essence and processes, but also in its purpose and method (although it does have a foundation in it). Its outstanding feature is represented by the newness and fullness of its aim, scope, and distinctive standpoint, and by the uniqueness of the totality of its method. Its comprehensiveness underscores its importance for the psychology of the human race. Its consequence and implications for the individual and collective life of man point directly to the perfection of mankind and the divinization of earth life.

In summary, Sri Aurobindo sets before us an aim and a goal—a spectrum and a panorama of achievement still to be accomplished, still to be achieved as a result of the preparation of Nature by all the past spiritual endeavors, though his own light belongs not "to the dawns of the past, but the noons of the future." The main points of difference new in Sri Aurobindo's yoga as compared with the old yogas can be best expressed in Sri Aurobindo's own words:

> 1. Because it aims not at a departure out of world and life into Heaven or Nirvana, but at a change of life and existence, not as something subordinate or incidental, but as a distinct and central object. If there is a descent in other yogas, yet it is only an incident on the way or resulting from the ascent—the ascent is the real thing. Here the ascent is the first step, but it is a means for the descent. It is the descent of the new consciousness attained by the ascent that is the stamp and seal of the sadhana. Even the tantra and Vaishnavism end in the release from life; here the object is the divine fulfillment of life.
>
> 2. Because the object sought after is not an individual achievement of divine realization for the sake of the individual, but something to be gained for the earth-consciousness here, a cosmic, not solely a supracosmic achievement. The thing to be gained also is the bringing

in of a Power of Consciousness (the supramental) not yet organized or active directly in earth-nature, even in the spiritual life, but yet to be organized and made directly active.

3. Because a method has been precognized for achieving this purpose which is as total and integral as the aim set before it, viz., the total and integral change of the consciousness and nature, taking up old methods but only as a part action and present aid to others that are distinctive. I have not found this method (as a whole) or anything like it professed or realized in the old yogas. . . .

. . . Our yoga is not a retreading of old walks, but a spiritual adventure.[8]

NOTES

1. *On the Tantra,* ed. M. P. Pandit (Pondicherry, India: Sri Aurobindo Ashram, 1970).
2. *Letters on Yoga,* Sri Aurobindo (Pondicherry, India: Sri Aurobindo Birth Centenary Library, Sri Aurobindo Ashram, 1972), Part I, Vol. 22, p. 73.
3. Ibid., p. 74.
4. Op. cit., p. 99.
5. Op. cit., p. 101.
6. Op. cit., p. 102.
7. All references to *Savitri* are from Sri Aurobindo's *Savitri* (with Letters) (Pondicherry, India: Sri Aurobindo Ashram, 1954).
8. Op. cit., pp. 100–1.

REFERENCES AND SUGGESTED READING

Aurobindo, Sri. *Centenary Library,* Vol. 22. Pondicherry, India: Sri Aurobindo Ashram, 1972.

——. *Savitri* (with Letters). Pondicherry, India: Sri Aurobindo Ashram, 1954.

——. *On the Tantra,* ed. M. P. Pandit. Pondicherry, India: Sri Aurobindo Ashram, 1970.

——. *Essays on the Gita.* Pondicherry, India: Sri Aurobindo Ashram, 1976.

——. *The Synthesis of Yoga*. Pondicherry, India: Sri Aurobindo Ashram, 1971.

Mookerjee, Ajit and Khanna, Madhu. *The Tantric Way*. Boston: Little, Brown, 1977.

Pandit, M. P. *Kundalini Yoga*. Madras, India: Ganesh & Co., 1959.

Shankaranarayanan, S. *Sri Chakra*. Pondicherry, India: Sri Aurobindo Ashram, Dipti Publications, 1973.

Tucci, Giuseppe. *The Theory and Practice of the Mandala*. New York: Samuel Weiser, 1973.

Woodroffe, Sir John. *The Serpent Power*. Madras, India: Ganesh & Co., 1964.

SIGNS OF AN AWAKENED KUNDALINI

Swami Vishnu Tirtha

When kundalini awakens, one invariably feels some involuntary movements of the body, which begin with trembling and shaking with an intensity varying with different persons. Some experience violent shaking of different kinds, as does a car before starting when the dynamo begins to work. Such physical movements are accompanied with a heretofore not experienced feeling of pleasure of spiritual intoxication. These are the first symptoms of an awakened kundalini and are followed by various signs and experiences too many to be enumerated.

Some characteristic symptoms of the awakened kundalini are here given below from *Mahayoga Vijnana,* a treatise on the subject in Hindi by Sri Yoganandji Maharaja, the author's revered guru. They are illustrative and by no means exhaustive:

1. When throbbing of muladhar begins, the whole body shakes, involuntary kumbhak (filling in of the lungs with air) starts beyond control, breath is forcibly exhaled out, without volition deep inhaling and exhaling of breath starts and the body gets uncontrollable, know then that kundalini has awakened. You then should give up your assertion and sit witnessing what happens.

2. When your body begins trembling, hair stands on roots, you laugh or begin to weep without your wishing, your tongue begins to utter deformed sounds, you are filled with

fear or see frightening visions, semen passes out, think that the kundalini shakti has become active.

3. When your posture becomes fixed, uddiyan, jalandhar, and mula bandhas come involuntarily, your tongue reverts back or rises up towards the soft palate and the whole body becomes so active that you are unable to sit still, your hands and legs stretch out forcibly, you ought to know that the divine power of the goddess kundalini has come into action.

4. When your posture becomes fixed and sight is attracted towards the middle point of eyebrows, the eye balls begin to revolve, you get automatic kewal-kumbhak, cessation of breath comes with no effort for inhaling or exhaling and the mind becomes vacant, void of all outward knowledge, understand that . . . the goddess kundalini has come into action.

5. When you feel currents of prana rising up your cerebrum within you, automatic repetition of Aum starts and the mind experiences waves after waves of blissful beatitude, think the universal mother kundalini has come into action.

6. When different kinds of nad [subtle sound] become audible, in your spinal column you experience vibrations, feeling of bodily existence for the time being is lost, in other words you feel as if there is no body, everything looks vacant, your eyelids become closed and open not in spite of your efforts, electric-like currents seem flowing up and down the nerves and you have convulsions, know that mahamaya kundalini has come into action.

7. When with the closing of eyelids your body falls to the ground, or begins to rotate like a grinding stone and breath comes not out, the body squatted on floor crosslegged begins to jump from place to place like a frog, or moves from place to place, or lies down like one dead, hands may not be lifted even if so desired, you feel contraction of nerves, you feel as if your life is passing away, the body undergoes convulsions like a dying fish, know that yogamaya kundalini has come into action.

8. When your mind gets influenced spiritually as if some spirit has taken possession of your body and under that influence different postures of yoga are involuntarily per-

formed without the least pain or fatigue and you feel increasingly buoyant, and simultaneously strange sorts of breathing exercises start, think that the divine power of kundalini has come into action.

9. When no sooner you have sat with eyes closed than in an instant the body begins to show activity of throwing out limbs forcibly, deformed sounds are loudly uttered, your speech begins to utter sounds like those of animals, birds and frogs or of a lion or like those of jackals, dogs, tigers, fear-inspiring and not pleasing to hear, understand that the great goddess kundalini has come into action.

10. When you feel vibrations of prana at different stations inside your body and feel its flow wherever you fix your attention and your nerves begin to show easy jerks like jerks of electricity as if passing through them, know that the goddess kundalini has come into action.

11. When all day and night you feel within your body some activity of prana and whenever you concentrate your mind, your body at once begins to shake or begins tossing and your mind remains filled with joy and bliss at all times, even when at call of nature, even during sleep you feel currents of prana rising up in your sahasrar and even in dreams you experience her presence, know that the joy-inspiring kundalini has come into action.

12. As soon as you sit for prayers your body begins to shake and in ecstasy of joy you begin to sing hymns in tones of music charming to hear and whose composition and poetry come out involuntarily, your hands giving a rhythmical clapping, and you pronounce languages you know not, but the sound ecstasizes your mind, know that the goddess of speech, Saraswati, has awakened into action.

13. When you feel intoxicated without taking any drug, while walking your steps fall majestically or like one drunk and you are unable to do any other work and you like to remain mute and dislike speaking to or hearing others and you feel like one drunk of divinity, know that your atma shakti kundalini, the power of Self, has come into action.

14. While walking, when your mind is filled with an im-

pulse to walk faster and your feet begin to run, you feel your body light like air and do not feel fatigued even having walked long enough, you feel buoyant and joyful, you are not unhappy even in dreams, you can keep the balance of your mind undisturbed in all ups and downs, and you acquire an inexhaustible energy for work, know that brahma shakti kundalini has come into action.

15. When in meditation you see visions divine and fall in a dreamy state of mind, have divine smells, see divine figures, feel divine tastes, hear divine sounds and experience divine touch and receive instructions from gods, then understand that the divine power of kundalini has come into action.

16. When you are in meditation and the future unfolds its secrets to you or the hidden meaning of scriptures, Vedas and Vedanta shine on your understanding, all doubts vanish, you acquire an insight into the abstruse meaning of the works on spiritual science even at their first glance, you acquire strange powers of oratory and feel not the need of approaching even Brahma, the creator himself, for knowledge and you acquire self-confidence, understand then that kundalini the bestower of siddhis (occult powers) has come into action.

17. When you are seated for meditation and your sight becomes fixed on the mid of eyebrows, your tongue rises up for khechari, breath stops altogether and mind plunges into the ocean of bliss, shambhavi mudra operates and you experience the pleasure of savikalpa samadhi, know that subtle power of kundalini is in action.

18. When at morning and evening hours punctually and automatically your body becomes charged with such of the divine influences, and body, mind, and prana become overpowered by her, know that the goddess kundalini is rightly functioning. . . .

KUNDALINI AND THE TANTRIC TRADITION

Swami Ajaya

There is a tendency in the West to treat yogic concepts and techniques independently of the system of philosophy and psychology from which they derive. This sometimes leads to considerable distortion in our understanding of yoga. When hatha yoga is taught independently of meditation and other practices, merely for its physical benefits, or when mantra yoga is taught separately from its spiritual context, the aim and purpose of yoga are misconstrued; for these techniques are meant to be used in a holistic context in order to help the individual grow toward self-realization in a balanced and integrated way. While an individual may derive certain benefits from these limited techniques, the true significance of the practice and its real fruits may be missed entirely.

I am introducing the topic of kundalini in this way because it too is often discussed outside of its proper context of tantra philosophy, psychology, and practice. And when kundalini is related to tantra, tantra itself is typically not understood properly. As a result, there is more confusion, speculation, and fantasizing about kundalini than about most yogic concepts.

Whenever I find mystique or mystery concerning some teaching it leads me to believe there is considerable ignorance of the subject among those perpetuating these attitudes. Since I come from a tradition that continues to preserve the principles and practices of the higher form of tantra yoga and teaches them in a pure, systematic, and scientific way, the misuse of these teachings seems particularly glaring and ludicrous. In the interests of encouraging others to be less fanciful about kundalini, I would like to briefly describe the context from which this concept springs.

There are several systems of Indian philosophy and psychology, each of which has a different focus. Yoga is one such system. Even within yoga there are many branches, each with a different emphasis. These systems do not compete with one another but rather focus on different aspects, which together make up the whole of the human being. Just as physics, chemistry, and biology specialize in explaining certain aspects of the physical universe and yet overlap in some areas, so do the branches of Eastern psychology and philosophy in regard to our internal processes. For example, the focus of Vedanta and jnana yoga is on understanding the *source* of this manifest universe. On the other hand, Patanjali's systemization of Samkya philosophy in the *Yoga Sutras* is the most thorough presentation of the practical psychology of yoga.

Tantra yoga is still another system. Tantra is a very practical science for systematically understanding and mastering the forces of the universe and traveling through the subtlest realms of existence to the very source of consciousness itself. Because the techniques of tantra might be misused by one who is not prepared—for example, one who is not selfless and compassionate—these teachings have been passed on only to close disciples. These days there are few worthy disciples and much of the teaching is being lost. Since the teachings of tantra are not readily available, a great deal of speculation based on fragmentary information abounds, particularly in the West.

Many people in the West mistakenly think that tantra is a rather loose philosophy that teaches that you can do whatever you desire—so long as you do it with the "right attitude"—and still progress toward spiritual awakening. But if we study tantra as it has been traditionally practiced in India, we find that it is a highly evolved science. In fact, certain forms of tantra are the most advanced of all yoga practices.

The tantric tradition has made unparalleled contributions

to understanding and mastering the finer forces of nature and attaining the most evolved states of consciousness. The use of mantra and yantra* toward this end has been systematically described in tantra. It is in the tantric scriptures that these are most thoroughly explained and coordinated. The detailed explanation of chakras, the transformation of subtle energy, and the kundalini concept also come to us from tantra. To talk about kundalini as some mysterious energy without properly understanding its connection to other tantric concepts—for example, the pathways through which energy travels—leads to all sorts of bizarre distortions. Only those genuine students of a valid school of tantra systematically understand and learn how to awaken and direct this potentially divine power within.

If we study the tantric paths, much of the confusion that exists concerning the awakening and experience of kundalini and the aim of tantra can be clarified. One of the first facts that we are likely to discover is that there are three clearly delineated approaches to awakening and directing the latent force within. The tantric scriptures have traditionally been divided into three groups. Though the followers of these three groups share a common understanding of the basic polarities conceived of as shiva and shakti, or the male and female principles, their depth of understanding of these principles and the subtlety of their methods for uniting these principles differ markedly. When the goals and practices of each is properly understood it becomes clear that much of the misinterpretation comes from confusing these approaches with one another.

Even more important than awakening kundalini is learning how to direct it so that it remains at chosen centers of consciousness. The practitioner's experience can be remarkably different, depending on where kundalini is directed. In fact, the differences among the three groups of practitioners can be most clearly comprehended by understanding not only their methods but also where the force of kundalini is directed.

* Yantra is the diagrammatic equivalent of mantra and is the yogic equivalent of the Buddhist mandala.

The three groups are called *kaula, mishra,* and *samaya.* Practitioners of the kaula group meditate on kundalini at the base of the spine. The mishra group awakens this latent force and leads it to the anahata chakra (the heart center). And the most evolved group of aspirants, those of the samaya group, learn advanced practices for directing kundalini to the thousand-petaled lotus, the sahasrara chakra at the crown of the head, which results in the final union and the highest state of realization. The realization of those in the first two schools is far from complete. In fact, their involvement in lower practices may provide compelling distractions and interfere with their progress toward self-realization.

The word kaula comes from the Sanskrit *ku* (earth). This refers to the practitioner's worship of kundalini at the muladhara chakra at the base of the spine, which is related to the earth tattva (element). In this group kundalini, though it may be awakened and release considerable energy, is not raised above this lowest center of consciousness. The kaula group uses external rituals. Sometimes sexual rites are used to awaken kundalini. Their practice is not spiritual but focuses on worldly concerns and the satisfaction of sensory pleasures. Black magic may be practiced to gratify one's selfish desires. The practitioners in this group do not understand the greater purpose to which the latent force may be applied but remain preoccupied with the achievement of psychic powers and power over nature. Their attachment to such powers diverts them from spiritual development in much the same way that the pursuit of sensory pleasures may inhibit the growth of the average person. This kaula group is considered to be the most inferior, though it is perhaps more widely known and more easily comprehended than the other groups. As a result, many Westerners tend to equate tantric practices with this inferior sect, remaining unaware of the more evolved tantric schools.

The word mishra means "mixed" and refers to that group of practitioners who follow the path that combines aspects of the lower tantra and higher tantra. Their accomplishments are quite different from those of the kaula group. The practitioner of this group follows a practical yoga aimed at fulfilling his duties in the world while transforming his worldly desires into spiritual ones. In order to accomplish this, the aspirant learns to lead kundalini to the heart center (anahata chakra). While the kaula group exclusively uses external rituals to awaken kundalini, the mishra group emphasizes internal worship. The aspirant may perform a ritual and repeat a selected mantra while concentrating on a yantra. After becoming familiar with the practice, he is asked to visualize the offerings, the mantra, and the yantra within. Through this practice the basic urges and base emotions become transmuted into feelings of devotion, love, and compassion. One may also achieve certain mastery in the world and mastery over the subtle forces of nature. However, this is not used for any selfish purpose, but for the benefit of others.

The samaya group of tantric texts is the most important. The word samaya means "he is with me" and refers to the ultimate union of shiva and shakti, the underlying polarities that make manifest this world. In this path shakti, the universal energy that brought the universe into existence, is worshiped in her most pure essence. Shakti in her form as kundalini is awakened by practicing certain austerities and using a mantra with internal visualization a fixed number of times at certain hours of the day. Shiva, the principle of divine consciousness, resides at the sahasrara chakra at the crown of the head. It is only by leading kundalini from the root center at the base of the spine successively through each chakra to the crown chakra that the polarities, shakti and shiva, unite. Through this union the highest state of enlightenment is attained. Those who follow this path liberate the soul from all material limitations and unite it with the universal Self. This internal union is true tantra and all other practices are mere preparation through mimicry of this divine union within.

The more advanced practices of tantra involve meditation on Sri Yantra. Sri Yantra is called the mother of all yantras because all other yantras derive from it.† This yantra is con-

† Just as all mantras derive from the mantra Om.

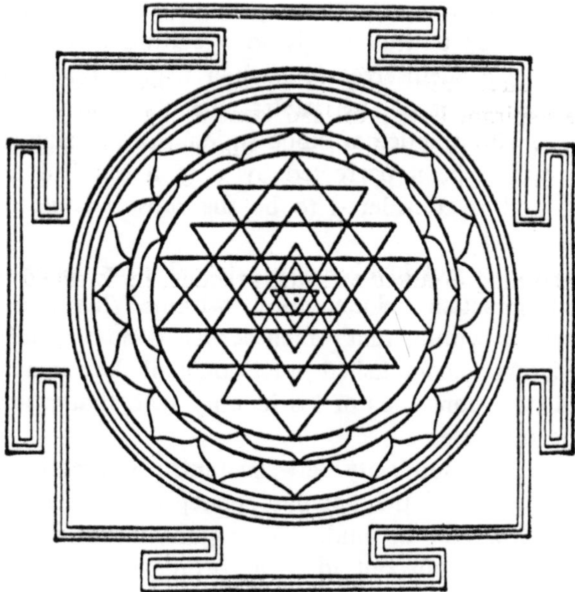

Figure 1. Sri Yantra.

sidered a map of the planes of manifestation. It is also known as Sri Chakra, for the intersecting triangles also represent the chakras as well as the realms (lokas) in the cosmos. According to tantra, all that is in the universe is also within the individual. Each chakra is related to a particular cosmic plane with its own quality and presiding deity.

Simply to concentrate on this yantra without a prescribed method is of little avail. But if one knows how to direct one's attention in a particular way using specified mantras, one is led to successively more and more primary or subtle levels of manifestation. Slowly the various facets of this spiritual jewel are known and the aspirant progresses toward the bindu (point) at the center of Sri Yantra. This bindu is the source of manifestation. Reaching there, the aspirant's consciousness transcends this manifest world and participates in the final union.

Among even those advanced aspirants who meditate on Sri

Yantra, most concentrate on simplified versions of the yantra, or have learned to travel only to a certain level. Very few have perfected themselves to such a degree that they have reached the center of this yantra, the abode of divine consciousness. The practice of bindu vedena, or piercing this central point, has been perfected by only a handful of living masters, and is considered to be the most advanced of all yogic practices.

Samaya does not involve any external worship or external rituals; the practice is done entirely within. When one masters that which is within, that which seems to be without is also mastered. The accomplished practitioner of the samaya group becomes fully conscious of his identity with that which manifests the universe.

There is little similarity between tantra as practiced in the samaya school and the popular conceptualizations of tantra and kundalini that abound. This higher form of tantra, in fact, does not at all contradict the principles of Vedanta. So pure and advanced is this form of tantra that Shankara, the great philosopher who established Advaita (monistic) Vedanta, and who founded the swami orders, is said to have given us this practice. The quintessence of these teachings is found in the hymn "Saundaryalahari" (The Flood of Beauty), which is attributed to Shankara. These beautiful verses of adoration are actually mantras, which are meant to be repeated along with concentration on selected components of Sri Yantra. In reading this divine poem, one would not ordinarily be aware that each verse contains a secret mystical practice that leads to mastery of some subtle aspect of manifestation. There have been several classic commentaries and explanations of these verses in Sanskrit, but the practices themselves can only be learned directly from that rare master who follows in the pure tradition.

We have seen that there is a wide range of practices for awakening and directing kundalini, some of which are not spiritual at all, and others of which are the most evolved spiritual practices to be found anywhere. We have also seen that there are clearly delineated schools that follow distinctive paths. It is hoped that the student will avoid those ways that do not lead to the center of consciousness, but instead end in disillusionment. Unfortunate are those who are misled or distracted from the true path of yoga. Fortunate are the few who through their own sincerity and purity of purpose attract a genuine teacher and travel the path of awakening kundalini and leading her to her final abode. "Among thousands of men perhaps one strives for perfection, and among thousands who strive, perhaps one knows me in truth."

IS KUNDALINI REAL?

Christopher Hills

For some years we have watched while various authorities have talked of kundalini and the yoga scene. Some have even started fashionable cults and built up impressive organizations of rather gullible but well-meaning people who have been promised that their kundalini will be raised by certain practices. Most of these, with two notable exceptions, have yet to show any remarkable internal changes or emphasis on detection of ego structures. We have seen great external changes in clothes, beads, and bells, but little of the real spiritual work on the quality of consciousness has come from these bringers of kundalini yoga to the West.

Alan Watts said to me once that yoga was all happening here at the grass roots and I looked around at the scene and wondered if he really knew! Yoga is not what passes for a current fashion or lip service or reading the right books, but something totally transforming, something which does not require us to look for spiritual crutches nor to make excuses for drugs. Consciousness is already the most powerful drug and a true yogin is already drugged and so intoxicated with it that all other drugs are superfluous. This is not to say that alcohol or sex are not good things but that an immoderate obsession with them shows that kundalini is not working its magic.

Experience Is the Test

So in writing about such things as kundalini I have come to see that many book writers and preachers do not necessarily demonstrate what they talk about except to the gullible and impressionable. When it comes to actual transformation of society or presenting some real original credentials to the world, we find these authorities and fashionable cults are lacking in depth and perspective.

When all the traditional words are said and done, what kundalini really is and what yoga really is may elude even the very elect. The evolutionary thrust is not toward explanations or "talking about" kundalini or for that matter speaking in anecdotes and second-hand knowledge of this and that. What the evolutionary consciousness is concerned with is something so scientifically verifiable that the laws of consciousness become as predictable as the laws of matter, or more so. The evolutionary force is not interested in any particular philosophy, religious tradition, or scientific method, but in more real ways of self-mastery.

In this sense all systems of religion and science which contain "essence knowledge" of kundalini can be said to be second-hand knowledge until it becomes validated by our own ignorance or insights of the systems. The tools of religion and science in the evolutionary sense are no greater than their users. One could say the same of kundalini or consciousness, just as a brand new set of chisels is not much use to an old widow who never learned carpentry.

It Can Be Dangerous

So from the viewpoint of an evolutionary kundalini force acting cosmically through man's vehicle, we are no further on until the potential state (which everyone has) becomes manifest. Without seeing its manifestation or being able to determine the shape, form, or content of its existence in the so-called material or external world, kundalini is as dangerous as it is enlightening, just as a kitchen knife is capable of cutting vegetables or of killing. Guns are not dangerous because they don't go off by themselves. They are only dangerous when human consciousness directs the bullet and pulls the trigger. Guns will stay harmless under your breakfast table for a hundred years as long as no one plays around with them. So with kundalini we are talking of the energy of consciousness when it burns away the dross of human dependence and raises man to wider levels of consciousness.

Heightening awareness of the cosmic relations that give us direct perception of psychic electricity is the only evidence that we can indeed evolve the biophysical structures we call a human body. But do we see this happening at the grass roots level or do we see the same preoccupations as our forefathers had with outward forms and exotic teachings? Is kundalini thrusting us irrevocably toward absorbing the history of gurus and the analogies and metaphors of ancient personalities?

Of what use is all this acquisition of ancient traditional religion if the evidence shows we are just as egotistical, self-seeking, personality-, fame-, and name-oriented and public relations-promoting for psychic income as any businessman is for dollar income? From the cosmic point of view, from the standpoint of eternal time, the promotional efforts of gurus to get the kundalini into action in the planetary sense may be sometimes seen as a considerable circus on a grand scale.

Surely nothing short of the Einsteinian revolution in science must take place in the spiritual sense of religious experience of kundalini manifestations. With man's very being becoming more threatened and more ominously blind, according to prophets Solzhenitsyn et al., with more countries of the planet falling to totalitarian despotism of small aggressive cliques of self-righteous know-alls, where is this so-called evolutionary power?

In the great monasteries of Tibet, the Chinese smashed in the faces of the great high lamas with rifle butts in front of thousands of Tibetan disciple lamas to show them that they really had no power at all and that their philosophy of superpowerful control of life-force was just a phoney myth. Millions of lamas and "believers" were disillusioned when their gods bled to death in front of their very eyes. What happened to the great tantric teachings about kundalini powers and the superhuman ideals?

We do not mention this to cast doubt on the ancient teachings of great traditions but only to remind ourselves that belief in such powers or for that matter kundalini, whatever it is, must be based on direct experience and not on some teacher's parroting of cultural brainwash. Hence methods of actually determining what kundalini is and how it works must now be outlined in some conclusive way, to enable us to experience its reality; some "thought experiment" similar to Einstein's physical concepts, which transformed the world of man with a power incalculable in terms of one man, or one all-knowing guru. The understanding of kundalini, in other words, must go beyond the "writing about" stage which is merely descriptive and allegorical, however interesting, to some real nitty-gritty things that we can do in our own backyard.

What Is Kundalini?

There seem to be so many people jumping on the kundalini bandwagon and including the word in their offerings to the public that I feel it's time to throw in my own two cents' worth and say what it is. We have heard a lot about kundalini energy but writing about something or talking about something is quite different from the actual thing itself. Judging by the number of claims made by ignorant people as to what kundalini really is and the loose talk which goes under its label, it might be wisest to start with some statements about what it is not.

Unfortunately, it is always easier to say what a thing is not, and a long list of what it is not would include practically everything on the spiritual path offered to the gullible as enlightenment. I propose instead to say that kundalini is not energy at all and that any attempt to understand it in terms of energy, orgone, etheric electricity, or in biophysical terms, is doomed to failure. In short, everyone has kundalini and it is not something special but something superordinary. In fact, you could not even read these words without kundalini coming out of your eyes and "seeing" the words in front of you.

Kundalini is basically *consciousness* and everyone has it. The only difference between a "seer" and an ordinary person is that kundalini is latent in one and manifest in the other when it moves out of its normal house in the bottom chakra and burns its way up to the higher chakras or psychic centers in man. How many young men have felt the burning sensation at the base of the spine when they become sexually aroused and frustrated through lack of a union?

Energy Is the Byproduct

This is caused when kundalini cannot rise and gets stuck at the barrier between the root chakra and the one above it. In some people it even gets stuck two chakras higher up and gives them a spinal weakness in the back. This burning sensation is the movement or the uncoiling of the kundalini which is there all the time being used for the ordinary purpose of living, mating, and feeling.

When it moves through the chakras, the kundalini burns like fire through the channels or nerve currents which carry it upward to the magnetic part of the mind and brain. Strictly speaking, what is burning and moving is not a chemical or an energy; but energy is the byproduct, just as light is completely unquantized until it is absorbed or impinges on something resulting in the release of heat and energy as a byproduct. So is consciousness the same as unquantized light. Only when it moves through the system can it be described as kundalini because only then do we become conscious of its existence as an ambrosia which melts and burns.

To describe kundalini in chemical or energetic terms alone is to avoid the real cause and look only at the effects. Without the light of consciousness moving through our receptors we would not see, smell, taste, hear, or touch anything. Yet we do not see kundalini described as ordinary consciousness but always as something special. Kundalini is a basic component of life and it is only when it moves from one place to another that we sense it or feel it as "energy."

To call it "kundalini energy" is therefore a misnomer. It is a prephysical state which merely becomes manifest when it burns its way through something. Then we sense it, but really it is asleep inside us all the time; it is there helping us to be alive, to sense the world through our eyes and ears, etc. and to imprint our consciousness with all its patterning. The mind-tapes we play have their counterpart in the habitual sensory responses of the body, which is no less a creature of habitual patterns than our emotions or mental states. These are the habitual states which block the rising of kundalini through the psychic electricity stations we call chakras. Kundalini is in everyone.

In my book *Supersensonics* I have described in detail what kundalini actually is and the way it works through the biophysical system, and I have linked its behavior to light and consciousness. However, I feel it is a great error to think of this as a concept of "energy" because that is merely mistaking the effect for the cause. Just as we feel pain when there is pressure on the cells of our big toe, so do we feel the passage of kundalini as a sensation of internal light. But just as the pain is really experienced in the brain and not the toe, as we prove by blocking the nerve current to the brain with an injection, so can we mistake the causation of kundalini moving through the chakras as kundalini energy when it is in fact only experienced in the brain and not in the root of the spine.

It is important to get this process crystal clear to understand kundalini. When I told someone who was making a deep study of kundalini that it was a psychic electricity he immediately mistook my statement and thought I was saying that nothing physical actually happened at the root of the spine and that it all took place in the head. Obviously there is a chemical and electrical energy which can easily be measured by supersensonic instruments not only at the base of the spine, but at all the chakras too, but as I said, this is only an effect and the psychophysical energy thus created disturbs the corresponding center in the brain. The cerebrospinal system is the seat of all experience in the body. Every center in the body has a corresponding energy center in the brain. Whatever happens inside the body or outside of the body eventually finishes up as electrical potentials inside the brain and thus eventually is recognized as a sensation in the mind-stuff which ultimately makes sense of it in our consciousness. The entire cerebral cortex is involved in the transformation of kundalini into the chemical, emotional, mental, and spiritual functions of each level of consciousness corresponding to the number of chakras activated in each person. The chakras are vortices of psychic electricity but like the nervous system they are only the biological prisms through which kundalini is differentiated from the whole spectrum.

Kundalini = Consciousness

When the chakra opens and the kundalini flows toward the brain, it is no different from the pain signal telling us through consciousness that something is happening to the molecules in our toes. The kundalini is actually made of consciousness and the actual sensation is merely a message of our consciousness passing through the psychic veil or skin which acts as a membrane between one world of experience and another. And thus it happens through all of the chakras, that our biological system is merely a physical replica of another system made of kundalini which is identical to consciousness, while we "experience" only the burning feeling and internal light that we call the cosmic fire.

In *Supersensonics,** which is Vol. III of the series "The

* See listing in Appendix. *Editor.*

Supersensitive Life of Man," I have written a full exposition of how kundalini follows the laws of consciousness and have shown how our invisible consciousness pours out of our eyes every second without our noticing anything unusual until we become enlightened. Then we see clearly that what we took for granted all along was really the priceless jewel of consciousness bouncing off everything, lighting up everything, enlightening everything, making all things light.

Consciousness = Light

Such is kundalini. We use it everyday, we have sex with it as often as we can, we use it for all the promiscuous activity of the mind, and we don't know it exists until we see lights inside our head! Just as the light we see inside our head as "brightness" is not the real light but only the psychic response of our receptors to light as it impinges on them, so is the burning sensation described by the sages only the passage through unaccustomed cells of a new level of consciousness functioning in a higher octave. Our body senses it in the biological vehicle because that is the antenna which receives it from the light of the cosmos, but it is our consciousness and brain which makes sense of these sensations in the psychobiological network.

To think of kundalini as something objective and separate from the experiencer is like separating the internal light of our consciousness from the external light of the cosmos. We think it can be done by closing our eyes. But without both internal and external light functioning together nothing objective can be seen or experienced.

Light only becomes energy when it strikes something material in space; until then it is unmanifest radiation unquantized and invisible throughout space to which the ancients gave the name *akasha,* meaning in Sanskrit the light that cannot be seen, as against *kasha* which means the light you see as brightness.

It would take a whole book to say what kundalini is and

that is why I wrote *Supersensonics* on it. However, I deliberately avoided the magic word "kundalini" in the title because of the false connotations placed upon it by half-baked seers who have obviously never experienced it for themselves. It is good to have Gopi Krishna come out and sound a note of caution and send out a clarion call for its proper investigation.

I hate to think what will be done in his name in the so-called biochemical research for the source of kundalini! He is one of the few who are talking sense, but I would like to see more rigor in getting from the "talking about" stage to the actual determination of its nature as consciousness moving through the structure of the psychobiological system and let us stop this nonsense term "kundalini yoga." All yoga is kundalini yoga. Yoga is meaningless without it. Let us stop referring to it as something special and begin to see its ordinariness as the fundamental supersensory sonic note of the universe.

Historical Background

Tantra yoga is sometimes referred to as "kundalini yoga" because it is the sadhana or path of the *prakriti* (defined as primordial creativity) through the dynamic aspects of life while the system of Shankacharya, which passively displaced Buddhism in India, is the sadhana of *purusa* (defined as "pure consciousness") which is accomplished without stress; it is the way of inaction or letting things *be*. Shankara taught that enlightenment is stability, peace, and joy of union with the inactive purusa which is the absolute total potentiality of existence, whereas tantra or the so-called kundalini path teaches that Truth is infinite power and dynamic manifestation. It is the creative utilization of all potential energy.

Shankacharya taught that the kundalini energy flows into endless potential states in which the manifested states of shakti and shiva (or positive-negative) are said to be annihilated and united in Brahman or Buddha who is One beyond all conceptualization of the duality of opposites.

There are many schools favoring the way of tantra or power which essentially is that path which predominantly seeks special knowledge of the kundalini within consciousness. There are fewer schools which seek the predominance of grace instead of power. Through the contemplation and enjoyment of uninterrupted bliss, these schools study pure being rather than manifestation of energy.

Don't Work for Powers

There are even fewer yogis and systems which seek to manifest kundalini power plus the total potentiality to be found only in grace and bliss. This elevation of "power" in favor of "being" involves the absolute control of the flow of consciousness in the void. Notably the Tibetans have absorbed both the tantra and the yoga of voidness or nirvana. Nirvana means nir (not) vana (flowing) and is a negative state, because it means not doing.

However, the number of persons who can do everything while not doing anything can be said to be those few who have become master of the creative forces of consciousness or kundalini. They are called *gunvana* in Sanskrit, or one who can control flow of kundalini through the gunas or creative forces. It is these three gunas or qualities which make up the prakriti or creative energy. Pra means primordial and kriti means creative so prakriti refers to kundalini before it becomes manifested.

The Samkyha yoga says that without mastery of purusa or pure consciousness, the control of kundalini at the pure creative prephysical level of prakriti is not possible except in our fantasies of life. This is simply because prakriti or kundalini in its primordial state can only imitate whatever has been put into the being in pure consciousness. Just as a seed can only bear fruit of itself, so the manifested creation can act on these potential powers only according to the true nature of the being.

When Proverbs 23:7 said, "As a man thinketh in his heart, so is he," it was merely stating the connection between the potential state and the manifested state which can only "act" according to its own true nature. Lao Tse observes the same thing when he says that all things are worked by the Tao and cannot act except in accordance with their ultimate true nature. "Kundalini yoga" adherents tend to forget this and work for powers and dynamic action, but as we see through the history of the world, the self cannot be conquered in that way.

Study the Nerve Currents

The first step toward the control of kundalini energy in the study of the tantras is the study of the path of the nadis or nerve currents which carry life-force to the divine spark of the soul which burns like a flame (*linga sarira*). This is achieved by balancing the polarities of the shakti female force on the left side of the sushumna (central spinal channel) with the shiva or male force on the right side through the ida and pingala nadis. Through breath control the prana (life force) springs up the central nadi from the *kanda* (plexus) at the base of the spine. Man is viewed as a divine instrument with the *meru danda* (cerebrospinal nervous system) as the axis of Mount Meru (the symbolic Mount Olympus) on which the gods reside. The Mount Meru is a symbol which refers to the top *padma* or chakra which expands into Brahman from the root word *Brih* (to expand). This tree of life in the brain expands to include all and pervade all. The path of the sleeping divine power residing in the chakra at the base of the spine is known as the uncoiling of kundalini from the verb root *kund* (to burn). Its movement is traced through the nerve plexus in the remaining six chakras or padmas. On reaching the sahasrara (highest chakra) the kundalini or burning fire unites with the magnetic part of the mind and causes the expansion of the self-sense into limitless selfhood. Each chakra has its own seed, its own orientation to subtle light energy called *tattwas* and is controlled by its own guna or kind of prakriti. The petals of the chakras or padmas depicted in so many pictures are merely its rate of vibration distinguished as subtle sounds.

Cosmic Perception Required

As the energy of kundalini passes upward like an ascending scale, the supersonic Aum manifests harmonic intervals between the resonant notes of each chakra. The sahasrara is sometimes called the *brahmarandra* or the opening of the top of the head. The null point or hub of the padma has its center in the "cave of Brahman" or the third ventricle in the brain. For the kundalini or energy of consciousness to keep on rising higher and higher, a complete purification of the self-sense through the direct perception of the cosmic intelligence is required.

It is known that certain elements and crystals resonate with the lower six padmas or chakras in the order of rising from the root chakra; they are lead, brass, tin, gold, copper, and mercury. The crystal lattices which correspond to the chakras are explained in my book *Supersensonics*. The wave length and beat frequencies are discussed in a later chapter, which also sets out the connection between colors and the chakras. Both show clearly the criteria of the different levels of consciousness caused by the movement of kundalini energy.

These levels of consciousness can only be directly experienced as one whole vibration by doing *samyama* (complete practice) on the "inner light of consciousness" which is the same thing as kundalini, except that kundalini is its active state of flowing into the cave of Brahman.

What Is a Real Yogi?

Only where we have direct perception of all these levels beyond the human personality or mind can we be illuminated and thereby directly understand the nature of the experience of consciousness. The windows of the soul are the eyes, but what makes sense of what the eyes see is consciousness.

In yoga or union anyone who achieves less than this supreme state of direct perception cannot be truly called a yogi. Only when the kundalini has risen and its manifestation has actually demonstrated this rising to other members of mankind, through a completely original insight or vision of the worlds of Being, only then can it be said that a human has become a yogi or seer and has transcended the human condition. For this to take place not only does the kundalini have to rise but the hidden evolutionary devices have to be activated, and it is these that spark off the visionary insights that penetrate the real structures of nature and give us the creative genius of the rishis or seers of every age.

The numbers of followers or the self-made claims are no use here because only a fresh vision of the world and the way laws of consciousness work in reality can contribute to real self knowledge. The acquisition or mere repetition of traditional knowledge which nowadays can be obtained through learning and scholarship or received second-hand from another is of no use in the control of kundalini forces. These subtle energies of prakriti are beyond the control of men until they become a gunavana through the direct experience within themselves of nirvana.

The Sky Is the Limit

This is the aim of all true yoga: to achieve this transhuman state and then communicate it to the universe. Until they can thus communicate their full vision and express it to another, they have not truly experienced the full control of kundalini energy. Only he who can map out the path of this energy and divine the causes for our human condition can truly be called a yogi or an avatar because all else is transitory, mere inherited comparative knowledge.

The true knowledge of consciousness is for all time—eternity—and is not transitory or comparable with anything else. Consciousness is beyond descriptive or intellective levels of communication simply because it is "pure," which means without any images or content. The form which holds the content can never exist without consciousness imaging its pattern. Therefore to teach of this content through forms, images or packaging of traditional information is not enough.

The consciousness which creates the "form" in all the manifested states is what we are after in supersensonics. Once this is experienced, the kundalini can take any form imaginable to man's faculties. Then the universal sky is the limit.

Yet the patterns of nature, including the form of man's being, its sensorial equipment, the nervous system of molecules are all kundalini. In this sense we answered our opening question, "Is kundalini real?" It is as real as your own consciousness is real.

Once a human being is enlightened this is not the end of the road as most people think, but only the beginning of a humiliating task. The job of communicating it back through all the levels from the highest inspiration of the imagination down through the conceptual mind and into the physical manifestation is no easy task. In fact, it represents the greatest challenge of the entire world, beside which all other tasks appear easy. It is easier to become president of a country or become a famous person than to speak one word from the level of the nuclear center and manifest it in the lives of others. The beings who have achieved this in the entire history of man, who speak to us through the minds of Christ and Buddha, Lao Tse and Krishna, are those who have this power to make the unnameable realm of God come alive in the heart.

ARE THE CHAKRAS REAL?

Ken Wilber

> When all the knots of the heart are unloosened, then even here, in this human birth, the mortal becomes immortal. This is the whole teaching of the Scriptures.
>
> *Katha Upanishad*

The ordinary human body, as Freud has extensively documented, is under sway of a well-organized tyranny—a tyranny imposed by a separate-self sense in flight from death and in flight from loving unity with the world of phenomena. Under these circumstances, the self does not consciously participate in the light and life of the Adi-Buddha, the Godhead, the Brahman, and is forced to retreat instead to the pale substitute of mental and symbolic forms, with a corresponding de-form-ation of the body. Hence, the being-consciousness-bliss of one's formless self is distorted and constricted, and under this tyranny appears in the restricted forms known as the chakras.

It is for this reason that the chakras are properly referred to by the terms *granthi* (knots) and *sankhocha* (contraction). In the *Chandogya Upanishad* we read, "In acquiring the traditional doctrine there is release from all knots." And in the *Mundaka Upanishad,* "He, verily, who knows that Supreme Brahman, becomes very Brahman. Liberated from the knots of the heart, he becomes immortal." Likewise, according to the *Surangama Sutra,* Sakyamuni Buddha explains liberation as the final dissolution of the "knots we have tied in the essential unity of our own Mind."

And yet, strictly speaking, final liberation, being the timeless and therefore eternal condition of all worlds and selves, is not so much the *result* of the *action* of untying these knots, but rather the tacit acknowledgment that these knots do not, and cannot, obstruct ultimate consciousness. Liberation, in short, is not the actual untying of these knots, but the silent admission that they are already untied. Herein lies the key to the paradox of the chakras: They are ultimately dissolved in the realization that they need not be dissolved.

Finally, therefore, the chakras are not real—in the sense that they do not pose a barrier to self-realization, nor do they constitute mandatory stages in an upward climb to liberation. In the last analysis, there are no stages in eternity—nor any ladder *to* the infinite that does not begin *with* the infinite. That the chakras in themselves are not real is the conclusion of most of the great sages, siddhas, mystics, and masters, such as Krishnamurti, Sri Ramana Maharshi, Shankara, Bubba Free John, and virtually all Ch'an and Zen masters. To quote but one, the illustrious Sri Ramana Maharshi: "Do not waste time meditating on chakras, nadis, padmas, or mantras of deities, or anything else of the kind. The six subtle centers (chakras) are merely mental pictures and are meant for beginners in yoga."

And yet—and this is the point to which much of our discussion must be directed—the chakras do *appear* real to the separate self who constructs these knots in his flight both from death and from a prior unity with all manifestation. The flight from death generates time, while the flight from unity generates space. Now, the self-created world of time-and-space is, by all accounts, the world of *samsara,* the ropes of our own bondage and suffering, and the chakras are but the knots in these binding ropes of misery. There are an enormous number of descriptions and explanations for the genesis of these knots in awareness, given, from several different angles, by the major metaphysical traditions. There are, to name some, the sefiroth of the Kabbalah, the vijnanas of the Yogacara, the kosas of the Vedanta, the hierarchies of the neo-Confucians, the kuei-hou intervals of the Taoists, the transmutation series of the Alchemists, and the energetics of the Tantras. All of these deal, in one way or another, with the apparent hierarchy of knots man has tied in his consciousness. But there is secreted in the works of Freud (and eloquently explained by the likes of Brown, Marcuse, and Lacan) an explanation–in the most rudimentary form–of the evolution of the chakra knots, an explanation that might be better suited to a Western readership, and therefore one I will briefly outline.

The infant, according to psychoanalytic observations, is under sway of "polymorphous perversity" and moved solely by the Pleasure Principle, which means that the child lives in a noncorrupted, blissful, and erotic unity with all of nature. For all practical purposes, its awareness is transpersonal, timeless, and spaceless. Very simply, its world is one of transcendent bliss, and for this reason alone Freud was quite right in announcing, much to the horror of his contemporaries, that children have a richer, more extensive, and more satisfying sex life than adults; for the infant takes equal erotic and blissful delight in all organs, surfaces, and activities of the body, and thus his entire cosmos is one of bliss, while the normal adult finds exuberance and bliss, if at all, in only one specific and narrowed region of the body–the genitals. Genital bliss can thus only be viewed, in comparison with the body's natural possibilities, as a constriction, a restriction, a cramp, a knot. Now it is *not* so much genital sexuality that comprises this knot, but rather the *restriction of bliss to only one specific region* of the body, excluding all others. This restriction of transcendent bliss is thus normal, but not natural. It is but one peculiar arrangement out of infinite possibilities.

How, then, comes this unnatural restriction of man's potential participation in transcendent bliss? According to the last formulations of Freud–which, alas, are carefully scrubbed out of all modern psychiatric texts–this restriction is engineered by a separate-self sense in flight from death and from loving unity with all objects; for the infant's earliest "identity" is literally with the cosmos itself—a type of immature "cosmic consciousness." He cannot distinguish his world from his actions upon it; nor differentiate self from other, subject from object, inside from outside. He knows nothing of the illusions of space nor of time, and thus, as Jung constantly emphasized, lives in a transpersonal and supra-individual world.

But as the infant learns to construct an irreducible barrier between self and other, between inside and outside, he forfeits his loving and blissful at-one-ness with the cosmos and centers his identity instead on his *personal organism*. He shifts from a Supreme Identity with the All to a personal identity confined to the boundaries of his skin. Thus Freud's famous dictum: "The ego-feeling we are aware of now is thus only a shrunken vestige of a far more extensive feeling—a feeling that embraced the universe and expressed an inseparable connection of the ego with the external world."

This shift in identity carries with it a host of unforeseen ramifications, for, identified almost exclusively with the personal organism, the infant is faced, for the first time, with the immanent fear of death. He suffers anxiety, and "anxiety is the ego's incapacity to accept death." Since he has identified his once transcendent self exclusively with his organism, the death of that organism seems to be an utter annihilation of his very self, a total subtraction that he cannot bear.

The infant, therefore, arrives at a fantasy solution to this illusory problem of death—a solution that eventually culminates in what is known as the Oedipal project. Now the Oedipal project is only secondarily the wish to sexually possess the mother and kill the father, for the infant's primary aim in the Oedipal situation is to abolish death by becoming the father of himself. He imagines, in his infantile fantasy, that he can gain a type of immortality by conceiving himself. As strange as this sounds, remember that even a typical adult will feel he can in some ways cheat death by leaving behind progeny, something of himself that will "survive death." Conceiving a child thus seems at least to touch immortality, and even more so to the infant's untutored fantasy.

The infant, therefore, attempts in fantasy to conceive himself, to become his own parent and thus assuage the anxiety that death presents to him. And by the time of the Oedipal project, the child's fantasies have centered around the genital area, as common sense and the analysis of children as well as adults disclose. But more significantly, the libido of the infant has also concentrated in the genital area, by and large to the exclusion of all other bodily regions. Now libido does not mean sexual, genital pleasure. Libido, in its undiluted form, is simply that capacity for overall bodily pleasure, for transcendent bliss, and in the earliest years of infancy it is distributed equally throughout all bodily organs, surfaces, and activities. The infant participates in transcendent bliss through any area or activity of his body.

But under the Oedipal project, this libido is concentrated in the genital region alone, driven there by the *fantasies* of overcoming death by uniting bodily with the mother. The libido is no longer democratically available to the entire body, but is now tyrannized by a single region. And the fate of this tyranny is sealed by what is known as the castration complex, for this complex—whose intricacies we need not detail here—smashes to pieces the Oedipal project, *but leaves the genital organization of the libido intact.* The Oedipal project continues its aims in other forms of fantasy, but the body itself remains deformed, with its libido, its transcendent bliss, diluted and restricted to only one particular area of the body. The body, in short, is left crippled with the constrictions and knots of infantile wishes. The ego becomes the dominant element in consciousness, and the genital the dominant element of the body and world.

And so it comes about that the normal adult's only access to transcendent bliss and ecstasy is through genital sexual release, a drastic and morbid reduction of the delight he enjoyed as a child. As Norman O. Brown put it, in infancy a person tastes the fruit of the tree of life, and he knows that it is good . . . and he never forgets. This is why Freud ultimately, unlike Ferenczi, Fenichel, Reich, and others, did *not* see full genital release as a cure for neuroses, because even the genital act itself is a necessary source of conflict, since full and unobstructed bliss is frustrated by its unnecessary restriction to a single, tyrannizing region of the body. But again I must emphasize that the "tyranny of genital organization" results not so much from genitality itself, but from the restriction of bliss to this region alone.

Now notice that with this restriction of transcendent bliss to the genital area, we arrive at . . . the first *major* chakra!* And notice also the path that original consciousness–bliss has taken in order to arrive at this first major knot: from a blissful, transcendent, timeless, and therefore eternal unity with all of manifestation, to a partial, fragmented, and abysmally restricted ego awareness stealing what bliss it can from a genital tyranny. From a cosmic body to a personal body—indeed, only a region of a personal body! This is the normal, but not natural, state of affairs for the ordinary person, and this is the state of affairs that kundalini yoga seeks to reverse.

It should be obvious, even from our brief and popularized Freudian discussion, that the processes that culminate in egoic awareness and exclusive genitality do not constitute a *single* event or a single step from a cosmic body to a deformed personal one. There are numerous intermediate stages, levels of identification, and bands of awareness that range in gradients from the Supreme Identity to egoic fantasy, forming what amounts to an *apparent* hierarchy of knots or chakras, each progressively "lower" knot being more restrictive and exclusive than its predecessor, with the entire process finally culminating in egoic-genital tyranny.

Kundalini yoga therefore wisely proceeds to reverse this tyranny of awareness and bliss step by careful step, untying the knots in what it sees as roughly the reverse of the order in which they were tied, until finally the chakras themselves lie dissolved—that is, fully "opened"—and transcendent bliss is returned to its prior and unobstructed condition, a condition

* For convenience, I am following the Vajrayana in grouping the first and second kundalini chakras into one major chakra, the first major chakra. Tibetan Buddhism recognizes five, not seven, chakras. The first and second, and the sixth and seventh, are combined.

essentially similar to the polymorphous freedom of the infant but now transmitted through a matured and fully developed personality. So we must emphatically point out that this process is not one of regression but of *involution,* a return to the Source and not to childhood. On the contrary, it is normal adult genital organization that is supported by regressive fantasies of an Oedipal nature that attempt to avoid death and secure an ersatz immortality. On the other hand, to live in transcendent bliss, timeless and eternal, is to yank every conceivable support from under the Oedipal complex, because it means tasting again, in a mature and developed form, the fruit of the Tree of Life.

The aim of kundalini yoga, therefore, is to free transcendent bliss (ananda) from its dilutions and restrictions, and to recognize it as boundless, oceanic, without limits in time or space. Each dissolving of a knot, each "opening" of a chakra, represents—and actually *feels* like—a return of transcendent bliss to a more oceanic and unobstructed state. And this fact leads to what first seems the most puzzling aspect of the chakras: their apparent *localization* in specific areas of the body. Even Ramana Maharshi—who otherwise discounted the reality of the chakras as far as spiritual sadhana was concerned—acknowledged that specific areas of the body seem best to *contain* the different degrees of "freed up" bliss. That certain feelings are best *contained* in specific areas of the body does not seem a fantastic proposal. For example, the genitals of a normal adult *contain* sexual bliss better than the feet, and in like manner, other types or degrees of feelings, vibrations, and energies seem to be best contained in other regions of the body, localizing around specific organs, surfaces, nerve ganglia, or muscle groups. Thus the "gut region" seems to contain "vital" or life-force bliss, and actually *feels* so to one who works through that chakra. So also, the heart-chest region seems best to contain and even radiate loving bliss; the head region, intellectual bliss; and the sahasrara, final ascending and transcendent bliss.

As we shall presently see, it is not *necessary* for liberation that consciousness–bliss travels through these particular centers outlined by kundalini theory. It is just that it might, especially if someone concentrates on the appropriate areas and in the appropriate sequence prescribed by kundalini yoga. In this connection, I don't think we need be confused by the reported fact that concentrating on a specific region-chakra, along with certain visualizations, can *evoke* the appropriate feeling and energy best contained by that specific region. Close your eyes, concentrate on the genital region, visualize two people making sensuous love, and see if an appropriate feeling and energy isn't evoked! Thus, at the other end of the pole, Ramana could say, "If one concentrates on the sahasrara there is no doubt that the ecstasy of samadhi ensues." The localization of the chakras, in general, seems to be one of their more self-evident features.

In this regard, it is not surprising that bioenergetics, the school of psychotherapy most alive to bodily feelings and energies, even in just their personal and nontranscendent forms, maintains that different feelings and cognitions are "located," or best contained in, certain well-defined segments of the body: one feels stability and groundedness in the legs and feet (and not, for instance, in the chin!); orgasmic ecstasy in the genitals; joy-vitality-laughter in the gut; openness-affirmation-love in the chest; intellection-insight in the eyes and head; and spirituality at the crown—a formulation essentially identical to that of the kundalini model, but without, of course, the latter's eye to the degrees of progressive transcendence accompanying these energies, nor their increasingly "subtle" character.

So I don't think there is anything mysterious about the location of the chakras. They are "there," they are "real," because 1) you can *feel* certain states or modifications of bliss and awareness at each major chakra, and 2) these feelings or energies just aren't appropriate to other areas of the body, as, for example, you cannot ordinarily feel an orgasm in your knee.

This, then, is the basis of the chakra system as presented in terms of feelings, vibrations, or *energetics* (prana, chi, ruh, ki). These energetics exist, they are "real," or rather, they are as real as any other feelings of joy or terror or excitement, and they take as their *terminals* specific centers, organs, muscle groups, nerve ganglia, or, as some maintain, endocrine glands. The most significant point, however, is not the localization of the chakras, but the modes of consciousness that take these regions as an appropriate outlet.

The chakras are *located* at specific areas or organs, but they are not *identical* to those areas. It is for this reason that kundalini yoga maintains that these centers deal primarily with the "subtle body," which is to say, with states of awareness and bliss that no longer recognize the conventional and illusory boundaries between the organism and the environment, and thus could hardly be localized *finally* in one or the other. It is just that, in the period of transition from a personal body to a cosmic one, the individual carries for some time the old and exclusive references to his isolated and personal body, and thus his insights might tend to take, as their *physical correlates,* certain terminals in the body. And as for the enlightened sages, even they walk on their feet, eat with their mouths, love with their hearts, and procreate with their genitals. These "localizations" hardly seem a mysterious affair. In other words, for the sage these localized centers remain, not as knots, but as appropriate and functional nodes of energy.

Thus far we have seen that the chakras represent both certain stages in a type of spiritual growth (steps in the freeing up of transcendent bliss) as well as certain locations of energies in the body. The usual controversy over the existence of the chakras—"Are they real?"—seems based on nothing other than an attempt to pit one of these characteristics of the chakras against the other. Thus, those who maintain that the chakras are purely metaphorical deny they have any "physical correlates" in the body, since this seems to drag spirit into the dirty realm of matter. This is an unnecessary concern, however, for spirit and matter have never been separated. On the other hand, those who claim that the chakras are purely physical—that is, *identical* to nerve plexes instead of *associated* with them—fall instantly into the Fallacy of Simple

Location, a favorite pastime of physiologists, and thus have the utmost difficulty in theoretically extracting a transcendent state of consciousness out of an endocrine gland.

I have tried to suggest that these two views are complementary. The fact that the chakras are symbolic does not prevent their association with particular regions of the body, and the fact that they may be more appropriately experienced in certain regions of the body does not rob them of their transcendent symbolism.

The chakras, as we have seen, are predominantly concerned with the apparent hierarchy of *energetics*—with vibrations, feelings, vital force, and bliss. Naturally, not all spiritual systems or disciplines emphasize this aspect of higher states of consciousness, preferring instead to emphasize, and work through, the *equivalent* hierarchies of insight, or absorption, or ontological world view, or cosmology, or awareness—all of which are perfectly valid. The Hindu points out that saguna Brahman is "characterized" by absolute being, consciousness, and bliss, and some spiritual systems and practices simply emphasize, and thus develop, one of these equivalent characteristics and its manifestations over the others. Thus the tantras deal with the samsaric hierarchy of knots in predominantly energetic terms and states; the Kabbalah works with the cosmological and ontological aspects; the Buddhists emphasize awareness and insight. These are all roughly equivalent expressions of a central truth: In the apparent world, "existence is graded, and with it, cognition," and, we would add, energetics and vibratory bliss. As far as spiritual practice is concerned, all of these honorable traditions point to a progressive dissolution of the constricting knots we have tied in our own consciousness.

To return to kundalini specifically: Many investigators, having some familiarity with Freud's work on sublimation, assume that kundalini yoga consists in the progressive sublimation or "forcing upward" of genital sexual energy. Further, some have proposed that laboratory studies would confirm this hypothesis, and that here we would finally have the pulling of the religious rabbit out of the laboratory hat. Being a biochemist by training, I am wholly in sympathy with any experimental thrust in this direction, even though we will then be faced with an extremely difficult dilemma should physiological tests show that certain neurological or hormonal changes do in fact occur as meditation proceeds through the chakras to higher states of consciousness. The dilemma: Is the higher consciousness the *result* of chemical changes or the *cause* of them? If the latter, then physiological changes are totally irrelevant to spiritual pursuits.

But this physiological line of reasoning has led some people to conclude that the energy of higher consciousness can be explained in terms of sublimated, genital sexual energy. Aside from the fact that genital sexuality cannot in theory be sublimated (the pregenital organizations alone provide the reservoir of libido that drives sublimations), I think the conclusion is precisely reversed. As I have tried to explain, genital sexuality is a constriction and a restriction of higher consciousness, and this is the state of affairs that kundalini yoga seeks to reverse. It thus *appears,* to an ordinary onlooker or researcher, that sexual energy is transmuting into higher states of consciousness–but it's really just the opposite. The higher consciousness is being freed from its chronic constrictions in "lower"–that is, limited and bounded–modes of awareness and energetics. God-consciousness is not sublimated sexuality; sexuality is repressed God-consciousness.

All in all, I think we can fairly conclude that each chakra represents both an appropriate center in the body and a particular stage in a type of spiritual growth. I say "type of spiritual growth" because there is much evidence in the orthodox traditions themselves (especially Tibetan Buddhism) that suggests that kundalini yoga is a valid but partial approach to even the energetics of higher consciousness, tending to ignore —with its exclusive emphasis on the ascending kundalini current–the equally important "descending" currents. Further, even the Hindu generally concedes that, except at its very summit, kundalini shakti is a phenomenon of the subtle body only. Hatha yoga addresses the gross body, and kundalini the subtle body, but it is jnana yoga that deals with the underlying reality of the causal body. Jnana yoga of Vedanta, Dzog chen and mahamudra of Vajrayana, chih-kuan and shikantaza of Zen—these simply investigate, through present awareness, any knot that arises in consciousness, and, finding it void of self-nature, are relieved of the burden of untying it.

Thus we return to the paradox with which we began this article—the chakras *do* appear to exist, and the chakras *are* knots. But the knots are illusory. Nothing binds us from the very start, but until we understand this, everything appears to. Nevertheless, kundalini theory, with its penetrating understanding of these shadowy knots themselves, offers sound, wise, and powerful advice on how to see through them, so that one may finally awaken, as if from a dream, to discover that the cosmos is one's body, and the sun one's solar self.

EXPLORING THE MYTHS AND MISCONCEPTIONS OF KUNDALINI

M. S. S. Gurucharan Singh Khalsa
[*with Yogi Bhajan*]

Meditation and yoga techniques have become accepted and integrated in many facets of our Western lifestyle. We are moving from being complete dilettantes to becoming a more sophisticated audience. If someone says, "I meditate," we now ask, "What form of meditation do you use?" We no longer think there is only one type of activity called meditation. We are slowly recognizing that meditations and yoga exercises have specific effects which differ greatly from technique to technique.

The Kundalini Research Institute was founded to study these differences and map out a science of consciousness which can be practically applied to daily problems as well as lead us to explore the deeper potentials of the human being. In current writings and teachings, there is great confusion about kundalini and kundalini yoga.

On one hand, authors say that kundalini is the most potent and powerful energy for changing consciousness. On the other hand, readers are either warned not to practice it, or the techniques are referred to in veiled secrecy. How can something as essential to consciousness change as kundalini be feared? Only gross mispractice of the technology of kundalini would be dangerous. The West has been very fortunate to have the master of kundalini yoga, Yogi Bhajan, teaching openly the ancient science. He has dispelled many of the misrepresentations and myths surrounding kundalini. His explicit teaching has given researchers techniques which can be tested.

Yogi Bhajan began teaching in the United States in January of 1969. He was, and still is, the only recognized master of kundalini yoga. Most teachers at that time did not discuss the kundalini. Many people warned against the practice. He taught the techniques and offered them to be tested. Now . . . the kundalini has become a popular topic. It has become an area of serious research.

Many of the teachers who would not speak of the kundalini now say they raise the kundalini energy if you just sit in their presence. Amrit Desai and Swami Muktananda both make such claims. Other yoga teachers identify the release of kundalini energy by the body jerks and hallucinations their students experience. Yogi Bhajan, when asked about this type of teaching, said "This is what we call jerk yoga! It is totally make-believe. The sign of the kundalini energy is the expansive consciousness, the compassion, and the practicality of the being who acts in humility before the Infinite Creator."

To dispel some of the myths about kundalini, let's look at some examples of where the distortions come from. The first problem is a lack of knowledge. Most writers are just writers. They have written things to sell and have not had the actual experiences they are writing about. They may be very honest in writing to share their knowledge, but they are only repeating what they have read from someone else who in turn is copying from someone before them.

Many times, the end of this chain of references does not lead to a master of kundalini yoga, but to rumor or misconception. Once the misconception is put into print, it gains a new power and reality which is difficult to erase. Most people prefer to read and quote rather than to test and experience. P. D. Ouspensky is a widely read philosopher and occultist who expounds the teachings of Gurdjieff. In his book, *In Search of the Miraculous,* the kundalini is seen as the hypnotist that holds mankind in illusion.

"In reality kundalini is the power of imagination, the power of fantasy, which takes the place of a real function. When a man dreams instead of acting, when his dreams take the place of reality, when a man imagines himself to be an eagle, a lion, or a magician, it is the force of kundalini acting in him. Kundalini can act in all centers and with its help all the centers can be satisfied with the imaginary instead of the real. A sheep which considers itself a lion or a magician lives under the power of kundalini.

"Kundalini is a force put into men in order to keep them in their present state. If men could really see their true position and could understand all the horror of it, they would be unable to remain where they are even for a second. They would begin to seek a way out and they would quickly find it, because there is a way out; but men fail to see it simply because they are hypnotized. Kundalini is the force that keeps them in a hypnotic state."

This view comes from a complete lack of knowledge. He has intellectually tried to put a new interpretation on the concept of kundalini without any technique or practice in it. This leads his readers to a close-minded attitude which prohibits creative inquiry.

Gopi Krishna has written a series of books about the kundalini. He very correctly says that it is the evolutionary force in consciousness and that its full development results in a spiritual and brilliant person. He also advises that research be done to find the biochemical changes which occur when the kundalini energy releases. But his writings confuse students when he describes his own "kundalini experience." He had no master or technique to raise kundalini. By haphazard meditation, he drew on the energy without physically preparing his body with breath or mantra. Consequently, he had a negative experience. In *The Awakening of Kundalini,* he says that when you are not attuned, the kundalini energy gives you a consciousness that is

> ". . . stained with complexes, anxiety, depression, fear, and other neurotic and paranoid conditions, which alternate with elevated blissful periods, visionary experiences, or creative moods. In the latter, it manifests itself in the various hideous forms of psychosis, in the horrible depression, frenzied excitement, and wild delusions of the insane. In plain words, the same life energy

> (prana) which, when pure, leads to the glorious visionary experiences of the harmonized mystic, when slightly tainted, can cause gloomy moods of tension, fear, depression, or anxiety and, when irremediably contaminated, creates the shrieking horrors of madness."

This statement puts fear into many students. A warning without a technique is valueless. It only creates insecurity and misunderstanding. In Kashmir, I asked Gopi Krishna why he wrote about such experiences without emphasizing that this is not the experience when actually practicing kundalini yoga. He replied, "I still do not understand the kundalini. The experience has been with me for twenty-seven years. I have translated the old texts, but they are written in a symbology code. So to this day, I cannot teach you anything, I can only encourage inquiry." He also wrote that celibacy was needed to raise the energy. So there are many young people who come to the Institute struggling with celibacy and searching for the great kundalini experience.

Another common mistake of writers is to limit the kundalini to a particular type of energy or physical nerve in order to give it physical or scientific validity. *The Mysterious Kundalini,* by Vasant Rele, identifies kundalini as "the serpent power which is the right vagus nerve of modern times, which supplies and controls all the important and vital organs." This tremendous failure of interpretation comes from a sincere attempt to explain the great physical benefits which accrue to practitioners of kundalini yoga. But he has totally misunderstood the unlimited nature of this energy.

Another common mistake is to take the symbolism of the chakras too literally. The symbols were created as reminders of the practical experiences and where the scriptures refer to the "turning of the lotus cup on the moon," it means "the secretion of the posterior pituitary gland has come in balance with the pineal gland and has produced a clear direct power of thought." When the "sphere of the stars" is referred to, it sometimes means the physical stars, but other times means the hemispheres of the brain.

Because of this gap between symbolism and meaning, a lot of unbalanced teachings are being sold to gullible students. Arthur Avalon does a fine job of translating in *The Serpent Power,* but is at a loss to make the writings practical. In a recent article in *Psychology Today,* the well respected scholar of symbolism, Joseph Campbell, wrote "Seven Levels of Consciousness." It described the symbols of the chakras, but gives absolutely no hint as to their real meaning or usefulness. Many readers think that visualizing the old symbols is the way to use them. This is not true. Ram Dass, in *The Only Dance There Is,* makes this mistake. He treats the kundalini energy lightly and says:

> It's called raising the kundalini. It's a very delicate technique.
> . . . I would do hatha yoga for a long time, then I would do pranayam which is a series of exercises. Some of them are like oxygenation, going on for some minutes . . . then you learn how to force your attention on the tip of your spine and to visualize right in from the tip of the spine, which is called in the Indian energy system the first chakra. You learn to focus on a triangle of flame in which there is a serpent wound with its head down three and a half times around a lingam or a phallus.

Meditation in this manner can only lead to difficulty. He is also an example of the common fallacy that when the kundalini energy releases, the practitioner becomes rigid and breathless.

> What incredible thing happens is that when you can take your attention away from the holding of the breath, you go into this state where you are not breathing and you are not holding your breath. Usually the awareness of that brings you back. You say, "My God, I'm not breathing" and that brings you down . . . you've flipped into this place where you're perfectly calm but there is no breath, and at that point you feel this energy pouring up your spine and into your head.

The kundalini experience does not mean you have gone into a deep breathless trance and are beyond this world or filled with inner lights. It integrates you more fully with reality and gives you a broader vision and sensitivity so that you can act more efficiently.

Not all writers or teachers have made these kinds of gross errors which have led to the myths of the kundalini. The great teacher, Swami Vivekananda, gives extensive instruction about the nature of meditation and yoga in *Raja Yoga.*

> When, by the power of long internal meditation the vast mass of energy stored up travels along the sushumna and strikes the centers, the reaction is tremendous, immensely superior to the reaction of the dream or imagination, immensely more intense than the reaction of sense-perception.
>
> Wherever there was any manifestation of what is ordinarily called supernatural power or wisdom, there a little current of kundalini must have found its way into the sushumna. Only, in the vast majority of such cases, people had ignorantly stumbled on some practice which set free a minute portion of the coiled-up kundalini. All worship, consciously or unconsciously, leads to this end.
>
> The man who thinks that he is receiving response to his prayers does not know that the fulfillment comes from his own nature, that he has succeeded by the mental attitude of prayer in waking up a bit of this infinite power which is coiled up within himself. What, thus, man ignorantly worships under various names, through fear and tribulation, the yogi declares to the world to be the real power coiled up in every being, the mother of eternal happiness, if we but know how to approach her. And yoga is the science of religion, the rationale of all worship, all prayers, forms, ceremonies and miracles.

Besides this understanding of kundalini, he points that there are eight limbs of yoga which must be practiced for proper balance. Concentration, mantra, physical exercise, and pranayama are part of these. Some popular groups such as

TM advocate meditation without concentration. They warn against breathing and kundalini.

Studies are beginning to show that meditation without concentration leads to an inability to work and to deal with emergency situations. That type of meditation leads to an overdominant right brain hemisphere which predisposes the meditator to fantasy. The teaching laid out by Swami Vivekananda and those given by Yogi Bhajan both emphasize the need for complete balance. The body, mind, and spirit must be dealt with in kundalini yoga.

The only difficulties that arise are when the practice is fragmentary. Swami Sivananda in *Kundalini Yoga* takes a clear and cogent position. He recognizes the spiritual qualities of kundalini and shares what practical techniques he knows. He also counters the idea that once you get a psychic experience the kundalini is fully raised.

> It is easy to awaken the kundalini, but it is very difficult to take it to sahasrara chakra through the different chakras. It demands a great deal of patience, perseverance, purity and steady practice. The yogi who has taken it to sahasrara chakra, is the real master of all forces. Generally yogi students stop their sadhana halfway on account of false satisfaction. They imagine that they have reached the goal when they get some mystic experiences and psychic powers. They desire to demonstrate such powers to the public to get reputation and fame and to earn money. This is a sad mistake. Full realization alone can give the final liberation, perfect peace and highest bliss.

The voices of the few knowledgeable teachers are heard infrequently over the clamor of teachers who struggle for fame and power. The teachers who are after personal disciples and bind them with secrecy obscure the beauty and simplicity inherent in the techniques of kundalini yoga. Many of these false teachers give an audience a psychic experience or a slight hallucination as evidence of their kundalini energy.

These are the deluded and misguided students Swami Sivananda refers to.

The Teaching of Yogi Bhajan

A real teacher will always focus you on your own self experience of the Self. He will have you measure that experience by your own stability, humility, ability to sacrifice, truthfulness, practicality, and your ability to know without speaking harshly. Yogi Bhajan was asked in 1969 to comment on the process and nature of the kundalini energy. His answer was clean and direct:

> I have recognized, with the blessing of my master, that it is possible to be healthy, to be happy, and to be holy while living in this society; but you must have energy so that your dead computer may live and pass on the signal to you and may compute all that you want to do in this society. We call this energy, in the olden science, the kundalini, which has been blocked in muladhara, the lowest of all chakras or lotuses.
>
> These are all imaginary things. Great big books have been written on them and these books also misled me for many years. Still I learned about it, and all these chakras (or circles as we call them in English), have put us in so many circles that we do not come out of it and we reach nowhere. There is a way we should set our computer to be in direct contact with Him, the Biggest Computer, and all things must then work automatically. That cannot work until the kundalini, the spiritual nerve, breaks through the blockage at the muladhara, and thus, travels up and reaches the stage so that you may have superconsciousness in consciousness.
>
> You must generate the pressure of the prana and mix it with the apana, and thus, when the two join together, you generate heat in the pranic center. With this heat of the prana, you put a pressure or charge on the kundalini,

the soul nerve, which is coiled in three and a half circles ('kundal' means 'the curl of the hair of the beloved,' it does not mean snake or serpent) on muladhara. This will awaken it so that it may pierce through the imaginary chakras and pass ultimately through jalandhara bandha (neck lock—the final blockage in the spine before the energy reaches the head).

Now let me define a few terms. Prana is the life force of the atom. Apana is elimination or the eliminating force. These are two forces, positive and negative, in us which are governed by pingala and ida; that is, right and left. When we join these two energies under the power and the science of kundalini yoga, we mix the prana with the apana and, under that pressure, bring the kundalini up. When it passes through the central nerve or sushumna, it reaches the higher chakras or lotuses, and thus man can easily look into the future. His psychic power becomes activated. He can know his total surroundings and he is a blessed being.

After one inhales the prana deep (down to the navel point) and pulls the apana with the root lock (up to the navel point), prana and apana mix at the navel center. This is known as nabhi chakra at the fourth vertebra. Heat is felt during the kundalini awakening and that heat is the filament of the sushumna or central spinal channel being lit by the joining of prana and apana. Below the nabhi chakra, the energy leaves the navel and goes to the rectum (or lower center) and then it rises. This is called reserve channels. It relates to your astral body.

Then, there are six more chakras through which the kundalini must rise—and it will happen all at once. Once you have raised it, that's it. The hardest job is to keep it up, to keep the channels clean and clear.

From the rectum to the vocal cord is known as the silver cord. From the neck to the top of the head is the passage. From the third eye to the pineal gland is the gold cord. To make the energy rise in these cords and passages, you must apply hydraulic locks. You must put a pressure. You live in California? You know how we take the oil out of the ground? Put a pressure and the oil will come out. Your spine is a staircase of energy. 1) Mulabandha brings apana, eliminating force, to the navel or fourth vertebra, the central seat of the kundalini. 2) Diaphragm lock takes it to the neck. 3) Neck lock takes it up all the rest of the way.

The pineal gland or seat of the soul, does not work when the tenth gate (top of the head) is sealed, but if the pineal will secrete (when the kundalini heat comes), your pituitary will act as radar, keeping the mind from negativity.

Yes, kundalini is known as the nerve of the soul. This is to be awakened. Your soul is to be awakened. When soul gets awakened, there remains nothing. What else?

In the practical reality, these chakras are imaginary and nothing else. This kundalini is just a kundalini and nothing else. It is not very important. These pranas and apanas are just there. Everything is set in us. We lack nothing. We use these terms simply to make the process clear so we can get on with it. It is very simple. After getting myself into the darkness for years together, I found that if I would have known on the first day that it was so easy, I could have saved myself a lot of hassle. When I found out that the kundalini really can come up like this, I was astonished. It was a surprise to me. I said, "That's all there is to the kundalini?" and my master said, "Yes."

All it is, creating the prana in the cavity and mixing it with apana and taking it down (as we give pressure to the oil) and bringing the oil up. This is kundalini. That's it. That is the greatest truth. Truth is bitter I know, so I cannot speak all the truth; but I speak indirectly and directly about the truth because I cannot speak something beyond truth.

I have realized the truth, and the fact is that you cannot breathe by your will. It is the God within you which breathes. Without that, you don't breathe. Now what is this breath business? I'll tell you. It is good information for the medical people. Under the eighth vertebra, there is a cavity. We call it the prana center. Good? In that prana center, with the breathing up to the tip of the tongue and on to the ida and pingala which adjusts the temperature of the body, we breathe pranic energy. Pranic energy is the life force of the atom. If fifty years ago I would have come and talked to you about atomic energy, you would have said, "Go away, we don't understand you." When I talk pranic energy, don't feel that I am talking something mystic. It is practical. This pranic energy is the life of the atom. We store it here (eighth vertebra down). We know certain actions through which we inhale this pranic energy and our pranic center is awakened. The pranic center supplies the pranic energy to the pranic nerve. The pranic nerve supplies the pranic energy to the muscles which are responsible for the beat of the heart and that of the diaphragm. We call it the "U" muscle because it is shaped like the letter "U." This "U" nerve is responsible for all this life current in you which is automatic and beyond your control. You know what yogis do? They create pranic energy reservoirs in that cavity and thus live on that reserve. They make that cavity active with certain exercises and thus they know how to control the pranic energy or prana-vayu, the life current. That's one part of it. The second one is apana which eliminates everything. It has a connection with the muladhara chakra. That is where that kundalini power lies. Now, when the pranic energy is in you, then the second part is that you can circulate it through your body. You can feel it and make people feel it. We teach people how to do it. It is a scientific thing which has nothing to do with mystics or something which I can't explain. It is so simple, it is practical. Thus, we circulate it.

In the circulation, we time it to go with the spinal cord. Then we make it hit the muladhara. Thus, we pierce through that bind or blockage before the kundalini power. The moment we do it, she has no option but to come up. The moment she comes up, you stand blessed. Then you will see; the computer will work. That's all.

Is it difficult? There is no secret about it. In twenty, thirty days, if you honestly practice it about one hour, two hours each day, you can be through with it. This is what I did.

Two cautions: You must practice neck lock. Pull the neck straight in, keeping the spine and neck absolutely straight with no bend of the neck. If you do not apply this lock, the higher flood of circulation will cause the cells of the brain to expand and people will get upset and crazy.

When you do yoga, please, for God's sake, remember you are playing with the energy which is the life force of the atom. You can well understand what you are doing. I'm giving you a word of warning. The prana has been described in the shastras (yogic scriptures) as that which makes the atom live. The voltage here in the wall socket is 110? And do you touch it without insulation? No! Then how can you play with the pranic energy? (Proper technique and preparation is the insulation you need.)

The fact remains that without having your kundalini awakened, your soul is not awakened. If your soul is awakened, what else do you need? If you will get into the actions that awaken the kundalini, the nerve of the soul, then this car of yours will be driven or chauffeured by the soul and not by the negative ego, and then you will have found the God in you. I shall be the greatest man on Earth if I shall be privileged to touch the dust of your feet if you have that state. Otherwise, you are a nut, and nothing else.

In a 1976 interview, Yogiji was asked several common questions about the kundalini.

Q: What is the kundalini?

A: It is the whole cosmos energy in the individual and beyond the individual. It is the energy of consciousness. Without the constant flow of that energy, you could not live. With a large flow, your mind begins to flow and awaken. You stop living in imaginary realities and you become very dutiful to the tasks and joys of this life.

Q: Is the kundalini dangerous?

A: Is money dangerous? It is just an energy. Kundalini is a latent energy that can be used for total consciousness. The only dangerous thing is the person whose kundalini is raised properly. That person is totally conscious. He cannot be lied to or cheated or politically swayed. The kundalini is essential. As long as you practice a total discipline or a complete and balanced kriya, there is no difficulty. In kundalini yoga, you will notice that every meditation and kriya has some form of mantra in it. This insures the channelization of the energy.

Q: What about people who have great visions and psychic experiences or whose bodies jerk and tremble after meditation? Is this the kundalini rising?

A: This is glitter at the bottom of the ladder. These hallucinations, psychism, and nerve weaknesses mean nothing. If a student practicing kundalini yoga is very blocked up in the spine and pranic nadis, he may have a one-time experience when the channels are cleared. But that is one time, brief, and does not disrupt anything. These other causes are when the nerves have not been prepared, there is no mantra, or breathing has not been practiced. The real measure of kundalini rising is your consciousness from breath to breath and courage you bring to your life. These momentary flashes brought on by weakness have nothing to do with kundalini.

Q: Is the goal for the yoga student to bring all the energy into the brain?

A: No! The energy of kundalini releases from the navel center, then rises to the top of the head. When it descends to complete its cycle of energy, the chakras open fully. By chakras opening I mean the talents of each chakra are consolidated into the character and behavior of that person. It does no good at all to fill a person with energy that he cannot integrate.

Q: Most kundalini yoga students let their hair grow. Is this necessary?

A: No. You can practice with any length hair, but the hair was the first technique to raise the kundalini energy. When the hair is at its natural full length and coiled over the anterior fontenelle for men or the posterior fontenelle for women, it draws pranic energy into the spine. The force of this downward positive energy causes the kundalini energy to rise for balance. This is why you always find grace and calmness in a person with uncut hair from birth if they keep it well. Actually the hair was so important that the word for consciousness, kundalini, actually derives from "kundal" which means "a coil of the beloved's hair."

Q: You referred to the chakras as centers of consciousness. Would you briefly describe the qualities each gives the individual?

A: There are seven nerve centers in the body. They are all in the spine. They each have a projected center or chakra. First is the rectum. Second projected center is the sex organ. Third is the navel center. When you pull the rectum and sex organ together, the energy projects to the third center of consciousness. Fourth is the center between the two nipples, the heart center. Fifth is the neck. Sixth is between the two eyes at the top of the nose. And the seventh is the last at the top of the head, corresponding to the pineal gland.

What is a human? Do these centers have some correlation with the man? Yes. A person whose consciousness dwells in the rectum is a homosexual. He will never have a straight sex relationship. A person whose center of consciousness is the second center will be a sex maniac or a sadist. He will enjoy giving pain in sex. He will define himself in terms of sex.

At the third center of consciousness a person can't overcome greediness. He may try his level best. Somehow he will like to get others' things. They may be useful to him or not. The fourth center of consciousness is the heart center where the nipples and throat form a triangle. Here a person gets knowledge. The fifth center of consciousness is at the throat. He may talk without flowery English, but his words will have that heaviness that goes right into the heart.

At the sixth center of consciousness, a person can know everything around him. He may use the knowledge or not. The pituitary gland gives him the greatest intuition. That person can forsee the time and what he sees is the correct thing. At the last center of consciousness, which is the highest center, a person becomes most humble. He has extreme humility. In the highest center the ego becomes a universal ego, so that person has no pain and no pleasure. What he says happens. That is the highest center of consciousness.

In a long deep meditation, you can know where your consciousness is. It can be seen and judged by assessing what your environments are and what the most important needs in your life are. You can know what chakras you are in. Now, knowing does not make any difference. Can you pull it up and change gears in such a way that you can come out of it?

There are three ways: having a faith and looking to your God or to your minister and trying to act on what he says. The second method is long meditation, to transcend oneself. One knows one's weaknesses, one goes to the root of this weakness and one has to fight them and thus eliminate them and then come out of it. The third way is: to make your energy and nerves so positively sound that the mind does not think of anything which is negative. These are the techniques known to this world.

Sexual energy should be controlled.

Q: Is it possible for a teacher to raise the kundalini of his students just by his presence?

A: The kundalini can be stimulated directly by a teacher. But that teacher is not much of a teacher! The students should be prepared, then given a technology to raise it themselves. Why should they wait at the feet of that teacher like puppies? They should go through the experience, then share the techniques with others. The techniques of kundalini yoga are so potent and beautiful that my main job as a master of that science is to keep the kundalini down and close the third eye!

Q: Does a student of the kundalini yoga have to be celibate?

A: The student should be a householder, except in special cases, raise a family and fulfill the obligations of a spiritual society. Celibacy actually means to be by yourself without abusing your sexual and regenerative abilities. A married person is by himself, for both people are merged as one. Even in marriage the sexual energy is respected and built up. A normal couple will find a frequency of one time a month completely satisfying if approached correctly. If you want to be celibate without ever having sex, remember to practice Sat Kriya each day so you can utilize the energy and not go nutty.

Q: When the kundalini rises, do you go into trance or become rigid?

A: A raised kundalini will give you grace of motion. Life fills every cell so you are able to move smoothly with an awareness of the rhythm and music of all your environments. The kundalini makes you alive and graceful, not rigid like some kind of death.

Q: Why are these teachings being shared so openly now? Is there a need for initiation?

A: The techniques belong to those who practice them. They are the heritage of humanity. I am just a postman with a lot of letters to deliver. You can open them and use them or not; that is your problem. But the world is going through a lot of changes. Your future generations will need these techniques to stay mentally healthy and physically strong. All these teachings will help humanity as it awakens from adolescence. I am sharing these teachings to create teachers and leaders for the future and to create a science of the total self.

II

A Handful of Personal Accounts

The sickness—the nausea—
    The pitiless pain—
Have ceased with fever
    That maddened my brain—
With the fever called "Living"—
    That burned in my brain.

And, oh! of all the tortures
    That torture the worst
Has abated—the terrible
    Torture of thirst

For the Napthaline river
    Of Passion accurst:—
I have drunk of a water
    That quenches all thirst. . . .

These lines from Edgar Allan Poe's poem *For Annie* present a puzzle for literary exegesis. A conventional explanation would assign them meaning in terms of conventional psychology. But when they are assessed from the perspective of the kundalini concept, a dramatic new dimension is added to the poem and, indeed, to Poe himself. If the kundalini experience is intimately connected with creativity—as one of the traditional names for kundalini, "Divine Mother," implies—then the creative impulse working in Poe and all other great poets would appear to be described quite literally here. The phenomenology of the kundalini experience will become clearer in later sections. For the moment, let us simply reflect on the well-known fact that Poe chose his words with greatest care. "Napthaline," the dictionary tells us, is a flammable, volatile, oily liquid used as a fuel, solvent, and illuminant–qualities that apply without exception to aspects of the kundalini phenomenon. Was Poe describing his personal experience with the awakening of kundalini? Such a possibility is only one of a multitude of insights–ranging from science to literary criticism–that await serious investigators of kundalini.

This section is intended to give a sense of personal experience–vicarious though it may be–through half a dozen firsthand accounts from people who have experienced the awakening of kundalini in various degrees. By no means is this section comprehensive. The accounts offered here are partial descriptions of initial or intermediate stages, and the stages themselves can vary greatly from individual to individual, depending upon many factors.

The experiences reported here range from the terrifying to the sublime. They are all dramatic in one way or another. However, it should be pointed out that the awakening of kundalini is not *inherently* a traumatic or theatrically glorious event. Rather, the spectacular inner phenomena so often reported–the brilliant lights, the blissful moments of self-abandonment, the Brahmic splendor (as R. M. Bucke put it in his description of cosmic consciousness)–are themselves evanescent and unstable experiences. They belong to the peaks, not the plateaus, of human consciousness. In someone whose "Illumination Quotient" is high from birth, such phenomena may be bypassed almost totally. Instead, the unfolding of higher consciousness may proceed with few pyrotechnics.

The point here is to de-emphasize any kundalini stereotype and the quest for "phenomena" as signs of enlightenment. The person who humbly and faithfully performs some menial function within a vast institution or organization, without seeking praise, reward, or even recognition, may be more illuminated than the person who proudly describes, in an eloquent literary style, the details of a relatively minor mental experience.

We begin with a brief account by a Westerner, Brian Van der Horst, who experienced a glimpse of the vast riches contained in the awakening of kundalini.

Next is an excerpt from the memoirs of Swami Muktananda Paramahansa, widely regarded as a living kundalini master. Muktananda's experiences, taken from his *Play of Consciousness,* go far beyond what is recounted here. The point of this selection is to demonstrate that sexuality can serve other life-supporting functions besides procreation. This insight, recognized from the most ancient times, is sadly debased today in the conventional attitude of various religions, primarily fundamentalist Protestantism and Roman Catholicism. What was once awareness of the evolutionary potential in people through properly controlled and properly directed sexual continence has degenerated into a puritanical harangue against all sexuality whatsoever, except within marriage. Muktananda himself had to unlearn the subtle attitudinal conditioning–that sex per se is wicked–that was preventing further unfoldment of the creative force within him. His frank account of this trying time in his life is a welcome corrective to the widespread misunderstanding of this aspect of human sexuality.

Paul Zweig's shaktipat experience is offered as representative of many that have been reported to occur due to the action of Swami Muktananda. In a similar manner, D. R. Butler experienced shaktipat through Yogi Amrit Desai. Butler's experience is still another confirmation of the positive aspect of the kundalini yoga tradition.

Kundalini in its negative aspect is presented through the accounts of John Scudder, a psychic healer with documented cures to his credit, and Gopi Krishna, a yogi-philosopher in Srinagar, Kashmir, whose autobiography, *Kundalini, the Evolutionary Energy in Man,* has done much to direct the attention of the scientific and intellectual communities to the kundalini concept. (See his article on kundalini research in the next section.)

Altogether these selections create a portrait of kundalini experience that can offer valuable guidance to both researchers and those on the spiritual path. However, it must be reemphasized that this portrait is a softly focused image, not a blueprint. The experiences described here by no means comprise an exhaustive list, and readers should be alert against blind acceptance of any rigid schema or stereotype for the phenomenology of the kundalini experience.

"SO THIS IS KUNDALINI"

Brian Van der Horst

I was practicing my lesson [from *A Course in Miracles*] at three o'clock in the morning. I suddenly felt some activity at the base of my spine. Previously I had ignored such sensations. I had it figured out that meditation should be something quiet. This time I said, what the hell, I'll just go with the flow. A feeling like shuddering, surging energy began traveling up my back. I felt as if every nerve trunk on my spine had begun firing. Each burst was as good as any orgasm I'd ever had. It kept climbing. I could feel vortexes of electricity around places that have been described as chakras. "Well," I thought. "So this is kundalini."

Then I began breathing quickly, spontaneously. First I was smiling, then grinning, then swept over with joy, ecstasy, rocking and quaking, my whole body aquiver. The fire climbed, and then shot out of the top of my head. "This makes celibacy look pretty good," I observed.

After a while I stood and walked over to a full-length mirror. My eyes relaxed out of focus, and my body appeared to vanish in the glass. All I could see was a shadowy radiant outline. Then I saw moving lights inside the outline which coalesced into a figure, a design I instinctively recognized as an energy pattern that symbolized my being. "Now I know I must be dreaming." I watched it for a while, noticed a half-hour had elapsed, and then went to bed, still glowing with an indescribable joy. It lasted for days.

Well, that was pretty advanced stuff, I assumed. Months

later I compared my drawing of the symbol I had seen in the mirror with one that Dr. H. had received years before in a sort of vision, representing a keepsake from her guide. We had never compared them before. They were identical.

A couple of weeks later I was walking through Swami Muktananda's ashram. Suddenly I saw my symbol hanging on the wall. I asked a disciple what it meant. "Oh, that's just Sanskrit for 'Om,'" I was told. . . .

SENSUAL EXCITEMENT

Swami Muktananda

Each day I had new experiences. It now so happened that my body and senses became possessed by carnal craving. What should not have taken place began to occur. I had, in fact, no desire for any sensuous object or enjoyment. I had traveled widely and seen the conditions of all classes of people, from the highest to the lowest, and I knew the final outcome of their modes of living. At Ganeshpuri all kinds of people came to my Gurudev, including wealthy tycoons, men of status, good artists, famous film actors, singers, orators, and important officials, as a great saint belongs to all. But each of them complained of some want or another in his life. Despite their wealth and possessions, each lacked one thing miserably—physical health. They would say, "Bhagawan, I have everything, but my heart is giving me trouble. The doctors permit me neither to move about nor eat my fill. Besides, my senses have lost their strength." "Babaji, my stomach aches terribly. I have been to England and America, spending thousands for a cure, but to no avail." "Bhagawan, I have no material want, but I can neither digest my food nor sleep at night. I have already spent two *lakhs* on treatment." Somebody had trouble with his eyes, another with his ears.

Thus all the miserable visitors narrated their woeful tales to Bhagawan Nityananda. Each suffered from some deficiency and wept pitifully. If he possessed wealth, he was poor in health or vice versa. Another was illiterate, poor in learning. A third was ugly, poor in beauty. A fourth was a widow, a fifth a widower, and a sixth was childless. Thus, whoever came was afflicted with some privation and would relate his pathetic account. I listened quietly. I considered what lesson I could learn from them. Truly speaking, I was in the same boat: poor in sadhana, self-knowledge, and self-realization. I regarded these people carefully. They were without brightness, equanimity, and health, frustrated in spite of their riches. Nor did they possess any strength or energy. New diseases were always attacking them. The reasons for all this were the waste of seminal fluid, sensuality, and an irregular life.

It is a strange irony that man regards himself as fortunate if he can enjoy sensual gratification. But he is only deluding himself, unaware that instead of enjoying pleasures, he is being enjoyed by them. As a result, he falls a helpless victim to all kinds of sicknesses. Even now people weep to me in the same manner. I keep seeing pitiful cases of new ailments. At that time, after constantly seeing the distressed condition of the many who visited Gurudev, I had only one desire left and that was for sadhana [spiritual practice].

Why should I be harassed by sensual craving when I was so vividly aware of its consequences? As I meditated in my hut at Suki, the red aura would appear. I would feel at peace, but not for long. A new occurrence soon filled me with a sense of shame. I should not even talk about it here. If I were to tell anyone about it, he would immediately brand me as indiscreet. If I told it to ordinary worldly people, they would say: "The sannyasi monks of today are quite dissolute and fatten themselves on charity. Doesn't it show that the life of a householder is much superior, since he can pursue his spiritual goal while still enjoying every pleasure?"

I am now going to tell my shameful story. My dear mothers! My dear sisters! You are all different forms of shakti. Please do not feel offended by my hateful account. Bless me, paying attention to its real purport. My dear readers! My dear seekers! Try to understand the purpose behind this description.

As I sat in meditation, the red aura appeared immediately.

I felt intoxicated, swaying, jumping, and frolicking around. I worshiped the guru. While I was engaged in meditation on the guru, within and without, chanting "Guru Om, Guru Om," and plunging into blissful *gurubhava,* my mind became filled with lustful thoughts. What shame! How disgusting! I still beheld the same red aura, though with a slightly different shading. It was of my size, glowing like the tender red morning aura in the east. As my mind was invaded by sensuality, I lost the ecstasy of love and also the Nityananda-*bhava.* I could not continue with the sublime guru worship either. Even the Guru Om mantra vanished and was replaced by a strong sexual desire. I was amazed. What secret lair did it emerge from? From where could so much life flow into my male organ, which was hitherto a mere lump of flesh? An acute lustful craving tortured me. Alas! Alas! This was worse than the scenes of dissolution on the first day. My sexual sense was pulled toward external activity.

I could think of nothing but sex. The only saving grace was that my meditative posture was not disturbed; my legs remained firmly interlocked. My whole body felt the stirring of lust. It is difficult to describe the agony of my organ. I tried to reason it out with my mind but could not succeed. As I closed my eyes I saw a ravishing naked maiden within the red aura. I tried not to see her, but seeing her was all I could do. I was full of fear and remorse. I opened my eyes and there she was —stripped of all her clothes. I could not avoid her whether my eyes were open or closed. What should I do now? To whom could I talk about such a disgraceful condition? I was greatly troubled, as this was being forced on me against my will. How powerful the craving of the organ! Only [guru] Bhagawan Nityananda or a seeker who has experienced this could understand what was happening.

My mind would be overcome with acute self-loathing when I recollected my sexual excitement and I could not meditate any longer. Feelings of fear, shame, and discontent afflicted me, affecting even my brain. "My present miserable condition must be the result of some grave sin in the past." Brooding in this vein, I was invaded by anxiety which mounted relentlessly.

I went outside and sat in the swing, still occupied with thoughts of disgust: "What is this new weakness in me? What has gone wrong? Alas! What shall I do now?" At noon I meditated again. The same nude female! Sometimes she laughed, sometimes smiled. At times she sat down, at times stood up. I was soon fed up with this sight. The other visions which had calmed and purified my senses, releasing the flow of love in my heart and imparting celestial delight, had vanished, being replaced by their exact opposite. My sexual organ became energized, excited, and restless. Other shameful things would follow, so I would get up immediately.

This condition was repeated during the evening meditation. I began to meditate. The red aura . . . mind delighted . . . heart gladdened . . . guru worship with faith and reverence . . . intensified gurubhava . . . bhava-samadhi. Then suddenly the scene changed. The same naked nymph was chasing me! She danced in front of me, a short distance away. She made peculiar gestures with her body and frisked around. When I opened my eyes she was still there. I was losing control of my senses. I was afraid that something regrettable would occur. I decided that I must reduce my physical vigor, so I stopped taking milk. Instead I drank a little water. I was unable to sleep until late at night because of self-loathing. Thinking of Ganeshpuri, I remembered Bhagawan Nityananda. I bowed to him and fell asleep.

I awoke early in the morning. Sometimes I would take a bath at 3 A.M. or simply wash my hands and feet. Then I would smear my body with the sacred ash, charged with mantras. I sat down to meditate. Immediately my meditation became dynamic. The red aura of my own size arose at once. I worshiped the guru. In a short while, as I went into bhava-samadhi, the same sexual desire became active. The naked woman pursued me, finally standing in front of me. She began to torture me excruciatingly with only one apparent objective: she wanted no other sacrifice save my sacred vow of celibacy.

Every man is pursued by some woman and every woman is pursued by some man. Such a woman is always after her husband, constantly harassing him with some demand or other. One pesters her man for food, another kicks up a row for clothes. One clamors for jewelry, another will have nothing to do with her husband's relatives. One attempts to keep her man away from friends and saints, another takes the life out of him, breaking his heart with bitter remarks. She complains, "I have fallen on evil days since I married you. My parents treated me with such love and care. I bathed in milk and drank honey. Each day I soared in the empyrean blue. You are a wretched fellow ruining my life. I have been utterly miserable ever since my first thought of you." With such acidic words, she drives her husband out of his wits. Such a one lacks true femininity.

I did not know from where that incredible woman appeared. This blessed siren would turn up even though I did not invite her or extend any courtesy to her. She did not make any overt demand. She only blasted my meditation, exciting my sexual organ. She tried her utmost to blow my vow of chastity to smithereens. What a trial! It was the most distressful phase of my life. I had never been tormented like this before. After a while, my meditation could not continue. I came out and sat on my cot. I brooded on the question: "What shall I do? How can I tide over this crisis?" I became more distressed, anxious, and deranged as time went by. I used to sit with a sad heart, afraid of women. I lost patience. I was afraid that I might indulge in licentious behavior. I remembered again and again the past seekers who had fallen from yoga, spirituality, and virtue. I cried as I remembered the stories of Ajamila, Surdas, and Tulsidas. I remembered one old story about the behavior of the sage Parashar in his boat. Recollecting numerous such incidents, I felt greatly troubled. I was afraid of the force of sexual passion. I thought I had made my organ lifeless and inert through mastery of the siddhasana. But it had sprung to life again. I was utterly astounded.

During the afternoon session of meditation, I again felt excitement in the sexual organ. I asked my landlord, whose wife cooked for me, to have my food cooked not by a woman but by a man. I subsisted on a small quantity of rice and gave up vegetables. Leaving my stomach half empty, I drank some water.

One day I came out of meditation thinking: "How can I escape this torture? Who shall guide me? When my organ, rendered inactive by the siddhasana, can become active again, what grace can save me?" While reflecting in this manner, I felt more desolate, concerned, and dissatisfied. The evening fell. There was a siddha called Hari Giri Baba staying at Baijapur, twenty miles away. He was very dear to me. I remembered him intensely. He must save me, otherwise tomorrow could prove fatal. I could not take anyone else into confidence about my secret misery. I wept bitterly; so much so that my head split and my ears deafened. Night came. I did not take any food. Babu turned up in a short while. He muttered something which I did not hear. I said to myself: "O my mind, do not get flustered."

I commenced my nightly session of meditation, keeping to my schedule. I meditated nobly. The red aura arose, which should signify good fortune for a yogi. As I looked at it, I was confronted by tiny refulgent saffron sparks. Then I performed the sublime guru worship. I was absorbed in guru-bhava. While numerous mudras took place and different feelings emerged, I began to hear an indistinct sound inwardly. I was overjoyed. But lo! The same female stood in front of me, unclad except for ornaments. The moment I saw her I opened my eyes, but she was still there.

Again my joy disappeared and the meditative posture was upset. I got up slowly and came out. I sat listlessly under the mango tree until midnight. Then I went to bed, but I could not find my usual peaceful sleep. I became quite crazy and confused. Sleepless, I tossed on my bed, right and left, until 3 A.M. I closed my eyes for a while, but finally got up and took a bath. I sat to meditate. I did not feel at all well. I was not physically sick, but I was disturbed and crazed. I bowed to all directions, mentally invoked all deities and began to meditate. At once I plunged into meditation, passing into tandra. The red aura began to shine brilliantly within and without. My body executed movements. For a moment my throat was blocked. The jalandhar and mula bandhas occurred, but soon unlocked. I heard a vague strain within. As my attention focused on it, I floated in bliss. An egg-shaped white light flashed. This new vision renewed my zest for worship and meditation on the guru. I attributed this to my invocation of all the gods and goddesses.

But the scene changed rapidly. The red aura turned another shade. What, again! The same damsel. I was taken aback. This time she was richly adorned, captivating me with her beauty. My mind shattered. My sexual organ reacted violently. If I opened my eyes, I saw her without. If I closed them, I saw her within. My loincloth was rent and the tip of my organ forcibly pressed up against my navel, digging into my navel pit. Who was driving me so forcefully? I was, however, fully conscious. Then I came out of meditation. I used to wear only a muslin loincloth for meditation. I was furious that it had been torn, so much so that I could not think clearly. It was 5 A.M. I got up and put on another loincloth. I came out of the hut. I considered going to a place where I was unknown. My mind was utterly confused. I was either going to become insane or act in a deplorable manner. Thinking thus, I sat outside. I was terribly worried about my passionate reaction.

Morning came. I sat calmly in the swing, brooding: "Where shall I go? My present condition is not at all good. It indicates neither success in sadhana nor the grace of God. This must be the evil fruit of some past sin." While occupied with such thoughts, I slipped into the tandra state. I went inside and began to meditate again. In a moment, I was absorbed in it. I began to roar like a lion. My tongue stuck out completely. I kept roaring for half an hour. I became more and more frightened. After three quarters of an hour, I came out of meditation. This time I was not clutched by the sexual urge. However, having escaped one enemy, I was gripped by another. It seemed as though I had only jumped from the frying pan into the fire, as the saying goes. My identification with a lion aggravated my self-disgust. I decided to quit that place. I will add here that all these emotional states were in fact the lofty workings of the grace of a siddha, the ennobling processes of siddha yoga. But being ignorant, I felt confusion instead of joy.

In a short while, I saw a tonga approaching the orchard. The driver was sitting in front, but I could not see who was sitting in the back. The tonga drove right up to the mango tree and someone stepped out. I recognized him. What a blessing! It was Hari Giri Baba, the great siddha yogi and unique avadhoot. He started calling me right from there: "O King! O Emperor! O Swami! Get up." Having uttered these words, he began to laugh heartily. I was beside myself with joy and got up from the swing. He was an omniscient saint, always laughing. He used to wander on the river bank, wearing expensive shoes, a number of coats, one over another, and a silk turban. Whenever he felt hungry, he would ask anyone for food, saying: "Give. Give me something to eat," and then ate. At once he would wash his hands and start off again on his jaunt. He was a saint of devilish disposition. He would collect tiny round pebbles from the river, look at one, then at another and mumble: "Yes . . . yes, coral, you are worth two million." He would talk like this, roaming around by himself. He walked at a flying pace. He would go to the river bank at 2 A.M. and return after dawn. If questioned about it, he would mutter an incomprehensible reply.

Hari Giri Baba came forward. I bowed to him. We loved each other greatly. I said, "Baba! I am in a sorry condition. I am feeling terrible."

He said, "I know what the matter is. I will explain it only if you give me two rupees." I was familiar with his jocular manner. Whenever he came, if asked about anything, he would demand money. I gave him the two rupees. Hari Giri Baba spoke again, "O Emperor! You are in a wonderful state. You are going to see much better times. You will become divine. You are suffering from a beneficial fever. Becoming infected with your fever, many people will overcome disease and sorrow. You will influence a large number of people." Having uttered these words, he walked away. I accompanied him a short distance, but on the way he said, "Go, go away. If one does not go, how can one return? Do not be afraid." Then he moved away. The neighbors began to run after him exclaiming "Hari Giri Baba has come."

I returned and sat in the swing. Once again my mind was in disarray, recollecting the sexual excitement of the morning and also the identification with a lion. I became more and more bewildered, since it is the nature of the mind to become like that on which it dwells intensely. It merges with its object of constant thought, assuming its qualities. I would quote a favorite stanza of mine:

The mind, always occupied with women, acquires their character,
The mind, constantly excited with anger, burns in its fire,
The mind, ever dwelling on maya, sinks in her bottomless pit,
But, Sunder says, the mind, continually resting in the Absolute, eventually becomes It.

These words of the poet-saint Sunderdas, who was established in Truth, are entirely true.

My mind was utterly befogged by those two disturbances. I said to myself, "I have been living at Yeola for a long time, commanding great respect. I am a self-respecting person. Why should I dishonor myself by letting them suspect my present predicament? I shall retire into a remote forest where nobody will recognize me." I resolved to leave at once. I got up and embraced the photograph whereby I worshiped my beloved Gurudev, saying, "Forgive me, but what can I do? I am helpless. You are a liberal giver, but I am unfortunate." I bowed to him repeatedly, and then put the frame down. I looked at the hut and said: "My dear hut, I don't know when I shall see you again. I spent a long period happily inside you. I bow to you." I touched the swing tenderly and also knelt to it. I hugged the mango trees, who were my dear friends, and said, "I spent many happy days in your shade. I have no alternative now, since I am utterly wretched. I must leave you."

I went inside the hut again. I took off my saffron clothes, tied them up in a bundle and left it to hang on a tree because I did not want to dishonor the garb of a sannyasi. Afterward I wore white clothes for a long time. I left the door of the hut open. I was wearing only a loincloth and a shawl over my shoulders. I picked up my water bowl and secretly set off eastward. I covered some distance and paused at a point from where I could still see the hut. I bowed again. My mind was full of intense grief and bitter remorse. I began to walk toward the Sahyadri range. I pushed on, walking between hills. I was determined to go far away and I would not have cared had my body collapsed on the way.

I continued my journey. From Daulatabad I reached Nagad via holy Ghrishneshwar. I stood on a Sahyadri peak and looked northward. From there I could espy a large orchard of oranges and sweet limes. There were also many mango orchards and sugar-cane fields of various sizes. Hunger was gnawing at me. I finally ended up in an orchard whose owner turned out to be quite wealthy. He was a practitioner of yoga, having great love for saints and sadhus. He was called Dagadu Singh. He approached and inquired after me. Then he took me with him and affectionately had khichari cooked for me.

As I looked around, I caught sight of a small hut intended for sadhana, where a certain yogi had practiced yoga previously. Dagadu Singh made arrangements for me to stay there. As I sat inside the hut, my legs locked themselves in the lotus posture and meditation began. The beloved red aura appeared before me. A voice called from within, saying: "Open that cupboard over there and read the book inside." At first I did not pay much attention to it. But when the voice spoke a second and then a third time, my meditation was disturbed. I opened my eyes and saw an old cupboard. I opened it, found the book and took it out. It opened automatically at the page that dealt with the process occurring in me. I read it and felt completely relieved. All my distress evaporated in a moment. I was no longer confused or worried. I realized that whatever had happened was a result of my Gurudev, Bhagawan Nityananda's bountiful grace. It marked a definite stage of the spiritual journey in siddha yoga. With my doubts at rest, I ate the khichari contentedly. Later I glided into a sound slumber.

I practiced meditation at Nagad for some time. Now I understood that the process which involved sexual excitement was, in fact, turning the flow of seminal fluid upward. One gains the power of shaktipat only after becoming an *urdhvareta.* The process was taking place in order to annihilate the sexual urge once and for all. As swadhisthan chakra is pierced, sexual impulses are aroused. But this happens in order to make an aspirant an urdhvareta, to expel sexual lust from his system forever.

When I realized that the sexual excitement was a great and significant event, I was delighted. How could I describe it? The previous joy flooded my being again. The vision of the naked woman had brought me so much distress because of my own ignorance, my erroneous notions. She was, as a matter of fact, the great Goddess Kundalini. I begged forgiveness of the Mother and recited a hymn to her. After that, I began to meditate even more deeply.

The next day, Mother Kundalini stood in the red aura again. But now I could perceive her celestial loveliness. She was the divine power of grace, ravishingly beautiful. As I saw her, I congratulated myself on my good fortune and bowed down to her. As I knelt down, the divine goddess merged in the red aura. From then on the divine shakti became my guru. She had looked naked to me because I myself was naked, lacking in true knowledge. My lustful reaction was because of my inability to see her as the great shakti kundalini. I had regarded her as an ordinary woman of this world. My suffering had resulted from my own ignorance. But now it was all over.

I went to see another saint I knew, Zipruanna, who was a great siddha. Though he remained naked and roamed through the village of Nasirabad, he was revered as a great soul by everyone, addressed as "Anna" by old and young alike. He preferred to stay in uninhabited corners, dilapidated houses or huts, far from the rural folk. He had attained a very high state in yoga. He was farsighted, being able to see into the distant past and future. His body had been so completely purified by the yogic fire that even when he sat on a heap of garbage he remained untainted. I was greatly surprised to see that he had raised even his body to such a high level. Just as the inner self of a yogi is never sullied by impurities, even so, Zipruanna's physical form could not be contaminated. The first time I went for his darshan he was relieving himself in a corner. As I approached him, he began to smear his body with his own feces! I sat near him. His body, amazingly enough, was emitting fragrance instead of foul stench. When I revisited him, I found him sitting on a pile of refuse without being polluted by it. I did not have the courage to go close, so I kept standing at a distance. In a short while he came down from the heap. I washed his feet. His limbs were exuding an aroma resembling that of ashtagandha (a fragrant herb). Zipruanna loved me greatly. To this day, I have not ceased marveling at the extraordinary state of this great saint. Once I asked him, "Anna! Why must you sit on such rubbish?" He replied, "Muktananda, inner impurities are far more revolting than this. Don't you know that the human body is a chest full of waste matter?" This silenced me. Zipruanna was a supreme avadhoot, the most precious of saintly jewels.

I went to see him then. He received me lovingly and sat down with his body pressed against mine. I told him about my experiences in the Suki hut. He said, "That is the grace, initiation, benevolence or shaktipat of a great saint. Such experiences are possible only because of sublime benediction. One envisions the great conflagration, ghosts, demons, demigods, cobras, kinnaras, and the spectral companions of Parashiva. This is exactly what you have seen." When I asked him about my sexual agony, he answered, "The sex organ's erection and its subsequent digging into the navel happens only in the case of a rare aspirant. This is due to the extraordinary divine grace of yoga. Do not underrate the phallus, which generates all and determines one's sex. Its absence makes one a pathetic eunuch. This highly worthy generative organ of man should be restrained and disciplined as much as possible. If, on touching the navel, it stays in that position for a while, the entire seminal fluid accumulated in the testicles starts flowing upward toward the heart. Then it gets purified by the gastric fire and moves on into the brain, strengthening all the sensory nerves and greatly enhancing a yogi's powers of memory and intelligence." Then he added, "O Swami! Such a one is called an urdhvareta. In the future, on the strength of this, you will achieve guruhood and bestow grace. As a result of this vajroli process which you have undergone, you will acquire the inner power of shaktipat. The great kundalini shakti has entirely uprooted your previous sexual appetite by means of the sexual torture which you had to endure. In the future, not the sexual urge, but pure love, will inundate your heart. The rays of your love will enkindle love in innumerable hearts."

I then referred to the naked female who appeared in my meditations, saying, "I always sat down for meditation after putting on Shiva's armor and sealing off different directions. How, then, could that naked woman make her appearance?" As I put this question, Baba Zipruanna brightened up and spoke in a serious tone. "O Swami! Who can penetrate your inner being, the radiant city of meditation? That is the refulgent land of Mother Chitshakti. None except Chiti, the chiti-endowed deity and the guru can ever gain admittance there. Your own idea of femininity was responsible for your confusion. What's the difference between a naked and a clad woman? The Mother assumes all forms. When you saw that nymph, you should have looked upon her as Goddess Chitshakti. Nobody else can enter there. The fruits that you reap correspond to your own attitude. From now on look upon whatever you see, whether good or bad, as different forms of Chiti. When you consider the naked maiden who arises from the inner heart to be the supreme goddess, her form becomes divine. Countless are the marvels of Chitshakti. She travels at an enormous speed. You must have seen how rapidly the red particles, subtler than the subtle, move within. You will see the infinite worlds existing in her. This Chitshakti, who assumes innumerable forms in a moment and reveals many in One, is the supreme maya, Mother Yoga Kundalini. O Swami! Whatever happened was for your good. Whatever happens in the future will also be for your good. Always remain aware of the true nature of kundalini.

"Another thing. The yogi on the siddha path should always remember that whatever he sees from time to time in the light of the inner heart, whatever emanates from Chiti, whether high or low, noble or ignoble, acceptable or rejectable, worthy or unworthy, beneficial or harmful, is nothing but Chiti in her fullness. None but Chiti can ever have a place there. The numerous visions and movements occurring there are entirely the Goddess Chiti, regardless of what you may take them to be."

Having listened to such sublime wisdom, I fell at the feet of "Zipreshwar," Lord Zipru. What wisdom! How true! What an authentic description of reality! "O my dear Baba!" exclaiming thus, I embraced him. He seated me on his lap. He licked my head, passed his hand over it and said, "Your glory will reach the highest heavens." Those days I used to suffer from acute headaches. From that day on that ailment vanished. Thus Zipruanna resolved all my problems. I had profound reverence and great faith in him. I loved him like my guru. It was he, in fact, who had sent me to Bhagawan Nityananda, saying, "You are going to reach the highest summit under his guidance. Your future with him is bright."

My dear students of siddha yoga! Listen carefully. Once you have been blessed by the guru's grace, you should discard all fears. Do, however, remember that in siddha yoga you must fully carry out the guru's orders. You should understand this essential truth: the guru's word alone matters. Fully bear in mind Anna's statement: "How can a full-grown woman enter the tiny cavity of the inner heart?" Can an ordinary woman pierce your armor, forged by mantra and tantra? You will be able to see everything in the red aura arising from Chiti Kundalini. Can you ever have such a vision without her wish? Think it over. Remember that the cavity of the heart is minute. None other than kundalini can penetrate it. Therefore, whatever happens within you, the visions you see and the movements you undergo, accept them all as the divine shakti's precious gifts and offer them all to her. Know that whatever happens is for your own progress. The forms Chiti assumes, the movements she motivates, the shapes or colors or states she reveals–bow inwardly to each, considering them her manifestations. This attitude will fill you with peace at once. If you look upon it otherwise, you will suffer remorse as Muktananda did.

After returning from my visit to Zipruanna, I began to practice sadhana with full faith, in my beloved hut at Nagad. The duration of my meditation increased automatically. I acquired various books since I did not feel satisfied unless I knew more about meditative states. I studied the *Mahayoga Vijnana,* containing experiences which are helpful for a meditator to know. I sent for other similar works such as *Yoga-vani* and *Shaktipat,* and studied them closely. In fact, maha yoga holds a special place in the Shaivite philosophy. Such works as *Shivasutras, Pratyabbijnahrdayam, Tantraloka,* and *Shiva Drishti* are written by experienced sages on the themes of shaktipat, the grace of a siddha and the dynamic play of Mother Kundalini. My stay at Nagad was solitary and fascinating.

SHAKTIPAT

Paul Zweig

I think of Walt Whitman sitting under an apple tree on Long Island at the age of thirty-six, drunk with the odor of crushed grass. I think of William Blake conversing with angels, and Jacob Boehme cobbling God's shoes. I think of Plato's *Symposium,* describing the ladder of universal love as an ascending current of knowledge mingled with delight. In that conversation between drunken friends, the wisdom of East and West mingle playfully, preparing future marriages.

I think of my own experience not long ago, sitting in a strangely decorated room, the air perfumed with incense. At one end is a seat draped with richly colored cloths. On the walls hang several greatly enlarged photographs of a dark-skinned man in a loin cloth, his body oddly smooth and glowing, his face expressing a combination of sleepiness and alert attention.

A few days before I had received a phone call from a friend I hadn't seen in quite some time.

"I've been in India for three and a half years, living in an ashram," she announced, "and now I'm in New York for a while with my guru. Why don't we get together?"

This was astounding news. Apparently my friend's life had taken some unexpected turns since I last saw her. I was embarrassed to admit I didn't know what an ashram was. My friend had gone to India to "shop around for a guru," she explained jokingly, and after some looking had found one. I didn't exactly know what a guru was either. Gurus had something to do with the wisdom of the East, I remembered ironically. They were some sort of wise men you went to when you had a question. I concluded I would rather ask my friends, or read a book.

Nonetheless, I was here to check out Odile's guru. We'd had coffee together the day before, and she'd talked about her life in India. She had always been a tough-minded person, and that hadn't changed. If anything she seemed tougher now, almost ominously solid. Whatever she'd been up to, it had somehow accentuated her personality, so that there seemed to be a kind of overflow in her movements.

She spoke slowly, pausing for a long time between words. I had the impression she had never talked about these things before, and that stuck in my mind more than anything she said. What sort of experience, I wondered, could a strong-minded, intelligent woman have been engrossed in for three and a half years, without ever having tried to explain it, even to herself? A few other things stuck in my mind. Her guru, Swami Muktananda, wasn't simply a guru, he was a satguru, the highest level of guru; so high, he had nothing in common with the pleasant-faced Indian gentlemen in white clothing one met presiding over yoga centers throughout America. A satguru was something else entirely. Not simply a teacher, but a "perfectly realized human being." I heard that expression in quotation marks, because it didn't seem to me it could be used in any other way. "Once upon a time there was a perfectly realized human being . . ." What do we mean when we use such an expression, I would ask my students? What in our psyches responds to mythic notions of this sort? After all, myths aren't merely a form of entertainment. They don't simply lie. Though, of course, I would add privately, they don't simply tell the truth either. But Odile wasn't talking in quotation marks.

"He's quite an unusual man," she said, smiling thoughtfully. "In India they call him a saint, but in a way, I think of him more as a warrior."

Muktananda's temporary ashram in New York was a lovely red brick school house near Riverside Park, where I was told, he took long walks every day before dawn. Consistent with his aura of sainthood, he had never been mugged. In fact, the idea was vaguely humorous. Later I would have dreams of violent young men running up in the darkness to throw themselves at his feet. He would bend over and thump them on the back, or walk by, playfully raising his eyebrows.

I had been ushered into a medium-sized room with large windows, where a number of people were already waiting. The curls of burning incense, the colorful chair, the exotic paraphernalia; people sitting expertly in the lotus posture, or leaning against a wall, or gathering their legs about them as best they could: the atmosphere was low key, yet vaguely expectant. An air of dormant obsession pervaded the room, making me feel as if I ought to pay attention, though I had no idea to what.

I didn't see the door open. He was simply there, quite suddenly. He walked across the room and sat down with a series of quick, fluid movements. Odile had warned me that he wouldn't seem very holy, and she was right. He wore an orange ski cap, dark glasses, and a gaudy robe that looked as if someone had raided a costume store. On the whole he bore a slight resemblance to a jazz musician, except that his face had a kind of feathery alertness, as he settled onto his chair, checked a clock, tapped a microphone to see if it worked, looked for a pile of orange cards on a side table, and sprinkled perfume on a wand of sumptuous peacock feathers. He seemed to be in perpetual motion, occasionally darting glances around the room at one person or another.

I had been startled when several people had touched their foreheads to the ground when he entered the room, but I didn't really pay much attention, mainly because I didn't feel concerned. I wasn't even there out of curiosity, I reminded myself, but simply as a gesture of friendship to Odile. I noticed that the man in the enlarged photographs on the wall was not Muktananda, and asked Odile about it. She said the photographs were of Muktananda's guru, Nityananda: a large-bodied, imposing figure, naked except for the loin cloth, and emanating a gruff, disturbing energy. He seemed quite different from the loudly dressed man moving around on his chair at the front of the room. There was a dark, almost demonic quality in the photograph, and a stillness which seemed to inhere in the figure itself.

Muktananda communicated through an interpreter, a lively young man dressed in orange robes, who sat cross-legged on the floor at his feet. The interpreter called the name of each visitor to come up and be introduced. Not much seemed to go into an introduction. You got to say your name and what you did, while Muktananda tilted his head graciously and smiled. His smile was crisp and restrained, yet benevolent in its way. However theatrical his clothes might be, Muktananda's face did not indulge in flourishes; on the contrary, even his wit had a quality of severity. My turn came early in the hour. I went up and, observing what appeared to be a practice, got on my knees while the introduction was made. Odile, to whom I had given copies of some books I had written, dumped them on the floor in front of Muktananda, who picked up the books and looked at them while the titles were translated. He asked if the word "emptiness" in one title, had anything to do with the Buddhist void. I answered that I had never thought about it. Did I want to ask him anything? That was the furthest thing from my mind. I said no, and the introduction was over.

More people were introduced. For the most part they were younger, and had been involved in the oriental scene in one way or another. Some had questions to ask about meditation, a few had been to India. The sorts of questions they asked rubbed me the wrong way: they seemed full of personal melodrama and inflated romantic excitement. "Sometimes I feel within me . . ." "I know in my heart . . ." "My inner awareness . . ." "My cosmic feelings . . ." I moved over to get a better look at Muktananda. For all his quickness and sudden changes of expression, there was a kind of distance in his face, an immobility not unlike the face in the photograph.

A young woman was speaking to him. She had lived for several years in Pondicherry Ashram. She gave Muktananda a drawing she had done, and in a high tremulous voice said she had a question to ask him. I found myself paying attention suddenly, not so much to what the woman said as to a feeling of vulnerability in her voice. When she meditated, the experience of silvery light was very intense, but then nightmarish forms came between her and the light, and she was frightened. Her voice became increasingly tenuous as she talked, and then it broke. I could tell she was crying. She had lifted up a hand, as if to describe the nightmares, and I saw that it was shaking. And suddenly I was shaking too. I felt as if I were rooted to the floor, trembling with intense feeling. I became aware that I had to make an effort not to cry, yet it wasn't simply crying, for my body had become buoyant and warm. I stared at the woman's hand sketching a movement in the air: it was pale, delicate. Even after the hand was tucked away in her lap, and Muktananda's voice had begun to speak an answer, I went on staring. My eyes seemed to be peering out of a deep, silvery tunnel, while the forms and colors of the room glided across their surface like paper cutouts.

The words, "afloat in tears," repeated themselves over and over in my mind. With no transition I seemed to be seeing my life from a new angle. An overwhelming idea had seized hold of me: all of us did our best against suffering and useless pain. Those nightmarish forms the woman had talked about were the element of my life, and everyone's life. All of us sitting in this room were on the point of crying out, for we existed far from the light. I had accomplished all sorts of things in my life. I had a position in the world; I wrote books; I was a discriminating person who cringed from the naive self-importance of these "kids." Yet nothing I had done meant a thing from the viewpoint of that light. I too was defenseless, full of longing; and we were equal, because we were human. Great clots seemed to be floating loose in my mind. Shapes so old they had come to seem part of the landscape were breaking up, and through the cracks in their ruin tears poured, like an imprisoned element suddenly set free.

As I stared at Muktananda's quick aimless movements, I was aware that my mouth was hanging open, but I couldn't seem to close it. For some reason I wasn't frightened; I was even pleased, though I couldn't say why. My jaws felt like great hinged gates into a cave full of tears. Muktananda had done this, but what had he done, and how? We hadn't talked much, and he had hardly looked at me. He was not especially charismatic: no great gestures or fixed, piercing glances. He moved around a lot, and played with his fingers. All the while I was holding back my tears by an effort of subtle attention. The tears seeped onto my face anyway, a few at a time.

Later in the hour I managed to stand up and indicate that I had a question after all. I marveled that my limbs still functioned as I made my way to the front of the room. The atmosphere was dreamlike and filmy, and I felt strangely dissolved in it.

"My question is the same one you asked me earlier. What *is* the connection between the experience of inner emptiness, the frightening feeling that at some level of my existence I'm nobody, that my identity has collapsed and, deep down, no one's there; what is the connection between this feeling, and the Buddhist void?"

"They are the same," he answered immediately, "but in the Buddhist void there is no fear."

Later on I thought about Muktananda's answer, although at the time I was too preoccupied with my emotional upheaval to think clearly at all. If anything, I felt vaguely disappointed, for what he said seemed like a non-answer. It was said offhandedly too, not as one ought to speak to someone whose life was breaking into warm, tearful pieces. I felt ever so faintly rebuffed, yet I was moved too. Until that very minute I had accepted mental pain as an ordinary part of life. I believed that my insufferable anxieties belonged to the fabric of existence; that in some way they were a good thing. This morning, sitting on a hard wood floor, looking at a dark-skinned Indian man with a large belly and an orange ski cap, a strange light had been driven into my gloom: the sickness can be cured, it has been cured. You are already free. I was experiencing the delirium of release.

It was very much like a delirium. My head had become increasingly large and feverish. My thoughts floated in a syrupy atmosphere to which the features of my face–lips, nose, eyes —gave an identity. Yet the thoughts, surging like sea creatures, were strong and sharp. They were not my thoughts at all, but residents of the heaviness in my mind. I was a fisherman, a swimmer. Words like happy or unhappy didn't mean anything: something was breaking open; something was bursting; something was spilling out.

Toward the end of the hour, a nervous redheaded man was introduced. He stood in front of Muktananda, and began talking in a voice full of forced arrogance:

"You people talk of bliss and liberation, but you ought to know that you're a tiny minority, a mere fraction. Most people don't see things your way. They suffer, and they hate. They work and they feel frustrated. That's reality. What would Anatole France say about you, I wonder?"

His body stiffened while he talked, and his shoulders hunched up defiantly. Every once in a while, he squeezed a laugh from his throat which resembled a cackle. He tried to get a cigarette to his mouth, but his hand was shaking too violently.

"What right do you have to announce that you're happy to people who are suffering? This is evil. Anyway, you can't prove it. How do I know you're not lying? You talk about love and compassion. You claim you're not afraid to die."

Baba cut in, "Just as you have the right to say you are unhappy and cling to your unhappiness, so I have the right to say I am happy. You love your unhappiness and I love my happiness."

He cackled again. Then, as if forcing himself to speak:

"Listen, I'm terrified of dying. What would you do if I pointed a gun at you right now, if I pulled a gun out of my pocket and pointed it at you?"

There was an undertone of violence in his voice that seemed almost crazy. Clearly the man was out of control, he might do anything, I thought. But Muktananda's interpreter did not seem at all nervous, although some visitors were getting ready to be scared, as I was. When the talk about the gun occurred, Muktananda answered:

"My love would still be coming toward you while you pulled the trigger."

I remember thinking: This is preposterous; no one can say such a thing and mean it. At the same time I was stunned by a thought which filled my mind as with a bright, vaporous whisper; yes, it's possible; such a response is possible. For an instant I glimpsed depths gaping under and around the frail island which I had confidently labeled human nature. I felt ignorant, a beginner crawling on a beach, an infant. Yet my ignorance was filled with happiness, because it seemed to me that something previously inconceivable was not only possible, but was happening before my eyes. It's odd, but I didn't ask myself if Muktananda was telling the truth at that moment. I was too overwhelmed by my discovery to even think of such a question.

The redheaded man seemed to collapse. He threw his head back and laughed, almost shyly. All at once he was hugging himself and turning his body from side to side like a little boy. Everyone was laughing gently, and the man seemed vulnerable, lonely. His fingers were caked with nicotine, and they still shook a little. With his talk of Anatole France, he reminded me of an uncle of mine: a nervous, frustrated intellectual. He reminded me of myself, or an aspect of myself: a frail, wiry individual who couldn't afford to be truly generous, who needed all his energy simply to stand still, at all costs, including inner paralysis, as if he were a rim around nothing, and had to expend quantities of passion simply to maintain the integrity of this rim.

Still rooted to the floor I shook ever so slightly and wept, staring at this awesome tableau which engraved itself on the surface of my attention. On one side, a nervous, vulnerable man emanating that self-intoxicating misery which I knew so well, because it had for years been my landmark in the desert, the sour liquid I gulped every day, on the theory that it was better to drink even foul water, than to die of thirst. Facing him, with an interested look, a brightly dressed black man sitting cross-legged, holding a wand of peacock feathers in one hand. Everything about him was intensely composed. He created a feeling of total presence which was so imposing that, without a word, I knew that he was the opposite figure of the tableau: impregnable, serene, existing on a plane of mental self-possession so remote, that words like pleasure, pain, longing and needing, could not be used to describe the activities of his mind.

Did I know this, or even think it at the time? Probably not. The trance of emotion which overwhelmed me during that meeting has, in retrospect, made the hour seem as whole and complete as life itself. I have often had the sense that everything I would ever need to know was contained in that hour, and needed only a certain amount of time to unfold its possibilities.

Muktananda glanced at a pop art clock on the table beside him. He said something in Hindi to his interpreter, and stood up, glancing around. The devotees bowed, and he walked briskly out of the room. His way of walking was unique, yet marvelous too. It would gradually become imprinted on my mind during the weeks that followed. He leaned backward a little and swung his arms in a long outward arc. This made his round soft stomach especially prominent. When I mentioned this to Odile one day, she smiled, and said that it wasn't really a pot belly, but a result of breath-retention. Most of the great Siddhas had round bellies. So did the Buddha.

After Muktananda left the room, we were invited downstairs and served lunch in what must have been an auditorium in the building's school days. I sat on the floor and thought the food into my mouth. When I wasn't thinking, my arms stopped, and a fullness heaved from some remote inner place, seeping out as tears. The people waiting for lunch chanted in a language I'd never heard before. Their chant was rhythmic and full-bodied, not at all like a church song or a religious hymn. It struck me that these people were having a good time. At the front of the room, a group played rhythmic accompaniment on a drum, a harmonium and a tall twangy instrument. Their music fed the mysterious intensity which came and went, making my body seem roomy and full. I had no idea what was happening to me, but for some reason I still wasn't afraid, or even curious. I was simply absorbed, as if I were singing or dancing with complete abandon. Yet I was sitting completely still, my face was expressionless. I might even have seemed sad to an observer.

I remember the afternoon in bits: trying to talk to people, but not able to say more than a few words before tears overwhelmed me; Muktananda's appearance a while later, wandering across the auditorium to his seat near the stage. I had become so absorbed in my experience it was a while before I noticed and hurried to sit near him, as did everyone else. Somehow he looked blacker, more solid. My eyes began to stare as they had that morning, tunneling deeply into themselves. I felt myself dissolving into the billows which broke warmly, silently in my mind. Everything was so vivid: Muktananda's wiry black beard and the moods flitting across his face; later, on my way home, the excruciating clarity of store windows, mounds of garbage, faces streaming toward me like separate pieces of a single awareness.

I remembered what a devotee had said to me during lunch: "It looks like you've got it."

What had I got, I asked.

"Shaktipat, a dose of Baba's shakti, his energy. That's what you're feeling now. Baba says that all of existence is a play of shakti, but that our personal shakti is dormant, as it is in external objects. Being intensely aware of objects is equivalent to awakening the shakti in them. That's what Baba does. He activates the dormant energy in us. It's like a lamp being used to light another lamp."

The explanation didn't really make any sense to me. Merely to follow it as an actual explanation of something that happened, like the law of gravity, required a wrenching of my mental habits which was quite beyond me. Nonetheless, I was dumbfounded. Apparently other people had had this experience often enough to give it a name: shaktipat. This thought alone was full of wonder for me. So I was not simply flipping out, according to some personal law, the end result of which was madness, however pleasureful. I was experiencing something real, something with a name.

At that moment, I glimpsed a mental trap I had lived in all my life. Despite being largely endowed with "inner resources" as the saying went, I had never fully accepted the reality of my feelings. An experience became real for me only when I shared it, giving it a name like tree, chair, or face. Without the name, it remained a little dubious, a little undependable. All my life I had read books, studied them, eventually written them, and the enveloping quality of my reading and writing had been a persistent anxious quest which no quantity of written words could satisfy, but which the acts of reading and writing themselves appeased while they were being performed: the quest for words capable of communicating to me the reality of my own feelings. Adam named the animals according to a technique which had, apparently, been lost to me, for his animals stayed named, while mine sank back again instantly, so that nothing was ever gained except the experience of naming itself which therefore could never be finished, and could also never be wholly satisfying.

All my life I had been convinced that my character had condemned me to a sort of inner impurity; that, for example, I could never keep a secret because, in my system of identity, secrets became empty and unreal when I refused to speak them. They became an actual menace to my integrity because when they dislocated in silence, I felt myself dislocating too. Secrets made me dizzy, and I did my best to avoid them, often by simple ignorance; I couldn't tell what I didn't know. The result was that I often knew nothing, especially about myself.

Even on that first day, walking home along Broadway in a state between dreamy relaxation and pure aerial energy, I sensed that my system had been overthrown, because what I was experiencing was simply irrefutable. This upheaval didn't need me to prove its reality. On the contrary, it was proving my reality, just as fear or erotic excitement are tremendous proofs of one's reality.

It occurred to me that I could keep this secret if I chose to.

The energy fusing from every part of my body sufficed to itself. It wasn't so much beyond words, as it was alongside of them, in some other realm. I liked that idea. In a confused way, it increased my feeling of self-respect. My secret sprayed itself through my body, and I reveled in the misunderstanding which made me seem different. My life was no longer subject to the universal law of suffering, or so it seemed. I had escaped by some miracle which I connected to a dark-skinned man in a ski cap, whose precise features, movements, and voice already seemed a little blurry; for that very moment, walking, filling the sidewalk with my presence, was so much more real than any place I could be coming from or going toward.

INSTANT COSMIC CONSCIOUSNESS?

D. R. Butler

Instant cosmic consciousness? Well, not really, but it seemed that way for most of the two hundred persons gathered for a week of camaraderie and intense yogic work at Watson Homestead near Corning, New York, for the 1973 ICSA* Yoga Convocation.

At that time my wife Pat and I, both in our mid-twenties, had studied yoga for five years. The convocation was an opportunity to devote an entire week to yogic disciplines and to associate with kindred souls.

The first two days were spent with ICSA director Margaret Coble who talked of the Divine Self within us all and told us that the primary goal for the week was to contact this inner self.

For the next three days Roy Eugene Davis, former student of Paramahansa Yogananda and head of the Center for Spiritual Awareness of Lakemont, Georgia, gave us intense instruction in raja yoga (meditation and mind control).

Then on Friday morning an unannounced guest arrived. He was Yogi Amrit Desai, a yoga teacher from Philadelphia of whom most of us had never heard. That afternoon, after summing up the various meditation techniques, Roy took a seat behind us on the floor and Yogi Desai went up front to speak or lead chants or do whatever was his "thing." We didn't know.

* International Center for Self-Analysis in North Syracuse, New York. *Editor.*

Clad in a flowing white robe and sitting on the table before us Amrit easily assumed the lotus posture, his body perfectly poised. He is a handsome East Indian in his late thirties with long black hair and intense dark eyes. He is younger than most yoga teachers but I soon learned he had unusual powers.

He led us into meditation, which is not unusual. Most yoga teachers begin with a meditation. Some chants in Sanskrit followed; still par for the course. I had my eyes closed and I felt pleasant currents of inner energy. Then, as Amrit led us deeper into meditation, I began to realize that something usual was happening to me.

The first thing I noticed was a wave of euphoria softly permeating my being. I felt intensely happy. I didn't know the reason for the wonderful feeling but I determined to relax and enjoy it.

Suddenly surges of energy—like electrical changes—streaked up my spine. These gradually evolved into a steady current of hot energy flowing from the tip of my spine to the top of my head. My impulse was to analyze intellectually what was happening but I quickly realized that the more I thought about it the less I felt it. So I stopped thinking and concentrated on *experiencing*.

Brilliant colors swirled inside my head; I thought I would burst with happiness. Nothing ever had felt so good! Suddenly a scream burst from someone in the back of the room, then another. In a few moments the place was a madhouse. People were crying hysterically, laughing uncontrollably, gasping for breath, even rolling on the floor. Apparently everyone was experiencing some manifestation of the same energy I was feeling.

I looked at Pat and saw tears rolling down her cheeks. When our eyes met, I knew we both were feeling the same. I closed my eyes and tried to resume meditation—or to experience as intensely as possible whatever was happening. I heard Roy Eugene Davis behind me reassuring various individuals, explaining that he had experienced similar feelings with Yogananda.

Suddenly the whole thing stopped as abruptly as it had

begun. The energy inside me subsided and the room quieted. Amrit began to explain what had happened.

We had just undergone what is known as a shaktipat initiation, he said. This is the awakening of the shakti or kundalini which in yoga is the primordial life force, the individualized expression of the Infinite which lies as dormant energy within each of us. The full awakening of shakti brings about cosmic consciousness; it is experienced physically as total bliss and serenity.

All forms of yoga and conciousness development aim at eventually awakening the kundalini force, but in shaktipat it happens immediately and spontaneously. The psychic energy is transferred directly from guru to disciple. Simply by being in Yogi Desai's presence we all had experienced to some degree the awakening of shakti.

How this comes about is somewhat mysterious. Yogi Desai explains that the astral body of the guru merges with that of the disciple; he also told us that the power came through him from his own master in India.†

I know that the person who is sufficiently developed to express himself on a certain energy level can cause a manifestation of that same level of energy in another. It might be called a manifestation of mind power–Yogi Desai *thought* and *knew* that the shakti in the group would be aroused and his concentration was so pure that it was.

Now that the room was quiet Yogi Desai explained that the ostensibly unpleasant manifestations some persons had experienced represented the cleansing of physical, emotional, and psychic impurities. Thus some had screamed and gone into hysterics when subconscious veils were lifted and they had experienced their true natures for the first time. Many persons later confirmed this, reporting that their experiences were ecstatic within, even if they had appeared to be suffering. Many also said that when it was all over they never had felt better in their lives.

Yogi Desai then announced that anyone who wished to

† Yogi Desai's guru is Swami Kripalvananda. *Editor.*

leave could do so. More than half of the gathering departed, many obviously shaken by what they could not understand. The rest of us stayed, wanting more.

When there remained only those who wanted to be with him Yogi Desai seemed to radiate even more intense energy than before. My body filled with a brilliant white light and I allowed myself to be absorbed in it. I felt that my life as I previously had known it literally came to an end. My ego identity became meaningless; there was no time; past and future did not exist. All that existed was pure light and pure bliss. I was content to remain in this state forever.

When I opened my eyes again I noticed that my body had bent forward; my forehead was touching the floor. I do not remember assuming that position. I was actually bowing down to Yogi Desai! I had never bowed to anyone in my life but some inner unknown force had prompted me—and I knew I wasn't bowing to Amrit Desai the person, but rather to my own higher self which he had helped me see.

He was surrounded by persons who only two hours before had never seen him but now sat on the floor around him, holding his feet, even kissing his feet, weeping unashamedly. Men and women of all ages and professions had found a part of themselves they never knew existed. I knew those people were feeling love and bliss and that Amrit himself was without ego. After a lifetime of practicing intense yogic disciplines he knew he was only a channel for transmitting the energy the others experienced.

At this point someone came into the room and announced it was time to eat. We all laughed uproariously, for food was the furthest thing from our minds. Who would consider leaving such newfound sublimity to put food in his belly? I was willing to leave my body forever if I only could retain that bliss.

Well, Amrit explained, there was more where that came from and we really should eat. My feeling of euphoria continued for several hours, however, and I knew I would never be quite the same again.

I wonder what would happen if those who turn to drugs

for glimpses of higher states of consciousness knew that the natural awakening of inner energies through yoga ultimately offers all they are seeking and much more. I wonder what would happen if all our political and religious leaders could spend only an hour or so with such advanced yogis as Amrit Desai. What changes would come over them and what wonders would they perform for the world?

A PSYCHIC HEALER EXPERIENCES KUNDALINI

John Scudder

My personal story begins on a night in April 1973, while I was teaching a class in esoteric healing. During the course of the evening, I began to feel ill. The first symptom was nausea similar to an upset stomach. When I returned to my home later that evening, the nausea became much worse.

I began to feel a sense of pressure in the crown chakra and the brow chakra—that is, the top of my head and my forehead. I spent a rather restless night and couldn't sleep. I was concerned about what was happening, wondered what disease it might be.

The following day, the pressure on my head increased still more, and after several days, with the pressure on the top of my head becoming progressively stronger, another phenomenon began to occur: a heat began to develop over my entire body. The heat did not come from any single location but, as I recall, my skin felt sunburned. There was no increase in surface temperature, however.

Shortly afterwards, I began to feel heat inside my body. It seemed to start with the blood. I could feel the flow through my veins as though my blood had turned into turpentine and was literally burning everything it touched.

Shortly after that, the organs in my body seemed to catch fire. I could actually feel each organ burning. During this period, the pressure on my head and brow became unbearable, as though I were walking around with a fifty-pound weight on both my head and brow. No matter whether I was lying down or walking, whatever I was engaged in doing, it was impossible for me to find any relief either from the burning sensation or from this tremendous pressure. The pressure inside my head then changed to a feeling of an energy flowing into my body.

As I recall now, this force very definitely came from my head, progressing down through my neck, chest, hips, and into my legs. There was nothing I could do to stop this force from flowing. It felt like I was standing under Niagara Falls, and it continued to increase until it became so frightening that it seemed as though my body would literally explode. I had this intense heat over my entire body—both inside and out—a tremendous pressure on the top and front of my head, and an energy force raging through my interior.

One Saturday night—it was actually two o'clock in the morning—I asked two of my friends to come to my home to observe the phenomenon because my heart had begun to beat so loudly that a person sitting alongside me could distinctly hear it. There was nothing they could do, of course, so after staying with me for more than an hour, they left. In church later that morning, it was announced that I had had a heart attack.

During this period, the best I could do for myself was to attempt to direct the force away from my heart. I was concerned that if it were made to withstand the full impact of this force, it would not be able to continue functioning. From the very outset, whenever I discussed my predicament with anyone who came to visit me, I would tell him that my life was hanging by a mere thread. The force, the pressure—it felt at any moment that I would breathe my last breath.

There were several other developments as the condition developed. I began to see and feel waves of force very clearly. It was like I was standing on shore, with the ocean's waves hitting me in my head. They just kept rolling in, rolling in, getting stronger all the while. As I recall now, when I first noticed the waves, they were purple in color. The color grew lighter, into a blue and then on up the spectrum until they were almost pure white. As the color changed, the force seemed to increase, until finally the whole experience seemed completely hopeless, as though, as I mentioned before, I was standing under Niagara Falls.

There was nothing that could be done for me medically, and there was nothing that could be done psychically. All I could do was hold on, waiting and hoping for an end to the terror. It was then that I thought of the *Book of Job:* "Though he slay me, yet will I trust him." I had no idea what kind of psychic attack I might be under. Two renowned psychics–very good friends of mine–came to visit. One was Olof Johnson, the author. Though he is an authority on occult matters, he thought I was just tired and overworked, that I was undergoing some sort of a nervous breakdown.

The other friend thought I was under a psychic attack, and she cleansed the house. But this did no good whatsoever. The force continued to grow, and the heat got even worse.

Another phenomenon which took place–it was sometime during the second week of the ordeal–was that my body became highly sensitive. If anyone was in the same room with me, I could feel his vibrations. If there were several persons in the room, I could feel each of their vibrations individually, and as they walked or moved about, I could easily sense the changes. One evening a healing group from my church came to help. There were six in the group, and they worked together as a healing circle. And I can remember very well still that despite all my troubles, I could feel each person's vibrations very distinctly. Later I remarked that I could evaluate each one's level and capability of healing.

My mind became so sensitive that I could actually sense the thoughts of anyone in the room with me. If there were more than one person, I could sense their individual thoughts. My third eye became so sensitive that even while sitting in my chair in the living room, I could see every room in my house as though the walls were made of glass. If my children were watching television downstairs or studying in their bedroom upstairs, I could see them without any difficulty at all.

The waves of energy also had another effect as the phenomenon continued. They became so strong it seemed as though I was being literally lifted out of my body; at least my consciousness seemed as though it were being lifted out and swept away. Try as I would, I could not resist.

One evening, while seated in the living room, I had a particularly unusual experience. The waves of energy were exceptionally strong and the color of gold, and I sat watching the energy flowing in. It grew stronger and stronger until it finally overpowered my will and I became dissolved into it. I lost consciousness.

The following day, while lying in my bed upstairs, I was told what apparently had happened. The healing group had been to see me again and after performing their work had left. Only my wife and our housekeeper were there in the room with me. I had gotten up from my chair and had walked into the kitchen and down into our family room—we live in a tri-level home, and one can go to the family room either through the kitchen or through the main entrance—and from there to my bedroom upstairs.

After nearly half an hour had elapsed, my wife came looking for me, since she had assumed that I had gone into the downstairs wash room and ought to have returned by then. She went through the kitchen and down the stairs into the family room and wash room, while our housekeeper took the other route, down the main hallway and on into the same family room. Not finding me anywhere, they stood wondering where I could possibly have gone. They had not heard the back door open, and had I gone out the front door, they would have seen me. Had I come back upstairs to go to my bedroom on the third level, I would have had to go through the kitchen or the main entrance in front, passing my wife and housekeeper before continuing up the stairs to the top floor.

To this day it remains a mystery to all of us how I managed to reach my bedroom without being seen. I can only remember sitting in my chair in the living room and then waking the following day in my bed. This was an eventful occasion for another reason: it was the first sleep I had had in nearly two weeks.

When my ordeal first began, I immediately did two things: first I stopped all work and remained home day and night, taking it very, very easy. Second, I had my wife buy a case of baby food, and every hour around the clock I would have a jar of it along with a piece of toast and a cup of coffee. I did not know what was happening to me, but both courses of action seemed to be necessary. Nobody could help or advise me. During this entire period of about three weeks—when my life seemed to be hanging on a string—I would not allow myself to become emotionally disturbed. I managed to remain completely calm all through the ordeal.

The description I've given thus far about the force, the pressure, and the heat, is wholly inadequate but the best I am able to give. It was beyond my comprehension. There is no way one can conceive of this force or the heat. There was no escape. It persisted twenty-four hours a day, whether I was lying down or walking, whether I was resting or active. It was like the ancient Chinese water torture in which the dropping water eventually drives a person out of his mind. The force, the heat, and the pressure—allowing absolutely no relief—had the same devastating effect.

One night I wrapped my head in a cold, wet turkish towel, but there was no let-up, no change whatsoever. All this while I had no idea what was happening to me. Although I had read many books on kundalini—the serpent power—they all described the phenomenon with the heat beginning at the base of the spine and moving up the back to the top of the head. This never happened to me. The heat began over my entire body and built in intensity. If there was any heat up and down my spine, it was insignificant when compared with the internal burning.

When it was finally over, after three weeks, there came a strange sensation over my entire body. It can best be described as "clean." Everybody has felt this clean feeling after taking a bath and putting on clean clothing; well, I had that same sensation, only much more so. But what was extraordinary was that the inside of my body as well as my skin felt this way—"clean." It was a very good feeling. And again, I had no idea what had happened to me.

Then one of my friends, a psychic and trance medium, asked her spirit guides what had happened to me. She was told that I had experienced an opening of the kundalini and that I should read a certain book published by the Theosophical Society. It was *Kundalini, An Occult Experience,* and I was to read page forty-five particularly. The book itself, however, does not do justice to the kundalini experience. Everything seems to be veiled, but it did refer to the "Kundalini Bath," and it explained that the word kundalini comes from the Sanskrit, meaning heat or burning.

Certain descriptions in the book did tally with my experiences almost completely, and I want to mention the phenomenon called the kundalini bath. Now, there were six of my friends who frequently came to visit, and afterwards, they reported that their hearts would begin to pound as if they were experiencing a heart attack. Two of them were so concerned that they had their physicians examine them. They had a feeling of nausea and dizziness to the point of fainting.

The reason that these disturbances were brought to my attention is that I had been active in healing for a number of years, and when my friends became ill in this way, they immediately called me to ask whether I could be of help to them. I had them write down their symptoms, and then I compared these with the symptoms of the kundalini bath as described in the book. They were identical. It was this that convinced me that I had experienced the opening of the kundalini.

However, from all the people who had told me that they had opened their kundalini and from all of the books I had read previously, I could only conclude that my experience was totally different. This, I think, was a very great injustice, because I was led to believe that the opening of the kundalini was a great and glorious occult experience. What I went through was absolute hell. If there is a hell, it could not be any worse than what I endured for three weeks. It never occurred to me, therefore, that my experience was even remotely associated with the opening of kundalini.

When I realized that it was the kundalini, I became very cautious, terminating all meditation and all healing activities. I would not meditate nor would I attempt any mystical practices while anyone was in my home.

Later, if everybody in my family was away, I would try a meditation, and gradually I learned that I could open my crown and brow chakras with some degree of safety. When some of my confidence returned, I also began my healing work again.

At this point the healing forces became much stronger. One evening I told my wife, who had become quite ill, that I would open the kundalini and give her a healing. I placed my hands on her feet, and within a few seconds she was unconscious. She regained consciousness in two or three minutes and reported that she felt greatly improved. Having a subject lose consciousness during a healing has become a common occurrence since my awakening.

I soon learned to open my kundalini at will–to a point–and then close it down again. But there have been occasions when, totally absorbed in my healing practices, I would forget the kundalini and it would get out of control. Then the same sensation–heat over my body and pressure on my head–would be felt. On these occasions, I again had to sit up all night, finding it impossible to sleep. However, the pain has never been as bad as it was during the initial three-week experience. Still, I am deeply concerned about what might lie ahead for me. Consequently, whenever I sense my crown chakra opening and the heat building up in my body, I immediately stop what I am doing and with all the will at my command close it down again.

During the summer–in July–my wife ordered a book through a friend who had recommended that I read it. It was *Kundalini, the Evolutionary Energy in Man,* by Gopi Krishna. I found it to be an absolutely exact description of the experience I had gone through. From that day on I have urged everyone who begins talking about the grand and glorious experience of the opening of the kundalini to purchase a copy of this book immediately and, regardless of anything else they have ever read on this subject, to read it through. It is the only literature that I know on kundalini that is absolutely true.

When I read that Gopi Krishna underwent the terrible ordeal on two occasions, the second time several years after the first, I began living under a dark cloud again. On several instances I have felt the kundalini beginning to open again in a manner similar to the initial experience, and I certainly don't want to go through that again. While it has helped tremendously in my healing and psychic work, I don't want to spend days and nights under the same torture as before. There's nothing pleasant about it. It's frightening, and there's nothing that can be done about it. There's no relief.

You may be interested in knowing that I have begun to experiment with opening and closing my kundalini to learn to what extent my will-power can bring the force under control. I've discovered a great deal through these experiments, and I believe I have developed the ability to open it to quite a degree and to close it at will. However, I can't say that I can open it to its fullest potential–the same as I had experienced that April–and close it down again. I'm approaching that point very gingerly, and it may be a number of years before I'll be able to say anything about this with any degree of authority or knowledge.

There are groups in this country that in their meditation purport to open the kundalini. I have talked to many of these people, and their concepts and ideas about kundalini and the experiences they have differ completely from the description Gopi Krishna writes about–and they are considerably different from anything that I have experienced.

In my lectures I often tell about Gopi Krishna's experience of seeing the earth floating in a sea of energy, an insignificant speck. Though I would describe it a little differently, I know the experience and it is a very elevating one. Though I have come through it alive, I definitely would not recommend that anyone fool with kundalini. It can be crippling and it can be deadly.

I may sound melodramatic, but if you have had the experience, you know that your life hangs by the thinnest strand of thread. It is as close to dying as a human can come and still survive. I strongly recommend that nobody attempt to open the kundalini, and I wish that more information could be given to persons interested in occult matters so that if they should have the experience, they will not be completely ignorant of what the real process is like.

THE SUDDEN AWAKENING OF KUNDALINI

Gopi Krishna

The sudden awakening of kundalini in one whose nervous system has reached the ripe stage of development as a result of favorable heredity, correct mode of living, and proper mental application, is often liable to create a most bewildering effect on the mind. The reason for it, though extremely simple, may not be easily acceptable to the present-day intellect, which treats the human mind as a finally sealed product, dependent, according to some, exclusively on the activity of the brain cells, beginning and ending with the body; according to others, on the responsiveness of the bone-shielded gray and white matter to the extremely subtle all-pervading cosmic mind or universal spirit; and according to still others, on the existence of an immortal individual soul in the body. Without entering into a discussion of the correctness of these hypotheses advanced to account for the existence of mind, it is sufficient for our purpose to say that according to the authorities on yoga, the activity of the brain and the nervous system, irrespective of whether it proceeds from an eternal self-existing spiritual source or from an embodied soul, depends on the existence in the body of a subtle life element known as prana, which pervades each cell of every tissue and fluid in the organism, much in the same way that electricity pervades each atom of a battery.

This vital element has a biological counterpart as thought has a biological complement in the brain, in the shape of an extremely fine biochemical essence of a highly delicate and volatile nature, extracted by the nerves from the surrounding organic mass. After extraction, this vital essence resides in the brain and the nervous system, and is capable of generating a subtle radiation impossible to isolate by laboratory analysis. It circulates in the organism as motor impulse and sensation, conducting all the organic functions of the body, permeated and worked by the superintelligent cosmic life energy, or prana, by which it is continuously affected, just as the sensitive chemical layer on a photographic plate is affected by light. The term prana, as used by authorities on yoga, signifies both the cosmic life energy and its subtle biological conductor in the body, the two being inseparable. At the very moment the body dies, the rare organic essence immediately undergoes chemical changes, ceasing to serve as a channel for the former in the previous capacity. Normally, the work of extraction of prana to feed the brain is done by a limited group of nerves, operating in a circumscribed area of the organism, with the result that the consciousness of an individual displays no variation in its nature or extent during the span of his life, exhibiting a constancy which is in sharp contrast to the continuously changing appearance of his body. With the awakening of kundalini, the arrangement suffers a radical alteration affecting the entire nervous system, as a result of which other and more extensive groups of nerves are stirred to activity, leading to the transmission of an enormously enhanced supply of a more concentrated form of pranic radiation into the brain drawn from a vastly increased area of the body. The far-reaching effects of this immensely augmented flow of a new form of vital current into the cephalic cavity through the spinal cord before the system becomes fully accustomed to it may be visualized by considering the effects of a sudden increase in the flow of blood to the brain such as faintness, complete insensibility, excitement, irritability, or, in extreme cases, delirium, paralysis, death.

The awakening may be gradual or sudden, varying in intensity and effect according to the development, constitution, and temperament of different individuals; but in most cases it results in a greater instability of the emotional nature and a greater liability to aberrant mental conditions in the subject, mainly owing to tainted heredity, faulty modes of conduct, or immoderation in any shape or form. Leaving out the extreme cases, which end in madness, this generalization applies to all the categories of men in whom kundalini is congenitally more or less active, comprising mystics, mediums, men of genius, and those of an exceptionally high intellectual or artistic development only a shade removed from genius. In the case of those in whom the awakening occurs all at once as the result of yoga or other spiritual practices, the sudden impact of powerful vital currents on the brain and other organs is often attended with grave risk and strange mental conditions, varying from moment to moment, exhibiting in the beginning the abnormal peculiarities of a medium, mystic, genius, and madman all rolled into one.

I had absolutely no knowledge of the technicalities of the science or the mode of operation of the great energy or of the spheres of its activity, as vast and as varied as humanity itself. I did not know that I had dug down to the very roots of my being and that my whole life was at stake. Like the vast majority of men interested in yoga I had no idea that a system designed to develop the latent possibilities and nobler qualities in man could be fraught with such danger at times as to destroy the sanity or crush life out of one by the sheer weight of entirely foreign and uncontrollable conditions of the mind.

On the third day of the awakening [in December 1937] I did not feel myself in a mood for meditation and passed the time in bed, not a little uneasy about the abnormal state of my mind and the exhausted condition of my body. The next day when I sat for meditation, after a practically sleepless night, I found to my consternation that I completely lacked the power to concentrate my attention on any point for even a brief interval and that a thin stream of the radiant essence, which had impinged on my brain with such vivifying and elevating effect on the first two occasions, was now pouring into it automatically with a sinister light that instead of uplifting had a most depressing influence on me.

The days that followed had all the appearance of a prolonged nightmare. It seemed as if I had abruptly precipitated myself from the steady rock of normality into a madly racing whirlpool of abnormal existence. The keen desire to sit and meditate, which had always been present during the preceding days, disappeared suddenly and was replaced by a feeling of horror of the supernatural. I wanted to fly from even the thought of it. At the same time I felt a sudden distaste for work and conversation, with the inevitable result that being left with nothing to keep myself engaged, time hung heavily on me, adding to the already distraught condition of my mind. The nights were even more terrible. I could not bear to have a light in my room after I had retired to bed. The moment my head touched the pillow a large tongue of flame sped across the spine into the interior of my head. It appeared as if the stream of living light continuously rushing through the spinal cord into the cranium gathered greater speed and volume during the hours of darkness. Whenever I closed my eyes I found myself looking into a weird circle of light, in which luminous currents swirled and eddied, moving rapidly from side to side. The spectacle was fascinating but awful, invested with a supernatural awe which sometimes chilled the very marrow in my bones.

Only a few days before it had been my habit, when in bed at night, to invite sleep by pursuing a pleasant chain of thoughts which often led me, without revealing the exact moment when it happened, from the waking state into the fantastic realm of dreams. Now everything was altered. I tossed restlessly from side to side without being able for hours to bring my agitated mind to the degree of composure needed to bring sleep. After extinguishing the lights, instead of seeing myself in darkness wafted gradually to a delicious state of rest preparatory to sleep, I found myself staring fearfully into a vast internal glow, disquieting and threatening at times, always in rapid motion as if the particles of an ethereal luminous stuff crossed and recrossed each other, resembling the ceaseless movement of wildly leaping lustrous clouds of spray rising from a waterfall which, lighted by the sun, rushes down foaming into a seething pool.

Sometimes it seemed as if a jet of molten copper, mounting up through the spine, dashed against my crown and fell in a scintillating shower of vast dimensions all around me. I gazed at it fascinated, with fear gripping my heart. Occasionally it resembled a fireworks display of great magnitude. As far as I could look inwardly with my mental eye, I saw only a brilliant shower or a glowing pool of light. I seemed to shrink in size when compared to the gigantic halo that surrounded me, stretching out on every side in undulating waves of copper color distinctly perceptible in the surrounding darkness, as if the optic center in the brain was now in direct contact with an extremely subtle, luminous substance in perpetual motion, flooding the brain and nervous system, without the intervention of the intermediary channels of the retina and the optic nerve.

I seemed to have touched accidentally the lever of an unknown mechanism, hidden in the extremely intricate and yet unexplored nervous structure in the body, releasing a hitherto held up torrent which, impinging upon the auditory and optic regions, created the sensation of roaring sounds and weirdly moving lights, introducing an entirely new and unexpected feature in the normal working of the mind that gave to all my thoughts and actions the semblance of unreality and abnormality. For a few days I thought I was suffering from hallucinations, hoping that my condition would become normal again after some time. But instead of disappearing or even diminishing as the days went by, the abnormality became more and more pronounced, assuming gradually the state of an obsession, which grew in intensity as the luminous appearances became wilder and more fantastic and the noises louder and more uncanny. The dreadful thought began to take hold of my mind that I was irretrievably heading toward a disaster from which I was powerless to save myself.

To one uninitiated in the esoteric science of kundalini, as I was at that time, all that transpired afterwards presented such an abnormal and unnatural appearance that I became extremely nervous about the outcome. I passed every minute of the time in a state of acute anxiety and tension, at a loss to know what had happened to me and why my system was functioning in such an entirely abnormal manner. I felt exhausted and spent. The day after the experience I suffered loss of appetite, and food tasted like ash in my mouth. My tongue was coated white, and there was a redness in the eyes never noticed before. My face wore a haggard and anxious expression, and there were acute disturbances in the digestive and excretory organs. I lost my regularity and found myself at the mercy of a newly released force about which I knew nothing, creating a tumultuous and agitated condition of the mind as the sweep of a tempest creates an agitation in the placid waters of a lake.

There was no remission in the current rising from the seat of kundalini. I could feel it leaping across the nerves in my back and even across those lining the front part of my body from the loins upward. But most alarming was the way in which my mind acted and behaved after the incident. I felt as if I were looking at the world from a higher elevation than that from which I saw it before. It is very difficult to express my mental condition accurately. All I can say is that it seemed as if my cognitive faculty had undergone a transformation and that I had, as it were, mentally expanded. What was more startling and terrifying was the fact that the point of consciousness in me was not as invariable nor its condition as stable as it had been before. It expanded and contracted, regulated in a mysterious way by the radiant current that was flowing up from the lowest plexus. This widening and narrowing were accompanied by a host of terrors for me. At times I felt slightly elated with a transient morbid sense of well-being and achievement, forgetting for the time being the abnormal state I was in, but soon after was made acutely conscious of my critical condition and again oppressed by a tormenting cloud of fear. The few brief intervals of mental elation were followed by fits of depression much more prolonged and so acute that I had to muster all my strength and will power to keep myself from succumbing completely to their influence. I sometimes gagged my mouth to keep from crying and fled from the solitude of my room to the crowded street to prevent myself from doing some desperate act.

For weeks I had no respite. Each morning heralded for me a new kind of terror, a fresh complication in the already disordered system, a deeper fit of melancholy or more irritable condition of the mind which I had to restrain to prevent it from completely overwhelming me by keeping myself alert, usually after a completely sleepless night; and after withstanding patiently the tortures of the day, I had to prepare myself for the even worse torment of the night. A man cheerfully overcomes insurmountable difficulties and bravely faces overwhelming odds when he is confident of his mental and physical condition. I completely lost confidence in my own mind and body and lived like a haunted, terror-stricken stranger in my own flesh, constantly reminded of my precarious state. My consciousness was in such a state of unceasing flux that I was never certain how it would behave within the next few minutes. It rose and fell like a wave, raising me one moment out of the clutches of fear to dash me again the next into the depths of despair. It seemed as if the stream of vitality rising into my brain through the backbone connected mysteriously with the region near the base of the spine was playing strange tricks with my imagination. Also I was unable to stop it or to resist its effect on my thoughts. Was I losing my mind? Were these the first indications of mental disorder? This thought constantly drove me to desperation. It was not so much the extremely weird nature of my mental condition as the fear of incipient madness or some grave disorder of the nervous system which filled me with growing dismay.

I lost all feeling of love for my wife and children. I had loved them fondly from the depths of my being. The fountain of love in me seemed to have dried up completely. It appeared as if a scorching blast had raced through every pore in my body, wiping out every trace of affection. I looked at my children again and again, trying to evoke the deep feeling with which I had regarded them previously, but in vain. My love for them seemed to be dead beyond recall. They appeared to me no better than strangers. To reawaken the emotion of love in my heart I fondled and caressed them, talked to them in endearing terms, but never succeeded in experiencing that spontaneity and warmth which are characteristic of true attachment. I knew they were my flesh and blood and was conscious of the duty I owed to them. My critical judgment was unimpaired, but love was dead. The recollection of my departed mother, whom I always remembered with deep affection, brought with it no wave of the deep emotion which I had invariably felt at the thought of her. I viewed this unnatural disappearance of a deep-rooted feeling with despondency, finding myself a different man altogether and my unhappiness increased at seeing myself robbed of that which gives life its greatest charm.

I studied my mental condition constantly with fear at my heart. When I compared my new conscious personality with what it had been before, I could definitely see a radical change. There had been an unmistakable extension. The vital energy which lighted the flame of being was pouring visibly inside my brain; this had not been the case before. The light, too, was impure and variable. The flame was not burning with a pure, imperceptible and steady luster as in normal consciousness. It grew brighter and fainter by turns. No doubt the illumination spread over a wider circle, but it was not as clear and transparent as before. It seemed as if I were looking at the world through a haze. When I glanced at the sky I failed to notice the lovely azure I used to see before. My eyesight had always been good and even now there was nothing obviously wrong with it. I could easily read the smallest type and clearly distinguish objects at a distance. Obviously my vision was unimpaired, but there was something wrong with the cognitive faculty. The recording instrument was still in good order, but something was amiss with the observer.

In the normal man, the flow of the stream of consciousness is so nicely regulated that he can notice no variation in it from boyhood to death. He knows himself as a conscious entity, a non-dimensional point of awareness located more particularly in the head with a faint extension covering the trunk and limbs. When he closes his eyes to study it attentively, he ends by observing a conscious presence, himself in fact, round the region of the head. As I could easily discern even in that condition of mental disquietude, this field of consciousness in me had vastly increased. It was akin to that which I had experienced in the vision, but divested of every trace of happiness which had characterized my first experience. On the contrary, it was gloomy and fear-ridden, depressed instead of cheerful, murky instead of clearly transparent. It seemed as if prolonged concentration had opened a yet partially developed center in the brain which depended for its fuel on the stream of energy constantly rushing upward from the reproductive region. The enlarged conscious field was the creation of this hitherto closed chamber, which was now functioning imperfectly, first because it had been forced open prematurely, and second because I was utterly ignorant of the way to adjust myself to the new development.

For weeks I wrestled with the mental gloom caused by my abnormal condition, growing more despondent each day. My face became extremely pale and my body thin and weak. I felt a distaste for food and found fear clutching my heart the moment I swallowed anything. Often I left the plate untouched. Very soon my whole intake of food amounted to a cup or two of milk and a few oranges. Beyond that I could eat nothing. I knew I could not survive for long on such an insufficient diet, but I could not help it. I was burning inside but had no means to assuage the fire. While my intake of food was drastically reduced, the daily expenditure of energy increased tremendously. My restlessness had assumed such a state that I could not sit quietly for even half an hour. When I did so, my attention was drawn irresistibly toward the strange behavior of my mind. Immediately the ever-present sense of fear was intensified, and my heart thumped violently. I had to divert my attention somehow to free myself from the horror of my condition.

In order to prevent my mind from dwelling again and again on itself, I took recourse to walking. On rising in the morning, as long as I possessed the strength to do so, I left immediately for a slow walk to counteract the effect of an oppressive sleepless night, when, forced to lie quiet in the darkness, I had no alternative but to be an awed spectator of the weird and fearsome display visible inside. On the way, I met scores of my acquaintances taking their morning constitutional, laughing and talking as they went. I could not share their enjoyment, and passed them in silence with merely a nod or gesture of salutation. I had no interest in any person or in any subject in the world. My own abnormality blotted out everything else from my mind. During the day I walked in my room or in the compound, diverting my attention from object to object without allowing it to rest on one particular thing for any length of time. I counted my steps or looked at the ceiling or at the wall, at the floor or at the surrounding objects one by one, at each for but a fleeting instant, thus with all the will power at my command preventing my brain from attaining a state of fixity at any time. I was fighting desperately against my own unruly mind.

But how long could my resistance last? How long could I save myself from madness creeping upon me? My starving body was becoming weaker and weaker; my legs tottered under me while I walked, and yet walk I had to if I was to rid myself of the clutching terror which gripped my heart as soon as I allowed my mind to brood upon itself. My memory became weaker and I faltered in my talk, while the anxious expression on my face deepened. At the blackest moments, my eyebrows drew together into an anxious frown, the thickly wrinkled forehead and a wild look in my gleaming eyes giving my countenance a maniacal expression. Several times during the day I glanced at myself in the looking-glass or felt my pulse, and to my horror found myself deteriorating more and more. I do not know what sustained my will so that even in a state of extreme terror I could maintain control over my actions and gestures. No one could even suspect what was happening to me inside. I knew that but a thin line now separated me from lunacy, and yet I gave no indication of my condition to anyone. I suffered unbearable torture in silence, weeping internally at the sad turn of events, blaming myself bitterly again and again for having delved into the supernatural without first acquiring a fuller knowledge of the subject and providing against the dangers and risks of the path.

Even at the times of greatest dejection, and even when almost at the breaking point, something inside prevented me from consulting a physician. There was no psychiatrist at Jammu in those days, and even if there had been one, I am sure I should not have gone to see him. It was well that I did not do so. The little knowledge of diseases that I possessed was enough to tell me that my abnormality was unique, that it was neither purely psychic nor purely physical, but the outcome of an alteration in the nervous activity of my body, which no therapist on earth could correctly diagnose or cure. On the other hand, a single mistake in treatment in that highly dangerous condition, when the whole system was in a state of complete disorder and not amenable to control, might have proved fatal. Mistakes were inevitable in view of the entirely obscure and unidentifiable nature of the disease.

A skilled physician bases his observations on the symptoms present in an ailment, relying for the success of his treatment on the uniformity of pathological conditions in the normal human body. Physiological processes follow a certain specific rhythm which the body tries to maintain under all ordinary circumstances. In my case, since the basic element responsible for the rhythm and the uniformity was at the moment itself in a state of turmoil, the anarchy prevailing not only in the system but also in the sphere of thought, nay in the innermost recesses of my being, can be better imagined than described. I did not know then what I came to grasp later on—that an automatic mechanism, forced by the practice of meditation, had suddenly started to function with the object of reshaping my mind to make it fit for the expression of a more heightened and extended consciousness, by means of biological processes as natural and as governed by inviolable laws as the evolution of species or the development and birth of a child. But to my great misfortune I did not know this at the time. To the best of my knowledge, this mighty secret of nature is not known on earth today, although there is ample evidence to show that certain methods to deal with the condition, when brought about suddenly by the practice of hatha yoga, were fully known to the ancient adepts.

I studied my condition thoroughly from day to day to assure myself that what I experienced was real and not imaginary. Just as a man finding himself in an unbelievable situation pinches himself to make certain that he is not dreaming but awake, I invariably studied my bodily symptoms to find corroboration for my mental condition. It would be a fallacy to assume that I was the victim of a hallucination. Subsequent events and my present condition absolutely rule out that possibility. No, the crisis I was passing through was not a creation of my own imagination. It had a real physiological basis and was interwoven with the whole organic structure of my body. The entire machinery from the brain to the smallest organ was deeply involved, and there was no escape for me from the storm of nervous forces which blew through my system day and night, released unexpectedly by my own effort.

III

Explorations in Kundalini Research

If there is wide agreement among spiritual teachers and those investigating mysteries of the mind that kundalini is a key concept for understanding psychic, occult, and spiritual phenomena, there is also serious *dis*agreement on various aspects of the concept. Thus, in the wake of increasing public discussion of it, a number of disputes have arisen about the philosophy, psychology, physiology, and methodology of kundalini. The previous sections have given evidence of this.

How might these problems be resolved? The primary means in the West is the empirical method. If the object of an investigation passes the test of scientific scrutiny, one has good reason for accepting the findings.

The chief advocate of kundalini research has been Gopi Krishna. Now in his seventies, Gopi Krishna has spent four decades observing kundalini at work in the laboratory of his own body. In half a dozen books he has given firm indications to science for a comprehensive research program into the phenomenon of kundalini. Since his autobiography was published in the United States in 1970, his work has drawn significant attention in the scientific and intellectual communities. *Psychology Today, Time, Harper's,* the *New York Times,* and a number of scholarly books have all recognized him as an important figure in consciousness research.

Kundalini, as Gopi Krishna presents it, is the bridge between mind and matter, psyche and soma. It is a unifying concept for the physical, biological, and social sciences. There is, he says, a direct but subtle psychophysical linkage between sexual and spiritual experience–the real "msising link" of human evolution–and this can be objectively demonstrated by empirical science to involve a microbiological transformation of the brain and nervous system that distinguishes an enlightened person from an ordinary one.

Gopi Krishna maintains that this formulation offers a *testable* field theory of psychophysical linkages among body, mind, culture, and cosmos, covering the entire spectrum of psychological, psychic, and mystical phenomena. As a hypothesis, it elegantly unites ancient occult/esoteric traditions with evolutionary theory and the transpersonal psychology arising from the traditions of Freud, Jung, and Maslow. It also explains, in a unified way, many mysteries of anthropology, religion, psychiatry, sociology, and biology.

More specifically, Gopi Krishna claims that (1) he has discovered that the reproductive system is also the mechanism by which intelligence is increased and evolution proceeds, (2) the religious impulse is biologically rooted, and (3) there is a predetermined target for human evolution toward which the entire race is being irresistibly drawn.

This knowledge, he says, has been recognized by all the world's major spiritual paths, genuine occult traditions, mystery schools, and hermetic philosophies. It is, in his view, the real secret behind yoga and all other systems of enlightenment that have produced mystics, sages, and saviors. In the words of Dr. Karan Singh, originator of the "Project Consciousness" research program to be carried out at the National Institute of Mental Health and Neurosciences in Bangalore, Gopi Krishna's hypothesis–central to "Project Consciousness"–is that "kundalini is not only some kind of vague spiritual power but a very definite quantifiable force which, when it reaches the brain, has a definite physical and chemical impact upon it which in turn causes a change in the level of consciousness."

In a private communication to me, Gopi Krishna summarized the uniqueness of his position with these words: "It is for the first time that the connection among insanity, genius, mystical ecstasy, psychic gifts, and other abnormal and paranormal states of the mind is being traced to kundalini. The research directed on the phenomenon is thus likely to lead to momentous results. The connection between kundalini and the paranormal and abnormal states of the mind has not even been suspected by most of the modern exponents of the serpent power."

A recent book, *Kundalini Yoga* by R. K. Karanjia, has a Foreword by Gopi Krishna in which he states succinctly why he is calling for research into the kundalini experience:

> I am so insistent on a thorough scientific investigation of the phenomenon because it would show to the thinkers and political leaders of mankind that the human brain is already designed for a supersensory performance, in the same way that the brain of an infant is already completely fashioned at birth for its performance during the whole of life. A wrong social or political environment can stunt or distort the evolutionary growth of the adult brain as surely as a wrong or adverse family environment can disrupt the harmonious growth of a child. Nothing about this ceaseless evolutionary activity of the human organism is yet known to science. But the knowledge is of paramount importance both for the individual and the race. When this fact is known, all social and political environments will have to be oriented to suit the evolutionary needs of every human being.
>
> I advocate the research because it would prove that talent and genius can be cultivated, as was done in India in the past. It would prove that human beings can reach a state of cosmic awareness in which the highest secrets of life and existence can be intuitively learnt. It would prove that nature has already provided a safeguard against the abuse of power in this age of highly advanced technology and science. This safeguard lies in the fact that knowledge of kundalini will tend to a recurrent crop of spiritual geniuses to handle the affairs of

> mankind. I advocate the research because kundalini provides the only avenue for a bloodless revolution in all spheres of human activity and thought to bring about those healthy social and political changes all over the earth which are absolutely necessary now to provide a congenial milieu for the collective evolutionary progress of mankind. Kundalini alone can officiate as the divine harbinger of a New Age and the architect of a war-free, united world in which the resources now wasted on mutual aggression, violence, and bloodshed would be utilized for the uplift of the weak and poor.

The potential scientific and social significance of kundalini research should be clear. But the research itself is no simple matter. For one thing, the necessary technology for detecting and measuring pranic energy exists only in rudimentary form. Conventional instruments for psychophysiological research should, of course, be used. These might include the electroencephalograph (EEG) for brain-wave measurement; immunoassay equipment for analyzing changes in oxygen level, lactic acid, sex hormones, etc., in the blood; Kirlian photography; and various other recording devices. However, the postulated bioenergy associated with kundalini phenomena would itself not be directly measurable through these devices —only inferable. My book *Future Science,* which examines the nature of life energies and the physics of paranormal phenomena, presents a number of devices that offer useful avenues of approach to direct detection and measurement of subtle forces. At the moment, though, sophisticated technology is lacking.

In the forefront of those inventive pioneers creating "spiritual instruments" is Christopher Hills. His decades of research into radiesthesia, science, and yoga have resulted in a large number of devices that he claims can demonstrate and measure biophysical effects arising from subtle energies. These instruments are described in his two masterworks, *Supersensonics* and *Nuclear Evolution* (see Appendix), and are presented separately in a short book, *Supersensonic Instruments of Knowing*. One instrument, the "Kundalini Roomph Coil," is said to "read off that point on the spiral coil where your kundalini energy is now focused" and then to allow the user to "tune this latent energy so that it safely proceeds in stages as each center opens gradually." Kundalini researchers will need personal experience with the energetic effects of kundalini arousal, and instruments such as the "Kundalini Roomph Coil" may be useful in this regard, as well as for measuring it in subjects.

The need for subtle-energy technology is not the only obstacle to advancing kundalini research. Another—perhaps even greater—is the serious disagreement on certain aspects of the kundalini concept among those who claim to speak with authority about it. Although many authorities consider kundalini a key concept in understanding psychic, occult, and spiritual phenomena, a variety of conceptual difficulties have arisen in the wake of increasing public discussion of kundalini.

The range of dispute can be illustrated through statements made about the nature of chakras. Gopi Krishna says they are primarily nerve plexes along the spine—major ganglia—and can be directly observed by scientific means to undergo changes upon the awakening of kundalini. The Indian sage Sri Aurobindo maintains that the chakras are primarily psychic energy points in the middle of the etheric body. The scholar Joseph Campbell said in a 1975 *Psychology Today* article (see Appendix) that the chakras are psychological teaching devices without any physical reality—merely metaphors. Yogi Bhajan maintains that they have multilevel reality as etheric energy transducers that interact with physical electromagnetic energy fields. They have physical connecting locations on the spine. The etheric vortexes, he says, project like cones from these spinal centers and from related glandular centers. However, he de-emphasizes the ancient symbolism of the chakras. When kundalini awakens, he declares, all the centers are integrated. Christopher Hills, in the excerpt reprinted in Part I, says it is erroneous to think of kundalini as energy. Kundalini, he says, is consciousness. The energetic effects experienced in the chakras and their associated psychologies are secondary byproducts, not kundalini itself.

Still further fuel is added to the controversy by Bhagwan Shree Rajneesh, a contemporary guru in India. In his book *Dynamics of Meditation,* he states, "Kundalini is not a life force by itself. It is a particular passage for the life force–a way. . . . The kundalini and its chakras (centers) are not located in the physical body. . . . The passage is in the etheric body and the centers also."

In defiance of all these authorities, Swami Agehananda Bharati, chairman of the anthropology department at Syracuse University and author of the recent book on mysticism, *The Light at the Center,* declares that kundalini is a lot of "claptrap." He points out that even Patanjali, who wrote the classic *Yoga Sutras,* called kundalini *kalpanantunka* (imaginary). In a 1975 interview with *Illustrated Weekly of India,* Bharati said, "The visual imagery of the series of chakras extending from the anus upward along the spine into the skull through which [kundalini] travels is latter-day nonsense."

A resolution to this dispute is offered by Ken Wilber in his article in Part I. By showing that many of these apparently opposed views can be assigned to various "levels" in the spectrum-of-consciousness model he has proposed in a book entitled *The Spectrum of Consciousness,* what were *op*posite become a *com*posite. The spectrum approach synthesizes them into a complementary whole, just as modern evolutionary theory has done with the once-competing views of De Vries (mutation theory) and Darwin (natural-selection theory).

Just as the reality of the chakras is disputed, so is the number of chakras subject to disagreement among authorities who accept their reality. There are different numbers of chakras given in different esoteric systems. People in the West usually hear that there are seven chakras, numbered in ascending order from the base of the spine to the crown of the head. But depending upon the text consulted, the number varies from five to thirteen major chakras, with thousands of minor chakras.

Assuming, therefore, that there are only seven major chakras and that they have some kind of physical reality or physical analogue, what can be said about the location of the seventh chakra? Some authorities identify it as the pineal gland. Others say it is the pituitary gland. Still others identify it with the anterior fontanelle—that small opening at the top of the skull—or, more generally, with the top of the head. It has also been described as the third ventricle of the brain. Yogi Bhajan says it is *projected* from its point of origin, the pineal gland, through the skull at the anterior fontanelle. And Gopi Krishna declares that the seventh chakra, properly speaking, is not a chakra at all. It is often pictured in literature as a thousand-petaled lotus, he says, because it is actually the entire cerebral cortex with all its convolutions. (He also maintains that the "opening of the third eye" is an expression referring not to the sixth chakra or to some specific organ in the brain, but rather to the transformation of the entire brain and nervous system, with a resultant higher mode of perception.)

These disagreements and others should make it obvious that if kundalini is central to enlightenment and spiritual unfoldment, as many claim, then scientific and scholarly research is needed to clarify differences and resolve contradictory statements.

The following section presents some recent explorations in kundalini research. None needs further commentary. It should be borne in mind, however, that these explorations—like all pioneering research and theoretical formulations—are tentative. They must be subjected to critical review by scientists, scholars, intellectuals, and spiritual teachers who must examine the data, the logic, and the conclusions. They must also, in the case of laboratory experiments and clinical observations, be replicated. Where the data differ from traditional views—as in the case of Itzhak Bentov's model and Lee Sannella's clinical findings, which require no "supernormal forces" to explain the phenomena—let the search for knowledge, for *scientia* be the standard. If, in the course of events, spiritual tradition meets the test of scientific investigation, so much the better for both. Whatever the case, though, let truth, not tradition, be our concern.

THE IMPORTANCE AND SOME IMPLICATIONS
OF A SCIENTIFIC INVESTIGATION OF

THE PHENOMENON OF KUNDALINI

Gopi Krishna

Study of the phenomenon of kundalini or the serpent power provides the only channel for the exploitation of prana, the channel through which the *illuminati* attain transcendence and geniuses extraordinary bloom of the mind. Kundalini is the natural inlet through which the human intellect can come into contact with the divine forces of creation.

The study of psychic phenomena or the practice of magical arts does not provide a safe avenue for this enterprise. The superphysical forces that cause psychic displays or lend potency to magic, if made amenable to human will, could place a weapon in the hands of the overambitious, the voluptuary, and the megalomaniac before which even the threat posed by the nuclear arsenals would pale into insignificance. Wars can be made to erupt telepathically and multitudes made abject slaves and puppets of a few.

But nature has provided safeguards which can make it impossible for any scientific investigation to know the nature of or to control the mysterious forces involved in these occurrences at the present evolutionary stature of the race. The reason for this is simple. We know what amazing devices protect life on earth. The whole drama of organic evolution from the beginning to this moment is a miracle of divine protection continued for billions of years against staggering odds: one chance against billions, repeated interminably. Yet that one infinitely slender chance succeeded, and humanity owes its existence to that.

We also know that there are defenses which act as umbrellas round the earth, the Heavyside layer for instance, that shield terrestrial life from the lethal effects of cosmic radiation. There are defenses that keep the forces of nature–flood and tide, storm and rain, heat and cold–from attaining a fury or a rigor fatal to life. There are defenses that allow us to live unconcerned and undisturbed while the earth whirls through space at terrific speed, with flaming oceans of fire storming and raging in her interior. There are defenses in our body that protect us from the deadly attacks of malignant bacteria time after time.

There are psychological devices, as there are devices in ants and bees, that rule the social conduct of human beings and form the instinctive background of every human social order. There are devices that bring the human fold back again to the path of evolution after every departure or digression, through the offices of religious teachers, revolutionaries and reformers.

There are devices that will come into operation at the time of a seemingly annihilating nuclear war to save the race from extinction, for it is meant to fulfill a glorious destiny. In short, we are miraculously preserved and protected from every side and at every moment. But how often do we admit to ourselves that all our life is spent at the mercy of forces of which we have no awareness at all? Often we even fail to realize that there is design in every fragment and every event in the universe. But the scale of its operation is so unimaginably vast in space and time that our poor sense equipment and puny intellect fails to grasp it. Another channel of perception is therefore needed to bring the intangible controlling forces of creation within our ken.

A decrease of half a degree during the last thirty years in the global temperature of the earth has made scientists concerned about the still unpredictable effect on the climatic conditions at different places, if the drop continues to occur. This shows what a delicate balance in the environment is necessary for life to survive on earth and that still unknown and unthought-of devices are operating to maintain that balance.

There are similar devices that will prevent the whole global body of science from penetrating into the mystery of the superphysical forces and harnessing them, as we have harnessed the physical forces of nature, because mankind must ascend yet another step on the ladder of evolution before this can become possible. The mastery might be gained when the precondition of a further rise in the evolutionary scale is fulfilled.

The twin products of an active kundalini, namely the illuminati and the men and women of genius and talent, have been the two main classes of human beings responsible for every advance made by mankind so far. It has long been known that heredity primarily accounts for the quota of intelligence and talent in human beings. This view has now been confirmed by exhaustive tests conducted on twins and other children at several places. In a recent article in the *National Observer,* Joan Rodgers writes:

> You may give a child excellent parental attention, a good home, fine schools and cultural experience, but if the youngster wasn't born smart, he will probably never be smart. It is an abhorrent idea to some but that is what several American and European scientists said in Rome at the First International Congress of Twin Studies. . . . There is an answer now, the scientists said, to the long-standing, often emotional question of whether it is genetics or environmental factors that principally determine one's learning ability. They say it is nature.

In support of this conclusion, Rodgers refers to the studies conducted by Dr. Joseph M. Horn, of the University of Texas, and other scientists. "Our studies and others clearly show," says Horn, "that individual differences in intelligence among individuals in Western culture are primarily determined by genetics. We know what is involved in making statements like that, but we have no choice. The data are there. . . . When one finds a trait such as intelligence substantially determined by genetic factors this does not mean we cannot design an environment to overcome it. But the evidence to date is that we have yet to find that environment and, what is more, we may be looking in the wrong places." Referring to the home and school environments that have been the traditional targets of manipulation by doctors, teachers, and psychologists, looking for the best environment for child development, Horn observes: "But what we need to do now is look elsewhere to other environments to alter." The manipulation of the inner environment before birth in terms of enrichment and prevention of defects, in the view of Dr. Horn, may do far more than manipulation of the external environment.

Kundalini provides the only avenue for overcoming the congenital deficiencies of the brain. The paramount importance of its study can be readily gauged even from this single fact. In this lies the only hope for the mentally retarded or the deficient. In the advanced stages of our knowledge about the mechanism, it might become possible for scientists to achieve what has been impossible so far: to bring hope, cheer, and the light of intelligence to millions and millions of mentally stunted human beings all over the world. It might also become possible to eradicate other congenital defects beyond cure at present. The evolution of the body and its immunity to death is based on this potentiality of the serpent power, which has a regenerative and recuperative effect on the system. But exhaustive research is necessary to devise safe methods for its arousal in keeping with its own laws.

The social aspect of research on kundalini is even more important. Revolutionary changes in the current thinking on social problems and political ideologies may result. The smoldering discontentment in some of the richest countries of the West and the strong curb on the freedom of expression in the Communist lands as a whole provide unquestionable evidence for the fact. There is hardly any country on the earth today which, under the surface, is not a seething caldron of unrest and disaffection.

Rings of fire and streams of blood mark at every phase the social evolution of mankind, from the dawn of history to the present day. There seldom, if ever, has been a peaceful transition from one social order or one political structure to another. So long as the basic reason for the need for change in the social environment of man is not understood, and mankind continues to be in the dark about this vital aspect of its evolutionary career, blood will continue to be shed.

Continued ignorance of this essential knowledge is fraught with the gravest danger for the race in the times to come. Within a few more decades all the countries with fairly large populations, and even the affluent smaller ones, will have nuclear arsenals to add to their security against the existing nuclear powers. Nuclear technology will make it possible to construct miniweapons for use by terrorist organizations and frustrated individuals. This can happen any day and lead to the plunging of the world into a nightmare of fear and anxiety at each small incident every day.

Deep-rooted instincts prescribe the social behavior of all other forms of life except man. The evolutionary dynamics of the human brain need a flexible social order amenable to revision from time to time. But conservative tendencies stand stubbornly in the way of needed change from one order to another. The counterculture in America and the revolt of youth in other parts of the world are all indications of the fact that the time of utility of the present order is over and a change is urgently called for.

Modern psychology is unaware of this resistless impulse in the human brain. The main actor in the drama of life is entirely missing in the learned dissertations on the human mind. The alarming increase in the psychic disorders is the outcome of obstructed evolution on account of unhygienic social conditions, but statistical data and study of abnormal mental behavior cannot help to bring this hidden actor to light. Another kind of study is needed to reach to the bottom of this mystery. The greatest potential for a complete revolution in the sphere of modern thought lies hidden in psychology.

Prophets, philosophers, and political revolutionaries have failed to bring about an era of lasting peace because the divine estate destined for man and divine mechanism designed to lead to it have never been empirically demonstrated.

Knowledge of the human body and the methods that could make this demonstration possible were never so advanced as they are now. But all the same, the demonstration constitutes a colossal enterprise. Once started it is likely to become an unending quest.

Research on kundalini is research on the very roots of life. The fossil data in support of the theory of evolution have been under investigation for more than a century. Still, the clinching evidence has not been found, and there is a difference of opinion about some of the most vital issues of the doctrine. The theory of gravity is another example. The constitution of the atom is another. Psychic phenomena provide another category where a clash of views has been in evidence for about a century now. It would therefore be too much to expect that research on kundalini or, in other words, on the cosmological forces of life, can produce decisive results in a day. It will provide a long and arduous quest.

But the stakes are high. Validation of the phenomena of religion and mystical ecstasy, evidence for the immortal nature of the soul, the purpose of life and the destiny of man, the force behind psychic phenomena, voluntary cultivation of genius, avoidance of destructive wars and bloody revolutions, insight into the causes of insanity, and illuminating answers to other problems of life will constitute the golden harvest yielded by this investigation bit by bit in the course of time.

Of all these categories, the most important and, at the same time, the most phenomenal, is the transformative prowess of kundalini. This sphere of its activity is so remote from our current conceptions that no exposition about it can convey the unthought-of possibilities inherent in it unless a case of this type comes actually under observation. A young Maharashtrian girl in Nagpur, it is reported, has been completely transformed into a Bengali-speaking shy housewife of more than 125 years ago. The girl, Sharada, as she calls herself, used to emerge for a short while and later gave way to the Maharashtrian girl. Later the spells lasted longer and the present one has continued for a month. The girl, who is highly educated, did not know Bengali before this transformation.

According to her parents, the change began about a year ago and the girl started to speak Bengali.

Transformation of personality, when it goes down to the very roots of an individual, betokens a transformation of the pranic spectrum. The change can occur sporadically, for short or long spells of time, or on a permanent basis. The phenomenon is well known to psychologists, but no satisfactory explanation has been found so far. I have myself witnessed every phase in the transformation of my own personality. There are many mediums and sensitives who evince the same trait on a sporadic basis. During the spells of their transformation they display extraordinary faculties of mind or show evidence of talents, ways of talk and behavior, or artistic gifts that are absent in their normal life. The phenomenon has been often repeated in history.

Specific areas or the still unused potential of the brain is used to build up the other personality. The architect is kundalini. Psychologists are content to treat such individuals as cases of double or multiple personality and let it rest at that. A complete metamorphosis, in which two entirely different individuals emerge from the same brain, is a phenomenon so astounding and so far in conflict with the current concepts about mind and the organ of its expression, i.e., the brain, that it is surprising so little attention has been paid to its investigation. This shows how narrow the frontiers of modern psychology are. There is no universally accepted explanation for any extraordinary or abnormal state of mind, including insanity. Yet psychologists, as a class, labor under the impression that they are academically competent to pass their judgments about the mental condition of the rest of the world in terms of their own nomenclature, which still lacks confirmation.

The process that occurs naturally in rare cases to build up a multiple personality can be set in motion voluntarily with the arousal of kundalini. In this lie the amazing possibilities of serpent power. There are well-known and well-attested cases of individuals who, in a trance or semitrance, bloom into great healers, clairvoyants, expounders of religious truths, prophesiers, oracles, and the like. With voluntary cultivation there is no end to the possibilities of the metamorphosis. With better knowledge of the mechanism and discovery of safer methods to activate it, the products of kundalini can bloom into prodigies in every sphere of human knowledge, into geniuses of the highest order, into prophets, seers, healers, and clairvoyants of surpassing stature, beyond anything we can imagine at present. They will be the leaders in every field of knowledge and activity in the future world.

The study can be divided into five broad parallel departments. *The first of these would consist of a thorough study of the oral and written tradition.* There are thousands of books on kundalini and yoga extant in India. The ancient esoteric treatises, including the Tantras, contain valuable hints about the serpent powers. The Vedas, the Upanishads, and the Puranas provide another fertile source. A study by a team of scholars can provide valuable material to initiate an empirical investigation of the phenomena.

Then there is a huge mass of literature formed by the self-revelations and other utterances of the medieval saints of India. It can also provide precious clues here and there and substantiate the information contained in the scriptural texts. The writings of the Western mystics, Sufis, Taoists, and Tibetan yogis should provide a valuable mine of information.

Religious lore of all faiths and the books on magic, alchemy, or the occult, existing from ancient times, can also supply valuable material bearing on the subject. Well-known documents on kundalini can begin the study, which can then be extended gradually to cover the sources available for this research.

The study of the oral tradition is equally important. The hint I, myself, received about the danger of an awakening occurring through the pingala or the solar nerve, was based on oral tradition. These facts are not generally mentioned in the books. The hints are transmitted orally by the preceptor to the disciple and acted upon in terms of need.

For instance, in the event of an awakening leading to the generation of a high degree of heat in the system, the remedy prescribed is to lay on a coat of wet clay over the body or to immerse it in a pool of water up to the neck. For the heat experienced at the crown of the head or the space between the eyebrows, the rubbing of sandalpaste is recommended. In fact, the mark applied by Hindus to the forehead is done as a sign of homage to the ajna chakra. It is only when kundalini enters this center that higher faculties of the mind make their appearance. The application of a mark to the forehead, which is such a common feature of worship or even adornment in India, and sometimes appears as a product of superstition to foreigners, carries a highly esoteric significance and an awareness of the physiological implications of the serpent power.

The second province of research would cover those cases in which kundalini is congenitally active. There are five categories of the individuals belonging to this class–the born mystic, the man and woman of genius, the prodigies, the mediums, and the psychotics.

Out of all these categories the last named are most easily accessible to research. Next to the cases of awakening due to certain disciplines or occurring spontaneously later in life, psychotics provide a most fertile field for this investigation. The old view of the psychoanalytic school that insanity is a subjective phenomenon arising out of repression or other similar causes, especially in childhood, is becoming increasingly obsolete. The latest studies show that schizophrenia, manic-depression, and other serious forms of insanity have roots deep in the organic soil of the body.

But often the roots penetrate to depths in the finer levels of the organism which are yet beyond the reach of laboratory study. And it has now been clearly established that some forms of psychoses show definite tracks in the brain. The horrifying visions and distracting sounds which the lunatics see and hear, it is now recognized, are not all mere figments of their imagination but can be maddeningly real with their roots in the excited and altered conditions of certain areas in the brain.

Even in the normal condition, our nerves are the generators and carriers of bioenergy or prana in its individual organic aspect. Modern biology or psychology has no inkling of this activity of the nervous system, as the medium involved is subtle beyond measurement by the instruments now in use. A beginning has been made with kirlian photography, but further advancement is needed to bring this elusive substance within the orbit of research. On the activation of kundalini there occurs a high increase in the production of bioenergy and also an enhancement in its potency. The ecstatic visions of the mystic, the creations of genius, the performance of the prodigy, the phenomenon of the medium, and the nightmares of the insane are all, without exception, the products of this enhanced flow of a more potent form of bioenergy into the brain.

In the case of the born mystic, the genius, the medium, and the prodigy, the brain cells are already attuned to the flow of bioenergy of a higher potency. But in the case of those in whom the power is aroused as the result of certain disciplines, a certain period of time is needed to accustom the brain to the altered condition of this force. This is the most critical period in the discipline of yoga and other spiritual exercises. Even in the case of individuals born with this peculiarity, crises continue to occur throughout life.

The susceptibility to mental derangement in the case of some of the most outstanding specimens of the latter, like Newton, is also due to this fact. Research into kundalini must make it possible to avert these crises in the lives of the most creative section of the race. The crises in the lives of the great mystics and saints–their tormenting desire for spiritual experience which sometimes goes to the point of mania–also owe their origin to the effect of this psychic radiation on the brain.

The mystic can attain such a state of absorption in his visionary experience that he can become entirely oblivious to the world and his surroundings. The very words "trance" or "ecstasy" denote this state of intense engrossment. This is also one of the characteristics of samadhi. The individual is lost to the world around him. To a lesser extent this is also the case with creative genius.

Intense absorption in the subject of study or the artistic production has been a marked feature of the creative mind. The anecdotes relating to the absorbed states of Newton are more or less applicable to other great geniuses also. In the case of mediums, too, the mental condition undergoes a transformation during the productive periods. There is often entrancement or signs of intense one-pointed mental effort during the performance.

In a different form the same symptom of withdrawal from the world marks the mental condition of the insane. The psychotic lives alienated from the world, completely engrossed in an inner experience which determines his external behavior also. But in this case the visionary or auditory experience is not alluring or absorbing. It is a phantasmagoria of disordered imagination, of erratic and absurd thought and act, fear, anxiety, and horror. The radiation pouring into the brain is no longer soothing and enrapturing. It is toxic, poisonous, and virulent, causing excitement or depression, frenzy or stupor, intense melancholy or insane laughter, and all the other characteristics peculiar to madness. The old personality disappears from the scene and a distorted one emerges lost to the norms of behavior and sense. The disoriented pranic spectrum now reflects a disfigured being completely or in part out of tune with the world around.

The studies carried out on mystics, now or in the past, and the revelations of mystics themselves, circle around halos of light, harmonies of sound, transporting visions, extraordinary insights, new depths of knowledge, glimpses of other planes of existence, or spiritual exaltation during the spell for which the ecstasy lasts. There also occurs an increase in creative activity, eloquence, and literary or artistic talent according to the mental aptitude of the subject.

With the flow of polluted pranic radiation into the brain, the lights become blinding glares, the sounds distracting noises and shrieks, the visions nightmares, deep insights become crazy whims. The glimpses of a new existence, the phantom-world of insanity and spiritual exaltation assume the form of grandiose delusions of rank and power. The increase in creative activity is translated into frenzied behavior, eloquence into raving, and increased literary or artistic ability into insane compositions and bizarre art.

I am positive about the fact that a morbid activation of kundalini can lead to psychoses in a variety of forms. I myself passed through phases akin to them during the period of my transition from one state of consciousness to the other. It took years for the new state to be stabilized. I have witnessed the same shifts toward a borderline mental condition on the activation of kundalini in several other cases also.

The extreme hazard involved in a forced voluntary arousal of the serpent power, which has long been known in India, stems from this possibility. The abortive cases turn into schizophrenics and manic-depressives, in some instances displaying remarkable psychic gifts. Research on kundalini is research on bioenergy and can lead to the causes responsible for vitiation of the psychic currents and their cure. Modern psychology clearly accepts the close association of sexuality with mental disorder but the actual mechanism is never indicated.

In order to understand the genesis of this form of insanity it is necessary to look a little more carefully into the mechanism of kundalini. As has been explained in my books, the activation of the mechanism marks the start of two new and different activities in the body. The whole vast network of nerves begins to manufacture a more potent form of psychic energy (prana) and pour it into the brain through the spinal duct. The most distinguished feature of this altered form of bioenergy is that it appears as a luminous cloud in the brain. The energy in the average men and women does not have this property. For this reason the visionary experience of mystics is almost always bathed in light.

This is the first important point to which any investigation into the phenomenon must pay attention. This is also the reason why kundalini is always likened to sun, moon, lightning, or fire. Flashes of light or other forms of luminosity, experienced by many people during the course of meditation, and sometimes even otherwise, are often due to a sudden, brief upsurge of the higher prana into the brain.

The other activity starts in the genital region. On the awakening, the reproductive juices in the form of radiation are sucked up in a mysterious way and poured into the spinal canal. How this suction is applied research will surely one day bring to light. This juicy stream rising through the spine represents the "nectar" or "ambrosia" repeatedly mentioned in the treatises on kundalini. It is the *soma* of the Vedas, *rasa* of the alchemists and *samarasa* of the medieval saints of India. The whole mystic literature of India is full of references to it. Its entry into the spinal cord, and later on into the brain, is marked by exquisitely pleasurable sensations even exceeding orgasm. This stream of organic essence is ramified into smaller streams, during the course of its ascent into the cranium, and these slender streams irrigate the visceral organs through the nerve plexes or the chakras.

The stream can be distinctly felt moving into the various organs, stomach, liver, intestines, heart, lungs, throat, and the like. A new channel for toning up the organs to meet additional needs, resulting from an increase in the area of awareness, now comes into operation. In this way the body and the brain are prepared for a more elevated manifestation of consciousness. The flow of more potent prana and this stream of fluidic secretions into the nerve-centers is known by the phrase "penetration of kundalini" as stated in the ancient books on the subject.

In the case of a morbid awakening the two movements do not start together, or there is imperfect coordination between them. The genital secretions for various reasons do not stream up and circulate in the system to adjust the organs and the brain to the flow of the high-potency prana, now operative in the system. Overindulgence or an unhealthy state of the reproductive organs can also lead to this condition. In such an eventuality the consequences can be terrible. Since the mechanism for preparing the tissues of the body for a greater output of psychic energy of a more concentrated kind fails to act altogether or in the right manner, the radiation pouring into the head lacks that degree of purity and excellence which is necessary for the healthy functioning of the brain in the altered condition. An impure, toxic current now flows through it creating a chaotic condition in the whole province of thought. The irritation caused in the brain cells by the contaminated pranic radiation is soon translated into anarchy in the thought and behavior of the afflicted individual.

It is no wonder that under the torment of this venomous current now flooding the brain the lunatic raves, shrieks, gesticulates, runs about wildly, laughs, foams at the mouth, resorts to violence, or lapses into frenzy in a manner characteristic of the mentally deranged. He has no perception of the radiation. What he experiences is a derangement in personality, thought, and act. The disoriented stream of prana gives rise to a disoriented human being. The suffering of the patient can be terrible. He may sink into a stupor, be entirely unable to collect his thoughts, lose all relish for food as the reflexes are deadened, experience agonizing loss of sleep, feel himself burning from head to toe, or experience other subjective, intensely painful and tormenting conditions.

At the present moment, psychic energy is beyond the probe of science, and there is absolutely no method to determine its purity or lack of it. Scientists faced with the actuality of mental disorder, yet unable to know anything about the subtle force responsible for it, continue to put forward ingenious explanations which take no cognizance of the mysterious agent at work. Insanity is a product of an impure state of pranic radiation, whether caused by the awakening of kundalini or otherwise due to the malfunctioning of the organism in its subtle levels involved in the production of prana. The somatic aspect of insanity is now becoming increasingly apparent to psychologists, but the basic factors are still unidentified.

There can be other variations. The pranic currents might flow through the ida and pingala causing awful, excited, or depressive conditions. The forms of insanity caused by a malignant kundalini and their varied patterns in different individuals comprise a subject so vast and so intricate that it would constitute a whole department of knowledge if the mechanism were to be empirically demonstrated. The subject will be dealt with in more detail elsewhere. Here it has been touched upon in passing to show its relevance to the research undertaken on kundalini. The observation of the sexual behavior of the mentally afflicted who belong to this category, and a close study of their reproductive organs, must in the course of time yield important clues for the identification of the mechanism responsible for the maladies.

It has not been possible for scientists to locate the real cause for mental and psychic maladies because of the fact that they have as yet no knowledge of bioenergy and no methods or devices to detect it. Kundalini provides the one natural channel for the exploration of this still unidentified force of creation. This exploration can be both subjective and objective, provided the mechanism is rightly manipulated. A great deal of research would be needed to define the parameters of the objective evidence. But with study and patience this can be done, leading to the emergence of a new science in due course of time. The benefits accruing from the cure of mental diseases through this investigation cannot be exaggerated. In the not-distant future, it might become possible to control mental disorders through the discovery of prana, as it has become possible now to control epidemics and infectious ailments through the discovery of the microbial origin of disease. Reich was right when he said that mental disorder is anchored in the somatic structure of the organism. This somatic anchorage is prana.

The pressures and tensions of modern life, especially in the more advanced, industrialized nations, seriously affect the delicate balance of prana, putting a heavy strain on the organic mechanism which insures its sensitive equilibrium. The result is that there are more patients suffering from mental disorder, seeking admission to clinics, than patients suffering from all other diseases taken together. This is an alarming situation pregnant with even worse possibilities in the future, for the tensions and pressures are still on the increase. Apart from the confirmed cases of mental disorder, there are millions upon millions of human beings, in all parts of the world, lacking in the power of adjustment to their surroundings. This results in untold suffering to their partners, families, and all those with whom they are in contact every day. For a control of these conditions also, the only natural mechanism is kundalini.

Genetic engineering, if it is ever undertaken, would ultimately lead to the same conclusions. It is the disorientation of the pranic spectrum which is responsible for all obsessions, fixations, perversions, and distortions of the mind. The channel to handle prana is kundalini. Since an alarmingly large proportion of the race is in the grip of a mental disorder or a twist or kink of some kind, or lacks in the proper degree of self-control and self-adjustment, the dimensions of research which can provide a panacea for all the ills of the mind and the nervous system can be better imagined than described. There is no other study so important for the peace and happiness of the race as the study of prana and the mechanism by which it can be handled and manipulated.

The third province of research can be provided by born mystics, geniuses, mediums, and prodigies in whom kundalini is more or less active from birth. The data obtained from the observation of the mental cases which have resulted from a morbid awakening of the serpent power can be put to use in drawing up a blueprint for the study of those born with it. Certain parameters of identity will always be there. The main targets of investigation should be the cerebrospinal fluid and the reproductive apparatus. In the case of mediums a tendency to orgasm during mediumship has already been noticed in some cases. The erotic nature of mystical ecstasy is fully recognized. The sex life of geniuses or men and women of extraordinary talent must provide indications of this type. The learned, as a class, are often unwilling to move out of the cloistered area of thought to which they are accustomed. But a few of them show a readiness to march into unknown territory. The ordeals undergone by those who broke through the fallacy of a geocentric universe are well known. The empirical validation of kundalini is sure to cause a revolution far exceeding in magnitude the one caused by Copernicus. But a tough battle will be necessary before scholarly prejudice can be overcome.

The modern concept of life is based on the assumption that a peculiar constitution and composition of atoms and molecules is at the bottom of the phenomenon. There is no conception of still unknown and immaterial forces in the universe. Although the very texture of thought and consciousness constitute a standing challenge to this erroneous conception, any attempt made to break through this barrier would always prove a tough undertaking. The difficulties inherent in research on kundalini must, therefore, be kept in mind from the first. The attempt is to break through the self-erected frontiers of modern science. A century of experimentation on psi phenomena by competent investigators, including eminent scientists, has not yet been able to cross this border. But properly conducted research on kundalini, in my opinion, is sure to perform this formidable task in less than one fifth of this period of time.

Once the underlying principles are known, the study of the individuals with an awakened kundalini should be easy to conduct and organize. There must be definite biological differences in the blood, the cerebrospinal fluid and the composition of brain matter in its subtler layers. The recent startling discoveries of new particles in the composition of the atom should make us cautious in allotting a limit to the composition of the organic cell. Its subtler layers are still beyond our probe. Our present day concepts are built on assumptions which any fresh discovery can prove to be wrong. There is a whole world of subtle energies lying hidden in every living organism. These energies, in their turn, subsist on subtle biological fuels which the organism produces and stores in every tissue and cell. This fuel is used by the cosmic life-energy or prana shakti to manufacture the individual prana or bioenergy. Neurons play an active part in this manufacture.

The accomplished yogis of India have been able to write with such assurance about the pranic currents in the body because in the heightened states of consciousness prana becomes easily perceptible. A scientific study of this subtle medium with instruments devised for the purpose can be of incalculable value to mankind. A painstaking study of persons with an active kundalini must at last furnish clues by which it would be possible to know the difference between the microbiology of a normal individual and a genius or mystic or any other specimen of this category. There can be absolutely no denial of the fact that there must exist some difference somewhere between the brain of an Einstein and that of a man of ordinary intelligence. But we know it only too well that this difference, in spite of repeated efforts made to this end, has not been found so far. The reason for this failure is that the extremely fine tissues involved have not come within the range of observation to this day.

The fourth province for study can be furnished by those in whom there occurs an activation of the serpent power later in life without in any way affecting the sanity of their mind. Those who have symptoms of this kind often pass through periods of suspense or suffering because of their ignorance of the factor responsible for them.

I have been receiving letters from people all over the world whom a study of some of my books made cognizant of the mysterious agency responsible for the strange and sometimes bizarre experiences they were undergoing or the unusual symptoms that they noticed in themselves. This activation can occur spontaneously, but more often meditation, yogic practices, or some other spiritual disciplines are the cause. The experiences can be sometimes elevating and sometimes distressful. They appear so varied that it often becomes difficult to trace them to the same cause.

For a study of cases falling under this category a widely publicized call for case histories can prove a good beginning. There is every likelihood that responses will come from all over the world. They will provide statistical data which, I feel sure, would be enough for an unbiased scientific mind to see the prevalence of the phenomenon. Out of the respondents some might even be prepared to volunteer themselves for further investigation. This can lead to the discovery of new avenues for the research. The vast variety of symptoms would also make the investigating scientists better informed about the multilateral effects of the force on different kinds of constitutions. The study can also provide hints for the investigation of insanity caused by a morbidly active kundalini. Since the accounts of the psychotics themselves would always lack clarity and precision, the borderline cases falling into this category can prove more dependable through a study of their symptoms also.

The fifth and most important area of research would be provided by those cases who voluntarily offer themselves for the bold exploit of rousing the serpent power. Among the ardent seekers after illumination in all parts of the world, there must be some who would readily lend themselves for an undertaking of this nature. This requires the establishment of a well-managed institution where the disciplines can be given.

A hundred well-selected candidates will provide the minimum needed to show results because the phenomenon is so rare. The institution should be located in a temperate region and should be well provided with all the amenities of life. It should provide an environment in which the nobler instincts in human beings find the highest expression. There must be competent scientists and dedicated yoga specialists in the governing body of this institution. An open-minded scientific approach, without the least tinge of dogma, should be made to all problems of the research.

The activation of kundalini in even one case out of this whole lot could be an illuminating experience. The body and the mind would suddenly start to function differently. There would be an increase in the metabolic processes, pulse, etc., to adjust the system to increased production and expenditure of the new form of psychic energy. The psychic fuel feeding the brain of a mystic during his ecstasies or a genius during his productive periods is not the same energy which nourishes the brain of an average individual. This is the basic feature which investigation into the phenomenon of kundalini is meant to establish.

In the case of a powerful awakening, there occurs a riot in the energy system of the body which is perceptible, both by external observation and also subjectively, to the individual himself. It is because of this highly accelerated flow of psychic energy in all parts of the body that the phenomenon has been designated as the awakening of shakti (energy) by the ancient authorities. A virtual tornado of psychic forces appears to be let loose in the system.

Besides my own, I have come across three other cases of this type. The symptoms are unmistakable and are a part of the oral tradition. A great deal of information about the bodily reactions on the awakening can be gathered from yoga ashrams and from those conversant with the existing literature and tradition relating to the subject. The period during which the system works at an increased tempo, under the stress of the newly released energy, can extend from months to years. In the successful cases there occurs a metamorphosis of consciousness and the initiate's mental faculties might attain a bloom which he had never experienced before. Even if this supreme consummation does not come to pass, as the result of some bodily flaw, the physiological processes set afoot by the arousal are of sufficient magnitude to throw a floodlight on the phenomenon.

This brief survey is, perhaps, enough to convey an idea of the stupendous nature of this research. There is no other area of study in the vast domain of science so pregnant with undreamed-of possibilities as kundalini. It is the divine mechanism for the transformation of the whole race, from an aimless crowd of jostling, fighting individuals, unaware of themselves, into a harmonious assembly of illuminated beings who have experienced the sovereign glory of the soul. There is no other knowledge that can bring peace and happiness to strife-torn mankind, at present balanced delicately on the precipice of war, like the knowledge of this mighty illuminative power. Kundalini provides the only way to settle the long-standing conflict between reason and faith, science and religion. There is no channel other than this to validate the truth of the major faiths of the world and make known the glorious possibilities inherent in the priceless yogic tradition of India.

The knowledge gained by this investigation will bring relief to untold millions affected with mental disability or disorder of some kind. It will yield the criteria on which mankind must build its social and political orders without bloodshed and violence. It also will provide the norms for the way of thought and behavior of those individuals who are in harmony with the needs of the evolving brain.

In the light of these facts, yoga provides the greatest enterprise known to man. It is in this light that it has been regarded so far. The finished products of yoga, the great sages and rishis of India, have always been allotted a stature higher even than that of kings. From the vedic times they were held to be the knowers of eternal truths on which depend the safety, peace, and happiness of the race.

It is a pity that during recent years, amid the growth of material progress brought about by science, the divine potentialities inherent in yoga for the mental and spiritual development of the race have been almost completely ignored. The priceless boons said to be possible with it in the spiritual lore of India–illumination, supernal wisdom, intellectual and artistic bloom, psychic gifts, and other rare faculties of the mind –have not even been considered in determining the steps so far taken to initiate research on this time-honored discipline.

Investigation on the merely curative aspect of yoga reduces it to the position of an unconventional system of therapy, like acupuncture or nature cure, and on the merely physical aspect, that is asanas and pranayama, lowers it to the position of a gymnastic exercise. This investigation has its own value but it fails to represent yoga in its true light.

The real aim of yoga is to open the door to the unused potential of the human brain. There is no doubt that an enterprise of this kind is beset with difficulties, but it is the only way to rescue this science from the oblivion into which it has fallen. It is the only way by which the sovereignty of this knowledge over all other sciences of the day can be firmly established. The other sciences deal with the body. This kingly science, as the *Bhagavat Gita* calls it, deals also with the mind and the soul.

It is only through patience and humility that success is possible in this undertaking. Investigation into physical phenomena is aimed at obtaining knowledge of the dead forces of nature, but the purpose of investigation into kundalini is to win access to the intelligent forces of creation. This investigation, therefore, imposes a great responsibility on those who would undertake it. The destined hour for the empirical study of this unique phenomenon and the disclosure of the, so far, secret knowledge relating to it, I feel certain, has arrived. But it remains to be seen who will win the crown of success in the effort. In the words of the Vedas, let us pray for divine guidance, for unity of hearts and unanimity of thought in this momentous task, because kundalini provides the only solution to the most burning problems of the day.

* * * * * *

(The following remarks were offered in June 1975 by Gopi Krishna in response to some critical comments made during a seminar on kundalini research. *Editor.*)

The view that "ananda" is the hallmark of a smooth awakening needs a little clarification. Ananda is not a hallmark of awakening, but of the transcendent consciousness to which it leads. The phrase "sat–chit–ananda" refers to Brahman or universal consciousness. It is only when, after the awakening, one is firmly established in the sahaja or jivan mukta state that there is a constant experience of ananda as an inherent trait of expanded consciousness. But when, due to mental or organic flaws, the awakening is unhealthy, then it leads to the anxiety state of neurosis or the terrors of insanity. I have made this point clear in my writings.

The awakening of kundalini, whether effected by yoga practices or spontaneously, is almost always attended by certain abnormal conditions of the body and the mind. It takes months and even years for the sadhakas to adjust themselves to the flow of the new pranic energy in the body. In fact, in all the representations of the goddess Kundalini, on which the initiates are asked to meditate, she is shown granting boons with one hand and dispelling fear with the other. This idea of dispelling fear has a profound significance. It is intended to convey an assurance to the initiate that the temporary state of maladjustment in which the sense of fear predominates, especially in the tantric sadhana, will vanish and that the goddess will be gracious to him.

I have not dwelt too much on the ananda side of the samadhi or mystical experience because then we reduce the whole phenomenon to a more or less selfish, individualistic hunt for happiness. This is what has happened in India. The cases of illumination are extremely rare, but thousands of aspirants attach the suffix "ananda" to their names. In actual fact, the present-day excessive stress on ananda does not occur either in the Vedas or the Upanishads or the discourses of Buddha or even the *Bhagavat Gita.* Arjuna is overwhelmed with awe and his hair literally stands on end when he perceives the universal form of the Lord. Contact with cosmic consciousness is a stupendous experience. "Ananda" is too tame a word to express it. Inspiration, unbounded wonder, supernatural awe, intimations of immortality, an overwhelming sense of thankfulness for the grace, utter collapse of ego and pride are prominent symptoms of a genuine experience.

Kundalini is not a magical force and her awakening does not signify a sudden landing in a fabulous El Dorado of bliss. It is a stern reality denoting a gradual or sudden change in the quality and volume of bioenergy in the body. In the event of a sudden upsurge, more common with hatha yoga practices, a flaming radiance literally circulates in the system. The hatha yoga manuals call it "lightning" and the Taoist volumes refer to it as the "circulation of light or fire." The experience can be frightening in the extreme.

It is easy to understand that a sudden change in the bioenergetic economy of the body can never be "smooth" or occur without causing severe psychosomatic disturbances in the whole system. No class of scholars can understand better than scientists that no transition of consciousness from one to another dimension, involving organic changes in the brain and nervous system, can be possible without causing an upheaval in the mind and body for varying periods. It is for this reason that several of the hatha yoga practices are intended mainly to build an iron will and to win control over the respiratory, digestive, and eliminatory organs so as to combat highly disturbed conditions of the system when they occur. There is otherwise no rhyme or reason for the hazardous practices of "shat karma." The exalted stature allotted to the accomplished guru rests also on the same reason. Taught by his own experience, he alone can guide the disciple to safety in the crises.

Another very common misunderstanding, prevailing even among scholars at present, is that mysticism is one thing and yoga another. Such a supposition makes transcendence not a lawful outcome of biological evolution, but a random affair varying with the method used to attain it. The uniformity of normal human consciousness must persist in the paranormal state also, if the brain and the body are an instrument in its manifestation. Otherwise we consign it to the realm of magic and sorcery.

The mystic literature of the world is full of stories pointing to the inner conflicts and unbalanced mental conditions of mystics during the period of readjustment until they become firmly established in their new mental state. Ananda is a characteristic of samadhi, that is, of superconsciousness, when the initial stages that lead up to it have been safely passed. The very fact that popular belief associates insanity with abortive hatha yoga practices confirms what I say. Any alteration in the psychic rhythm of the body cannot be an easy affair. This is what a scientist cannot fail to recognize.

The symptoms attending the awakening of kundalini must, therefore, be present to a greater or lesser extent in the case of mystics, Sufis, and Taoists. If there is no such uniformity, it means that one law is not operating in all cases. But a study of the lives of Christian mystics, Sufis, Indian yoga saints, and other illuminati makes it abundantly clear that psychophysical stress and storm is a part of spiritual adventure. Where it does not occur, we deal with autohypnosis, autosuggestion, or hysteria in a disguised form.

It is because yoga has been isolated from mystical ecstasy that there is such a great misconception about the discipline in the West. The present-day misrepresentation of this hoary science at the hands of professionals has the same cause. In actual fact, yoga represents various systems of exercises, developed in India during the course of centuries, to induce mystical ecstasy. A thorough study of mystical literature, both of the East and the West, is therefore absolutely necessary for scientists who would embark on the investigation of the phenomenon of kundalini.

I am advocating a scientific investigation of kundalini because it would, in the long run, lead to the formulation of a symptomology of the awakening. This in turn would tend toward the discovery of the force responsible for mystical experience, samadhi, or ecstasy. The lives of Plotinus, Saint Catherine, Saint Teresa, the Sufi poets Jami and Rumi, Paramhamsa Ramakrishna and others provide a clear testimony to what I say.

The modern writers on mysticism have not failed to notice this characteristic of mental or physical unbalance among the mystics as a class. We can even trace its ramifications among mankind's great geniuses. Commenting on this aspect of mystical life, Evelyn Underhill writes in her well-known work on mysticism: "If we see in the mystics, as some have done, the sporadic beginning of a power, a higher consciousness, towards which the race slowly tends, then it seems likely enough that where it appears, nerves and organs should suffer under a stress to which they have not yet become adapted and that a spirit, more highly organized than its bodily home, should be able to impose strange conditions on the flesh. When man first stood upright a body long accustomed to going on all fours, legs which had adjusted themselves to bearing but half his weight must have rebelled against this unnatural proceeding, inflicting upon its author much pain and discomfort, if not actual illness." It is at least permissible to look upon the strange "psychophysical" state, common amongst the mystics, as just such a rebellion on the part of a normal nervous and vascular system against the experiences of a way of life to which it has not yet adjusted itself.

Most writers on mysticism are agreed on this aspect of mankind. In comments on this aspect of mystical life, which lies shrouded in mystery, the crises encountered in mystical life have been variously explained without reaching the factor at their base. The psychosomatic disciplines of yoga provide safeguards against and methods to combat the crises when they occur, but even so the period of adjustment to the higher force of life is often full of travail and suffering. This is also one of the reasons why attainment of higher consciousness has been compared to rebirth.

As regards Dr. [B.]'s questioning of my view as to whether the chakras are purely symbolic, it is enough to say that the chakras are, in fact, the nerve clusters or plexes commanding the various organs. What is symbolic are the lotuses with a specified number of petals, gods and goddesses, and the letters of the alphabet associated with them. These highly colorful picures of the chakras can be seen in any book on hatha yoga. *The Serpent Power* by Arthur Avalon contains diagrams of all of them. I have discussed this issue at length in *The Secret of Yoga.* To believe in all that the ancient treatises say would be to carry the science of kundalini into the realm of fantastic myth. The psychic force released on the awakening is felt distinctly moving in the nerve clusters and the motion is often circulatory. This gives the impression of a wheel or chakra. Further light will be thrown on the phenomenon during the course of the research.

I agree that present-day science is not yet really in a position to register more than the grosser aspects of the process. But the symptoms are so peculiar and the resultant transformation of consciousness is so striking that a new sytem can be developed on the psychosomatic syndrome characteristic of kundalini awakening. That is what every lover of science should welcome. Once it is established that the human organism behaves in a certain characteristic way on the awakening of this power or, in other words, on the flow of sublimated reproductive energy into the various organs and the brain, it will mark the beginning of a new science which can grow with the passage of time. It is to this end that I am striving. . . .

About the comments of Prof. [E.] that kundalini is said to

belong merely to the "subtle anatomy" of human beings, it may be stated that both the subtle and the gross anatomy are involved in the experiment. If only the subtle anatomy were involved, then it would have no repercussions on the gross anatomy of the body. In the human frame the gross and the subtle, that is the psychic forces and the material flesh, act and react on each other in a mysterious way. We have not been able so far to determine how this interaction comes about. The reproductive essence is a compound of concentrated nerve energy and a gross substance manufactured from the blood. On the arousal of kundalini the nerve energy is transformed into radiation and the gross material into a subtle, tonic substance which nourishes the brain cells and the nerve centers in the various organs to adjust the whole system to the circulation of a more potent form of psychic energy. It is a remarkable phenomenon and can be understood rightly only when a subject in whom the awakening has occurred is kept under observation for some time.

It is a favorite theme of many writers on kundalini yoga to say that the phenomenon belongs to the subtle anatomy of the body, and therefore cannot be investigated by the methods known to science. This is often said in the false belief that all that is written in the ancient treatises on the subject is correct to the last detail. In actual fact, the ancient writings, in conformity to the notions prevailing at the time, are a compound of fact, fiction, and myth, and it is only through properly directed research that the precious bits of accurate information contained in them can be separated, like grain from chaff. If the phenomenon is observed and studied even in one case, the findings recorded would be much different from what is contained in the ancient books. We can frame a rough idea of this difference when we compare the ancient recipes for healing drugs and potions or works on alchemy with the modern standard books on pharmacology and chemistry.

As regards the point raised by Sri [D.] about the utility of the research on kundalini, I can only say that this important issue will be dramatically decided with the first experiment on an awakened subject. If it is found that there is an evolutionary mechanism still active in human beings, both in the individual and the race as a whole, and that any violation of the laws of this evolutionary process recoils sharply both on the individual and the race, like violation of the hygienic or organic laws of the body, the highly important nature of the investigation will then at once become apparent.

Apart from the issue of nutrition, in which a worldwide study of yoga can prove beneficial, there is another field of research in which the results achieved can be even more important for mankind. We know that one of the characteristics of samadhi is said to be a sense of supernal peace and calm. In fact, a well-known Sanskrit verse characterizes cosmic consciousness as a symbol of serenity. Every Sanskrit prayer ends with a note of "shanti" (peace). It is a well-observed fact, verified by the study already done on meditating yogis, that certain healthy types of meditation tend to create a sense of repose, relaxation, and peace even in those who have to work under heavy pressure for many hours in the day. A calm and composed condition of the mind is the opposite of tension, worry, fear, and anxiety, which are common features of the average mind today.

The alarming prevalence of psychopathic conditions and psychosis, especially among the advanced industrial nations of our time, is well known. Any preventive methods or disciplines that can bring peace and serenity to the tormented multitudes should, therefore, be the primary concern of a world health organization. If supernal peace is a marked feature of samadhi or mystical ecstasy, and if yoga or other spiritual disciplines tend to calm the restlessness of ruffled minds, it clearly betokens that there is something in these practices which has a salutary effect on the nervous system and the brain which results in the calming down of agitated states.

It is needless for me to reiterate that this calming effect is exercised by the bioenergy released by kundalini. Even if the power is not awakened as in the case of the illuminated, the radiation let free in the system by means of meditational exercises acts to cause a calming effect on the cerebrospinal system. It is the lack of knowledge of the evolutionary process and of the mode of life which it demands that is responsible for the present-day hectic conditions of the human mind. Nature does not intend man to be a bundle of uncontrollable complexes and compulsions, tormented by fear and anxiety, but a serene, happy being at peace with himself and the world at large.

The connection between genius and insanity has been noticed from very early times. Aristotle made a clear statement of it when he said: "Famous poets, artists and statesmen frequently suffer from melancholy or madness as did Ajax . . . Such a disposition occurred in Socrates, Empedocles, Plato and many others but especially in our poets." Lombroso unequivocally labeled genius as madness. "The paradox that confounds genius with neurosis," he said, "however cruel and sad it may be, is found to be not devoid of solid foundations." George Pickering in his recent work, *Creative Malady*, ascribes the outstanding work done by some of the great geniuses of our time to psychoneurosis. He writes: "My examination of the personalities here considered, their achievements and their illnesses, has led me to conclude that the world is indebted to their illnesses for the great contributions they made to their own times and to posterity." Most writers on genius are agreed on the borderline mental condition of high talent.

The connection between delirium and prophecy has also been noticed from very ancient times. Plato affirms this in his *Phaedo*. The idea that insanity and clairvoyance are interconnected is still prevalent in India and the Middle East. Psychopathic clairvoyants are regarded with awe and veneration by the masses at many places. There are words in Hebrew, Sanskrit, Persian, and Arabic which apply both to God-intoxication and madness.

These facts make it clear that for some inexplicable reason mystics on the one hand and men and women of genius on the other are much more prone to mental aberration, neurosis, or insanity than the average people. If to this is added the fact that mental and nervous disorders are on the increase in the advanced nations, the conclusion becomes unavoidable that increased sensibility and intellectual advancement tend to critical mental conditions in the mystics and geniuses and to a greater incidence of psychic disorder in the average people for some reason which is unknown to us at present.

The great Shankaracharya refers to the often observed unconventional behavior of the awakened in these words: "Established in the ethereal plane of absolute knowledge, he wanders in the world, sometimes like a madman, sometimes like a child and at other times like a ghoul, having no other clothes on his person except the quarters, or sometimes wearing clothes or perhaps skins at other times." Such a mode of conduct does not appear abhorrent or abnormal when enlightenment is regarded as union with the Absolute, demanding withdrawal from the world and freedom from its binding customs and conventions. But if enlightenment denotes a rise to another level of consciousness–the future normal awareness of human beings–then any kind of abnormality needs to be viewed in a different light.

In that case the inference would be that expanded states of consciousness impose a strain on the psychosomatic organism which it is not fully equipped to carry, resulting in derangement and disorder both mental and physical. Reared in religious traditions, we are often prone to regard the enlightened as superhuman beings in possession of miraculous powers or as supernormal siddhis. But a dispassionate survey of this lofty class of human beings cannot fail to show that they were as much exposed to the pressure of circumstances and as vulnerable to disease and decay as other mortals. Shankaracharya passed away at the young age of about thirty-two years as the result of an intestinal disorder. Two other great saints of India in our time, Rama Tirtha and Vivekananda, also died young, the former by drowning in the Ganges. On the other hand, the far-famed Ramanuja, who basically differed from Shankara's monistic philosophy, and founded his own system of Visistha-advaita, breathed his last at the advanced age of one hundred and twenty-five years.

I am entering into these details to show that a realistic approach to the phenomenon of mystical ecstasy or illumination cannot fail to reveal certain points of basic similarity between the illuminati and the other types of genius. Mental aberration or abnormal behavior is one of these points of resemblance. A passionate, single-minded pursuit of one idea, one aim, or one line of inquiry is another. Extraordinary insight or inspiration is the third. Variable moods—productive spells and barren periods in the case of geniuses and ecstatic intervals followed by return to banality in the case of mystics—is the fourth. Intense absorption in creative work in the case of the former, and in the contemplation of inner realities in the latter provides still another point of resemblance and there are others besides.

It is evident that mystical consciousness is an advanced form of genius, but genius nevertheless, and shares both its disabilities and its benefits. In the vast majority of cases the great prophets and mystics known to history were either born with the gift or had a natural predisposition for a contemplative life. They excelled the other geniuses in the possession of psychic or so-called "miraculous" powers and in the illuminative contacts with transcendent realities beyond the reach of normal perception. In other words, the two groups represent the same phenomenon in a more or less developed form.

Contact with transcendent realities does not carry with it the guarantee that one can become all-knowing or all-powerful or can overrule the biological limitations of the body. Transcendence can be a lopsided development with superconsciousness at one end, and a childlike ignorance of the world at the other. The same disproportionate structure we often see in genius also. This is the reason why geniuses in science succeeded far better than the illuminati in transforming the environment and the temporal life of man and why individuals of ordinary ability but sound common sense often fared better in the battle of life than the geniuses, in spite of the great difference in their mental endowment.

The religious lore of mankind has emanated from the spiritual geniuses in the same way as the original works on art, science, and philosophy emanated from the geniuses in these departments of knowledge and culture. There is only a difference of degree between "inspiration," "revelation," or "flash of discovery." The basic mechanism is the same. All systems of yoga are designed to bring about the ecstatic state of the born mystic, even in those not born with the endowment. But in spite of the fact that millions take to the various disciplines, drawn by the lure of the occult, success in the enterprise is extremely rare.

The accomplished yogi, according to the criteria laid down in the *Bhagavat Gita* and other scriptural lore of India, must be an embodiment of serenity, inner happiness, and supernal wisdom (*jnana*). But this ideal is seldom, if ever, realized. The disciplines are oriented to create such a condition, but the biological factors and survival instincts combine to create a conflict which finally results in the emergence of a lopsided or emotionally unstable personality. The great task lying in front of the illuminati of the future would be to make the transition from the normal to transcendental consciousness as smooth and safe as possible. The accomplished products of this culture would be the real progenitors of the "superman" to come.

Can we not draw the momentous conclusion from all this evidence that there is some latent common factor in mystical ecstasy, genius, and the sociocultural advancement of nations which expresses itself in certain aberrant mental conditions or in their increased ratio in some populations? If this is accepted, it would mean that it is not "civilization" which is to be blamed for various kinds of neuroses, as held by Freud and some other psychologists, but our own ignorance and defiance of a biological law which is at the root of civilization itself—that is, the law of organic evolution.

If both these points are conceded, does it not mean that modern science is up against a still-unresolved enigma in the human body which is responsible not only for mystical experience, exceptional talent or psychosocial evolution of humans, but also for the creation of unstable mental conditions, especially in the first two categories? This enigma, I affirm, is kundalini. It is clear from the old esoteric volumes on this fabulous reservoir of bioenergy that the psychic effects we have discussed were known even to the ancient authorities. Considering the fact that mental health, especially among the leading personalities, is of incalculable value for the peace, happiness, and survival of mankind, it is high time that a wide ranging program of research on yoga and kundalini should be undertaken. If this is done there is every possibility that methods would be found to combat and control these conditions. The critical situation of the world at present and the possibilities of total destruction through modern technology make this investigation even more imperative.

Kundalini is still a fringe subject, shrouded in mystery and myth, and it will take a good deal of time and labor by dedicated savants to put the whole phenomenon on a scientific basis. But even so, inner transformation will remain beyond the reach of objective study. It is only through the inspiration and the utterances of the illuminated subjects that transcendental knowledge of mind and consciousness will become available to the race. There is no other channel to reach the ineffable.

KUNDALINI ENERGY

M. S. S. Gurucharan Singh Khalsa and Sadhu Singh Khalsa

During the last twenty years the Western world has developed a growing interest in self-induced, non-chemical, altered states of consciousness, and in the controlled application of these states of consciousness for the promotion of physical, mental, and spiritual growth. The source for many of the techniques used to induce these ASCs is the Eastern spiritual tradition. Among the most outstanding methods of this genre is the practice of yoga and meditation. As meditation has grown in popularity, the need to understand its effects in Western terms has greatly increased.

Yoga is a vast field of knowledge. To properly understand the structure of consciousness via the study of the altered states induced by yoga, an investigator might practice and test techniques for a lifetime and still fail. Fortunately there are a number of approaches, schools, or paths that can be taken to gain an optimum result with a minimum of perfectly executed effort.

All yogas ultimately deal with the same basic theme—the raising of kundalini. How different systems approach this and how they refer to kundalini will differ according to the contents and environments the teaching emphasizes.

If we want to know more about the process of change that yoga brings about, then we have to experiment with the techniques and try to understand the energy and structure of the change process itself—that is, the kundalini.

In studying the kundalini energy, we commit ourselves to

the study of the whole human being. We cannot simply concern ourselves with isolated parts of individual consciousness, but we must deal with the integration of the entire range of human potentialities. Furthermore, our study is not restricted to the cultures of the East, since the kundalini has also been referred to in the myths and methodologies of many ancient Western cultures. It is recognized in the tribal lore of North and South America as well as in the scriptures of the Far East. The psychologist Jung, an expert in the study of cross cultural symbols in relation to the individual, considers the process of kundalini to be a universal archetype (energy) in the growth of the psyche.

The kundalini is said to be the primary essential energy underlying consciousness and its integrative transformations. Without understanding its myths and mysteries, the depth of human potential will remain largely untapped. Yet, it is only since 1969 that the wealth of secret technical knowledge that can lead to this understanding has become available in an undiluted form. At this time, Siri Singh Sahib Bhai Sahib Harbhajan Singh Khalsa Yogiji [Yogi Bhajan], a master of kundalini yoga, began teaching in the United States. As we separate myth from scientific facts in testing the ancient claims he has presented to us, we can learn to use the kundalini technology to enhance our life and improve our understanding of the fundamental energies of the cosmos.

Although interest in meditative states has grown rapidly, there are many obstacles to systematic scientific studies of those states. The needed methodologies through which we can approach the subject remain largely undeveloped. A common language in which we can define our terms and state our hypothesis has not yet been created. The techniques of meditation themselves have been hard to acquire. Objective measures for states of consciousness that we can describe subjectively are not available. Nor has a clearcut avenue of approach yet been established: some investigators are testing exceptional individuals, while others are exploring specified techniques that apply to everyone. In trying to solve these and other methodological problems, the field of consciousness research is making its transition to a new self-awareness and validity. Until it reaches a more stable point in its evolution, even the results attained with reliable "standard" tests must be accepted only tentatively. This is the time for pioneering efforts: it is time to learn how to apply our old scientific tools in unfamiliar territories, and develop new tools for the understanding of consciousness. Ultimately, we have to develop "state-specific sciences" that will take into account the consciousness of the investigator as well as the data derived from the subject of the experiment.

In the late nineteenth century, the founders of psychology spoke freely of such things as "consciousness," "will," "desire," "soul," etc. William James, in his classic *Varieties of Religious Experience,* gave several descriptive accounts of altered states of consciousness and psychic research in the exploration of the human mind. The comparative study of altered states of consciousness was considered valuable in understanding the basic nature of the mind and the structure of normal waking-state consciousness. The phenomenological descriptions that arose, however, were clumsy and unscientific. In response to this imprecision, the materialistic attitudes of behaviorism were pushed into the forefront of psychological research. With these ideas came new attempts at developing a more precise language for dealing with the mind and its energies. This language excluded most "internal experiences" and "states of consciousness" in favor of outwardly observable behavior. Along these same lines, many advances were made in the study of physiological psychology. Investigators turned to neural chemistry for more scientific explanations of human consciousness.

From the experience of these years, scientists became much more sophisticated in their approach to a terminology of consciousness. With the availability of altered states of consciousness for study within the drug culture of the 1960s, and the popularity of meditation of the 1970s, the language has been further refined. Writers such as Charles Tart of the University of California at Davis have been stimulated to create new paradigms for researching consciousness. On the basis of these paradigms, we can formulate meaningful questions and expect meaningful answers. Yet, even greater sophistication must be attained before we can expect to make sense of our findings. We are faced with a conundrum similar to that classic problem encountered by a group of investigators while studying the language of the Eskimos. Many Eskimo statements seemed superstitious, irrelevant, or nonsensical until the researchers realized that Eskimos are sensitive to things that we are not. They can sense subtle differences in the quality of snow that have functional implications and meaning for them, but are not even distinguishable to outsiders. Consequently, they have more than a dozen words for snow, many of which seem redundant to us, but which are necessary to distinguish the many subtle states of snow. Similarly, the native traveler in altered states of consciousness may report subtle changes or invent terms that are not meaningful to "outsider" psychologists whose paradigms relate to nothing but stimulus, feeling, and response. What is needed is a language that is sophisticated enough to distinguish between very subtle states of consciousness, yet can also communicate the differences in measurable terms.

Even with Tart's excellent start in developing a more sophisticated language, we are still faced with the problem of finding reliable units of measure to work with. Even if we could define a state of consciousness in terms of space/time perception, identity, exteroception, memory, kinesthetic sensation, and certain other psychological measures, it would be difficult, if not impossible, to measure these parameters without disturbing the state of consciousness we are trying to study. To obtain the information needed to form a reliable scale of measurement, we would have to change the state that gave rise to that information.

Another related problem is the difficulty faced in trying to induce the same altered state of consciousness in a group of test subjects. To deal with this difficulty, many investigators have chosen to test exceptional individuals. Others have taught standard techniques for experiencing a particular altered state of consciousness to ordinary individuals and then measured the final states attained. Such an approach has been well established by practitioners of kundalini yoga.

The standard techniques used to induce a particular altered state of consciousness in this method are called *kriyas.* A kriya is a sequence of physical and mental actions that affect body, mind, and spirit concurrently. These sequences of action may include only meditation, or exercise, or both, but in any case, the combination must constitute a complete stimulation of all systems relevant to a particular change in consciousness.

In each case the kriya has specific claims associated with it. Every form of exercise is not a kriya. To shift gears in a car you do not randomly push the clutch, pump the gas, and move the gear shift lever. To change gears you must sequentially go through each step and you must coordinate the engine speed, the clutch, and proper sequence of changing gear ratios. Similarly, to shift the state of consciousness a number of systems, both physical and mental, must be stimulated and coordinated to create a stable change. Kriyas code these particular combinations in an extremely subtle way and control how the various energy systems interlock. There are kriyas associated with each area of human potential. The ancient designers of kriyas did not conceive of a "single" mystical state. There are many stable states other than the norm of a particular culture.

Each kriya will produce a different effect. Some kriyas bring understanding and illumination, others produce fear and depression, others create physical and mental stability, others develop sensitivity, and still others lead to rapid changes in identity and physical condition through a direct awakening of the kundalini energy.

Because of the range of these effects, each kriya must be tested by itself. We must be careful not to presume that there is only one state, called "meditation," that is a common effect of all kriyas, or else we will fall into the same bind as the researchers of Eskimos who could not differentiate between the numerous states of snow. Fortunately, it is possible to train large numbers of subjects in each kriya, or one subject in several. This allows us to make comparative studies between kriyas and to factor out the individual differences.

If the data from an experiment is to make sense and if duplication is to be possible, then all the parameters that define a kriya must be specified. It is not sufficient for scientific reports to say the subject practiced kundalini meditation or TM or Zen. The exact posture, breathing, concentration, imagery, mantra, duration, time of day, etc. must be specified.

It must be emphasized that not all meditations or exercises taught by various organizations and traditions are kriyas. Consequently, the results of the practice are not always predictable or stable. Each kriya, when mastered, gives the practitioner easy and immediate access to a particular state of emotion or consciousness. Paramahansa Yogananda followed this concept and offers a few well-defined kriyas to test. Certain exercises in Zen such as breath counting exercises with a point of concentration are kriyas but other Zen exercises are not. Once a kriya is understood it can be critically used to adjust temporary "problem states" in consciousness. For example, some mantras used in TM are real "bij" or seed mantras, others are not. Of those that are (such as *hum, sohang,* or *ainga*) some potent effects are possible. Almost none of the TM techniques are kriyas because they are not integrated with breath, concentration, visualization, etc. Consequently, partial effects sometimes get established. Also, the techniques of a particular teaching group may move people to a state with different physiological characteristics, but what state those changes really represent is a very open question. It may be a state of ecstasy, of withdrawal, of integration, or of disintegration. Because of its sociopsychological implications, the answer to this question will be a major aim of investigators in the next decade.

In pursuing the approach of specifically defined parameters, there is reason to believe that comprehensive paradigms can eventually be developed that will adequately encompass the entire range of consciousness change using kriyas and their effects as a central construct in the models.

Ultimately, this will have to be done if we are to understand the human consciousness in its full range of manifestation.

Any methodological limitations that we are likely to encounter stem from our conceptual models of the universe. How we approach the study of consciousness depends upon our conception of what consciousness is. Most psychological experimenters understand reality as an interaction between matter and energy that occurs within well-defined boundaries of space and time. The strong materialist-reductionist philosophy that was popular at the turn of the century still tends to restrict our study of consciousness to the matter/energy dynamic of neural chemistry. Within the framework of this conceptual model, consciousness is reduced to a mere epiphenomenon that results from more basic electrochemical interactions. As Tart points out:

> An almost universal theory in western scientific circles, sunk to the level of an implicit belief and thus controlling us effectively, is that awareness is a product of brain functioning. No brain functioning, no consciousness.[1]

In effect, it is our conceptual paradigms that create a major stumbling block to our scientific investigation of mind and consciousness. In a similar vein, Davidson discusses the plight of the experimentalist who

> feels compelled to limit himself to considering physical or behavioral variables in order to comply with the dominant physicalist-reductionist paradigm of modern science.[2]

This type of bias leads to research efforts that define states of consciousness solely in terms of physiological parameters. Although physiological changes that accompany some altered states of consciousness are certainly relevant to research, *they are not sufficient in themselves to define the specific states we are trying to study*. Physiological factors simply reflect some of the many relationships that exist between the various levels of systems on which awareness encodes itself.

Even in these reflections there is an inherent ambiguity in

interpretation. The famous experiments by Singer and Schacter proved that two opposing emotional states could be precipitated with the same physiological change if the cognitive set was different. So the mind and the cognitive understanding of experiential events is a critical and irreducible element in what determines the final state of experience and consciousness.[3]

It is probable that in addition to the relations that are reflected in the physiological variables, there are other relations that can only be reflected in more subtle dimensions, not measurable by our standard instruments. There can be changes in radiant energy fields, in elementary particle structure, in the aura, etc. There may even be dimensions of consciousness that cannot be put into any of the terms of the classical approach of physical materialism. So research should proceed wholeheartedly but with caution against claiming too many conclusions on simple material changes. At best we are looking at fragments of complex organic changes that affect all levels of the human being's existence.

The possibility that awareness is not just an epiphenomenon of neural chemistry is now being seriously considered by many physicists, biologists, and some psychologists. According to Tart, the reason for this new open-mindedness is

> . . . the existence of first-class data to suggest that awareness may be something other than a product of the brain. I refer to excellent evidence of parapsychological phenomena like telepathy—evidence that shows that the mind can sometimes function in ways that are impossible in terms of our current physical view of the world.[4]

While scientists are just beginning to open up to reality that transcends the physical, it is interesting to note that yogis and mystics down through the ages have considered the merely physical universe to be nothing but an illusion, the play of maya. The conceptual paradigm that is based on this illusion is simply the result of relating to finite limitation rather than infinity. As Yogi Bhajan says, "The first principle is Ek Ong Kar—a complete interconnectedness between everything in the cosmos." Lama Govinda, a Tibetan Buddhist, puts it this way:

> The external world and the inner world are for the Buddhist only two sides of the fabric, in which the threads of all forces and of all events, of all forms of consciousness and of their objects are woven into an inseparable net of endless, mutually conditioned relations.[5]

In this view of the world, consciousness is an integral part of the cosmos that helps to create and define all other parts. It is not limited to space/time structures, but also serves to encompass realities that are not determined by space and time considerations.

But the realization that consciousness extends beyond the confines of the universe of matter/energy dynamics is by no means limited to Eastern philosophies. Penfield, a great Western neurophysiologist, studied the brain thoroughly in all its patterns and physiological mechanisms trying to relate consciousness to brain functioning. After decades of research, he concluded that physiological brain mechanisms cannot explain the mind. He questioned:

> Can reflex action in the end account for it (action of Mind)? After many years of studying the emerging mechanisms within the human brain, my own answer is "No." Mind comes into action and goes out of action with the highest brain mechanism, it is true. But the mind has energy. The form of the energy is different from that of neuronal potentials that travel the axon pathways.[6]

The conceptual framework of nineteenth-century physics does not prepare us to deal with such a possibility. However, with the emergence of modern quantum physics, Western sciences have begun to move toward the same conclusion that the yogis and mystics have accepted all along. The emphasis is no longer on particular units, individuals, or particles, but on relationships. Werner Heisenberg describes the universe from this view:

> . . . as a complicated tissue of events, in which connections of different kinds alternate or overlap or combine and thereby determine the texture of the whole.[7]

Modern physics is now laying a conceptual framework that parallels the idea of interconnectedness taken for granted by the yogis when explaining the nature of energy and consciousness. For those familiar with these ideas, paranormal phenomena is no longer seen outside the realm of rational explanation. A survey by *New Scientist* revealed that 67 per cent of responding readers (mostly scientists) consider ESP to be an established fact or likely possibility, and 88 per cent thought the investigations to be legitimate.[8] A recent paper by Stanford Research Institute offers the conclusion that:

> . . . these phenomena are not at all inconsistent with the framework of modern physics . . . [the] often-held view that observations of this type are a priori incompatible with known laws is erroneous in that such a concept is based on the naive realism prevalent before the development of quantum theory and information theory.[9]

Along with this evolution in our understanding of energy relations, we are also witnessing a major re-evaluation of the role of consciousness in the overall scheme of things. What was once considered an epiphenomenon is now becoming a central focal point of interest with its own indisputable reality.

The implications of this new understanding echo to the core of the scientific method itself. John Wheeler, a leading theoretical physicist, points out that because of the nature of consciousness, the observer and his involvement in an experiment is a determining factor in the outcome of that experiment. He even suggests replacing the term "observer" with "participant" to remind us of how central and active the effect of consciousness is. Eugene Wigner, Nobel prize winner in physics, says:

> It seems more likely that living matter is actually influenced by what it clearly influences: consciousness.

> The description of this phenomenon clearly requires the incorporation of concepts into our laws of nature which are foreign to the present laws of physics. Perhaps the relation of consciousness to matter is not too dissimilar to the relation of light to matter as it was known in the last century.[10]

To modern physicists, then, consciousness has acquired a significance greater than that which is attributed to it by most psychologists.

In recent work, physical theorists such as Helliwell, Tiller, and Hettel consider some of the higher mechanisms of the mind in terms of elementary energy particles, such as neutrinos, photons, and tachyons. A neutrino is a chargeless, massless particle. A photon consists of a neutrino and its opposite, an anti-neutrino, which is capable of passing through matter at the speed of light. With these characteristics, such particles could conceivably serve as carriers for clairvoyant images. The tachyon, which moves even faster than light, could also conceivably carry information from the future. N. Kozyrev has proposed a theory that time is related to an energy density that is affected by rotating masses and other active processes. With such a conceptualization, it is possible now to explain how psychics can be affected by catastrophic events taking place miles away or in the future.

While theories such as these remain only educated speculations, they serve to show the emergence of an advanced modern approach to a type of energy phenomenon that is closely linked to an understanding of the mind, the higher brain functions, and human consciousness. These theories give courage to the psychological researchers of consciousness who would deny the physical reductionist view of the world and offer new approaches that take consciousness as a valid, important, and real phenomenon worthy of serious study. It is in the light of this newly emerging attitude toward consciousness that the necessary methodologies will soon develop.

The study of kundalini as an energy and a primary force in the structure and transformation of consciousness provides a particularly promising avenue of approach in the development of such languages and methodologies.

In theory, the kundalini energy can provide a tangible link between conscious experiential states and physiological variables. One of the keys to this link will be found in the proper study of the many kundalini kriyas whose structures, processes, and effects lead to specific and repeatable altered states of consciousness.

Review of Some Pilot Studies

With these conceptual foundations in mind, we have begun a number of pilot studies to determine avenues of inquiry that might prove worthy of investigation. What follows is a brief discussion of these studies and their implications for the direction of future research.

STUDIES IN BIOENERGETICS

Since quantum physicists are comfortable with the possibility of higher energy fields, and since this area could add perspective to all our other efforts, we decided to look at a few experiments that may relate to these energies. The experiments we did focused on "laying on of hands," energy exchanges that are induced by certain yogic kriyas, and the phenomenon of kirlian photography.

The yogic sutras, as well as most popular works on yoga, claim that certain exercises or meditations can help to develop the ability to consciously transfer healing energies to other living systems. As this concept has become more plausible to those in mainstream science, a few good investigations have been done that support the existence of these healing energy exchanges. M. J. Smith found that trypsin, a digestive enzyme, decreased its rate of activity when it was damaged by ultraviolet light and increased activity when exposed to a high intensity magnetic field. She further discovered that when a solution of water and damaged trypsin was held between the hands of some recognized healers for up to seventy-two minutes, the rate of activity would increase.[11] One possible explanation for this effect is that the structural damage might have somehow been repaired or compensated for by an exchange of energy from the healer. The same effect was seen on the undamaged trypsin and was comparable to the effects of the increased magnetic field.

Rather than determining the physical mechanisms behind such an occurrence, or measuring physical changes in chemical structures, we chose to test a biological response to the hypothesized energy exchange resulting from the practice of a yogic kriya. We were encouraged in this direction by the excellent experimental work of Bernard Grad, a physiologist at McGill University. Grad did a series of well controlled double blind experiments which showed that the percentage of germinations and the growth heights of barley seeds could be significantly increased by using water "treated" by the hands of a known healer.[12]

Hypothesizing that it might be possible to observe a biological response to healing energy, we selected a kundalini kriya that is "known" to produce such energy in its practitioners. In place of Grad's measures of germination percentages and changes in height we measured the percentage of cells in onions that showed mitotic activity. At the beginning of the experiment, R. Yaeger and G. S. Khalsa randomly mixed onion sprouts into control and experimental groups. An experienced yogic practitioner performed a breathing meditation* for fifteen minutes. He then held his hands in a fixed position about two feet from the experimental plants for another fifteen minutes. At a different place on the same floor of the building, a control subject sat at the same distance in the same position relative to control plants, but did not do the kriya. Both people were told that we were investigating the reaction of plants to their presence.

After repeating this treatment for four days, the onions

* Details of the meditative procedures used in this experiment are available upon request from the author.

were soaked in a 1 per cent colchicine solution. Colchicine is a chemical which stops the mitotic process by interfering with the spindle mechanism. By staining the cells, it is possible to detect this stoppage. The root tips of both the experimental and control group onions were carefully sliced and put on slides. A standard counting procedure gave a measure of the percentage of cells that had divided in each sample. The results were analyzed statistically with the test, indicating a significant difference with $p \leq .001$. The experimental group showed an increase in cell divisions of 108 per cent.[13]

From this experiment, we cannot infer what mechanisms were operative, nor can we say for sure that this kriya was critical in producing the effect without doing more experiments. The biological response in onion mitosis witnessed in the performance of this kriya must be compared with that of other kriyas performed in the same situation to determine if the critical factor is the kriya itself or simply a certain cognitive set.

We did another study in which an inexperienced subject performed the same kriya and held his hands over flasks of sealed water. This time, the kriya was done for ten minutes in one session only. The sealed water was mixed with flasks of untreated water in double blind fashion and administered to an experimental and control group of plants. Again, we saw an increase (>30 per cent) in the plants receiving treated water but the significance was not as high ($.1 < p < .15$). This experiment needs to be done with more people in repeated sessions to give clarity to the results. If it is in fact possible to obtain significant results with untrained individuals, then it is also possible to train individuals to heal! The fact that basic cellular processes can be affected by the practice of a kundalini kriya gives us an indication that physiochemical measures of healing activity can be developed by future research. Other investigators have also seen evidence for this. D. Dean, for example, has recorded a shift in the infrared spectroscope and an increase in surface tension of water treated by healers.[14,15]

Another area of research that has stimulated much interest,

speculation, and controversy in the realm of energy studies is kirlian photography. Kirlian photography is a process that creates photographic images via high voltage, high frequency discharges through a target object. The electrical coronas created by this technique are visually exciting and seem to show unusual characteristics that correlate to some subjective and emotional states of consciousness. If this technique did in fact produce a measurable parameter that correlated uniquely with subjective states, it would be a great leap forward for investigators of consciousness. Unfortunately the initial speculations about this possibility have been effectively countered by the extensive research of W. Tiller at Stanford.[16] He has shown that the current state of the art in kirlian technology does not yet provide such a measurable parameter. He can produce a wide range of kirlian coronas by altering finger pressure, frequency, film type, electrode, and angle of pressure. Before a reliable standard of measurement can be developed, all of these and other variables need to be controlled. A wave of newly improved instruments may open this possibility again in the near future.

Much of the interest in kirlian photography comes from the close parallel between the properties of the electrical coronas and the properties of "auras" reported by yogis and psychics. The aura is an intermediate energy field that surrounds and penetrates the physical body. It purportedly reflects physical and mental changes and is a medium through which many mental phenomena can be explained. The Russian researchers have termed this energy field "bioplasma." This bioplasma is not considered to be a simple byproduct of cellular activity, but something more fundamental.[17]

One experiment that supports this theory is the lost-leaf effect. The Russians reported, and it was duplicated by T. Moss in kirlian photographs, that the electrical coronas of leaves that had 10–20 per cent of their tips removed, did not follow the cut edge but instead followed the outlines of the whole leaf! The energy field for the leaf tip was evident even though the cells of the leaf were not there to give rise to it.[18] H. S. Burr and others have proposed that it is this surrounding energy field that supplies information to the living system about how to grow and define its shape.[19]

Although all of this must remain speculative for now, kirlian photography offers the promising possibility of working with the radiant energy fields of living systems. Although much better instrumentation must be developed, this technique is a potential tool for dealing experimentally with new field concepts. Recognizing the difficulties inherent in developing sufficient controls and interpreting the results obtained with such new techniques, we conducted several experiments to look for effects of kriyas on the surrounding energy fields of the body/mind.

Rama Kirn Singh and Shama Kirn Singh did an experiment in which they looked at the kirlian photographs of patients in a psychiatric ward of a state hospital. They explored the characteristics of the fingertip coronas of depressed and manic patients in drugged and undrugged states using a portable kirlian device. The observable differences between drugged and undrugged states obtained in this experiment provided a reference standard for comparison that could then be used to measure other differences in states of consciousness as indicated by the particular device they were using.

Next, they then took photos of students from kundalini yoga classes before and after exercising, and of people attending a tantric yoga course taught by Yogi Bhajan. The students from classes showed a wide range of effects. Although changes were noticeable, there was no good base for interpretation. The participants in the tantric course consistently showed a large, even increase in their blue-white coronas, compared to no increase in non-participants at the same event.[20]

At a conference at California State College at Sonoma, Yogi Bhajan verbally guided both an experienced meditator and a conference member who was new to meditation through several states of meditation. Both subjects showed large changes in the structure and size of the kirlian coronas, and reported themselves to have attained significant alterations in their conscious state. It is interesting to note that the beginner's final kirlian photographs from meditation were similar in structure and size to the initial photos of the experienced meditator. As the experienced subject was instructed to go into different states, the changes in the corona were outstanding. Although the circumstances did not allow for extensive controls, its results combined with the other pilot studies suggested that we should look more carefully at the possibility of observing differences between kriyas in kirlian coronas.[21]

In another study, G. S. Khalsa selected seven meditations that were different in their physical requirements and that reportedly produced different effects. Five subjects were asked to do each of the seven meditations in mixed order, while five controls were asked to simply sit quietly. The subjects sat in the isolated chamber at Moss's laboratory at UCLA, while J. Hubacher assisted and took the kirlian photographs.

Controls who just sat quietly in the chamber showed a slight overall increase in the size of their coronas (an effect that is commonly associated with relaxation) but exhibited no other major structural changes. Six of the meditations produced expansions and structural changes much greater than shown by the controls. Since we photographed all ten fingertips we were also able to notice a fingertip-specific effect. Each kriya would expand the corona of some fingertips and decrease the corona of others. The effect varied for different individuals. The corona changes induced by each kriya were generally similar for all five meditations, but not consistently.

The most interesting result was obtained with the seventh meditation. It was presented just as the others were, but it gave results opposite to the rest of the kriyas. The yogic claim for this meditation is that it would create a temporary state of negativity of depression in order to expose certain subconscious elements in the cônscious mind. In three out of five subjects, the corona almost disappeared. The remaining two showed diminished structures. Their photos resembled those of depressed patients.[22]

The results suggest there exist real differences between the states created by different meditations. Before we can count kirlian photography as a useful technique in exploring these differences, however, we need better equipment, tighter technical controls, and more precise measurements of verbal and nonverbal cues that induce cognitive set.

PHYSIOLOGICAL STUDIES

In the yogic system, it is claimed that the rhythm, depth, and form of breathing can be used to alter consciousness, promote healing, and increase physical capacities. The acceptance of distinct differences between right and left nostril breathing, for example, is central to the conceptual structure of kundalini yoga as a healing system. The yogis claim that although the nostrils both lead to the same major air pathway, left and right nostril breathing have opposite effects on the body and consciousness. They also claim that each individual has a regular biorhythm in which the predominance of breath flowing through any one nostril at any one time alternates. The time period given for this nasal cycle varies with the source that lists it. Swami Vishnu Devananda claims a 110-minute rhythm, whereas Yogi Bhajan claims that a two-and-a-half-hour cycle (or 150 minutes) is most conducive for a balanced, healthy individual.

Western professionals in general have taken little notice of breath as a major determinant of consciousness. Some psychological approaches such as bioenergetics use breath as an emotional release mechanism but the techniques used are much less sophisticated than those of the well-developed kundalini yoga system. Breath has been used only slightly in the more traditional Western psychologies because very little research has been done to relate breath and consciousness.

To begin a systematic study of breathing in kundalini yoga, we first asked a dozen volunteers to note every fifteen minutes throughout a normal day whether they were breathing predominantly through one nostril or the other, or equally through both. These subjective records showed several things: 1) all three conditions (of left nostril, right nostril, and equal dominance) were observed to exist; 2) the state recorded least was equal nostril breathing; 3) breathing dominance did not randomly switch back and forth (L equals R); 4) environmental conditions such as an accident or eating a large meal seemed to correlate with the nasal cycle shifts; 5) the time period of these cyclical shifts varied from one and a half to three hours; and 6) most subjects tended to show a predominant left nostril breath at sunset, and a right nostril breath just after sunrise or after awakening.

In searching the literature we found seventeen significant references dealing with the nasal cycle in the period from 1895 to 1975. The investigators unequivocably establish the existence of the nasal cycle in humans and report an average cycle time to be two and a half hours. This agrees with the kundalini yoga literature which points out that the cycle in each nostril is not triggered by the cycle of the other as a reflex. Instead the controlling area is deeper in the central nervous system. J. T. Connell, a clinical researcher, noticed nasal resistance could be altered by changing the light intensity directed to an eye.[23] There were no connections made, however, linking the nasal cycle to states of consciousness, to hemispheric dominance, to perceptual styles, or to the stages of sleep and its related phenomena. None of the authors dealt with yogic-related ideas, nor did they attempt to alter internal physiological or psychological states by regulating this external cycle.

To check whether the nasal cycle continued in sleep, we observed one subject during a night's sleep for a period of five hours. The airflow through each nostril was measured with thermocouples. The thermocouples were connected to a Beckman dynograph and the airflow through each nostril recorded on EEG graph paper. The nasal cycle was observed in this particular subject to oscillate every two hours.[24]

The results of this preliminary study were encouraging. We are now conducting several well controlled experiments with much better equipment and computer correlation.

In another pilot experiment conducted by Khalsa and Raynor at UCR, the nasal cycle in a subject was measured simultaneously with changes in sleep state to see if any relationship could be found between the periodicity of these two cycles. The experiment showed tendencies for the nasal cycle to shift at the onset of each new REM period. Since only one subject was observed we cannot form any definite connections about the actual relationship, but these preliminary results strongly suggest the value of further experimentation in this area.[25]

Another yogic claim related to breath is that left and right nostril breathing activate different areas of the brain, and create different subjective experiences. Yogi Bhajan has said, "Actually, we have two souls, a left soul, and a right soul. The brain is divided into four parts: the front, the back, the left and the right. When the left nostril works, the right brain works; when the right nostril works, the left brain works. They work alternately in two and one half hour cycles to keep the body temperature normal." This mention of left and right "soul" is in line with the current trend in psychology to talk about hemispheric functions. Ornstein in his book *Psychology of Consciousness* writes that the words "feminine or moon" (associated with left nostril) and "masculine or sun" (associated with right nostril) can be correlated respectively to the right and left hemispheres of the brain. The tendency to separate these brain functions is found in many cultures. The Hopi Indians, for example, say the right hand is for writing and the left is for making music. Ornstein relates this cultural observation to studies on epileptic patients. When the two hemispheres of the brain were surgically separated in these patients, it was found that each hemisphere tended to have a different cognitive mode of operation. The left hemisphere tended to be verbal and analytic compared to the right hemisphere which tended to be spatial and musical.

If the results of these studies are valid, then left nostril breathing should stimulate activities associated with the right hemisphere, and right nostril breathing should stimulate activities associated with the left. To examine the possibility of an extensive study into these correlations, Khalsa and Raynor measured the muscle tone on the left and right sides of the head. The tension was predominant on the side opposite to the nostril being used in breathing. The results of this experiment lent support to our hypothesis.[26]

In another approach we used a test developed by Ornstein to measure preference for verbal or spatial cognition. First, we tested naive subjects, who were randomly assigned to breathe through either their left or right nostril for six minutes, and compared their test results to a control group. There were no noticeable shifts in the thirty people tested. Then we took into account the yogic injunction that "the mind will begin to shift after fifteen minutes of this breath" and that the time for the effects of this kriya to be completely observed is thirty-one minutes. Six volunteers were selected and randomly assigned to left or right nostril breathing. When the test was administered to this small sample group, a statistical analysis of variance showed the subjects who did left nostril breathing to be more spatially oriented, while the right nostril breathers were more verbally oriented. The probability of this happening was less than 10 per cent. To confirm the results of this experiment, however, we need to repeat the test with a larger group and attain a probability of less than 5 per cent. The results are suggestive, however, and certainly sufficient to warrant further study of the relationship between hemispheric dominance and the nasal cycle.[27]

Several studies on the chemistry of rhythms are being conducted by G. Singh Goodman in conjunction with the Kundalini Research Institute. He did a study of the breath technique used in kundalini yoga called "breath of fire." It is used extensively with various postures and exercises, and is practiced anywhere from thirty seconds to twenty minutes at a time. The average length of practice is three minutes. The technique involves a rapid pumping motion (one and a half pumps per second) at the navel point. The breath goes out as the abdomen moves back toward the spine, and the breath enters the lungs as the abdomen goes forward by an equal amount. The breathing is done through the nose, never through the mouth.

A frequent criticism from non-practitioners is that this technique is actually clinical hyperventilation, and that the feeling of energy that students report is nothing more than vasodilation. Goodman, in a 1974 study under Tart at the University of California at Davis tested several subjects with an eight-channel electroencephalograph (EEG). These results were compared to those of controls, and to the standard EEG of clinical hyperventilation. He could find no relationship between the two conditions. The resultant brain waves after three minutes of breath of fire showed increased amplitude, and an increase in the percentage of alpha that spread from the occipital (back) to the frontal areas of the skull.[28]

These results relate favorably to a preliminary research note by G. S. Khalsa and S. K. Khalsa, who tested the pO_2, pCO_2 in arterial blood from the fingertips of nine subjects who had done either five or ten minutes of breath of fire. They noted the pO_2 increased slightly, then reduced and remained stable but above normal. The pO_2 did not reach the level reported for hyperventilation.[29]

If breath of fire is not hyperventilation, yet produces a temporarily stable state of metabolism that deviates from the normal, it should be an interesting phenomenon to investigate. The yogis claim it cleans the blood, remagnetizes the blood cells, expands the lung capacity and improves the circulation, but these claims have never been scientifically substantiated. Perhaps these types of breathing exercises have been overlooked because of cherished yet biased paradigms. We know that hyperventilation exists, is well documented, and can produce various physical and mental effects. To someone unfamiliar with the many forms of breathing common to yogic practice, forms other than the "normal" would tend to be grouped together—as either hyperventilation or hypoventilation. So they would not bother to test the state since apparently their model already includes the phenomenon. This is another case in which our current models do not discriminate or have a language for all the subtle states we wish to investigate.

The technique known as the electroencephalograph (EEG), mentioned earlier, is another example of the gap between theory and methodology. The EEG has been helpful in recognizing major brain disturbances such as epilepsy or tumors and in noticing major changes during states such as sleep. There is much doubt, however, of the EEG's usefulness for identifying unique altered states of consciousness. It is possible that the subtle changes of meditative states may be reflected in individual neuron pathway variations that do not appear in the averages recorded by EEG. Using the EEG, scientists can only look at a small range of the potential frequencies on which the brain can operate.

Regardless of these limitations, many investigators began experimenting with EEG in 1957 when Wenger and Bagchi reported unusual EEG patterns in yogic meditators.[30] The most commonly observed change in these experiments is an increase in the alpha rhythm (brain waves occurring in the eight to thirteen hertz range). J. J. Banquet, a physiologist, observed that the dominant alpha frequencies were recorded from broader areas of the brain during meditation. These findings were further supported in a study by G. S. Goodman in which he tested a student of kundalini yoga in meditation. He observed the expected increase in amplitude, and that alpha waves along with other waves at lower frequencies were measured from all major areas of the brain.[31]

These findings concerning alpha rhythm have been popularized because of the development of biofeedback training procedures. As a result, many people mistakenly identified meditation with the ability to produce alpha. It cannot actually be concluded, however, that alpha is a primary characteristic of meditative states, nor that those who produce alpha are in meditation. J. J. Lynch, for example, points out that the maximum alpha is produced in a normal waking state when the eyes are closed and the EEG is recorded from the occipital area of the skull.[32] In other words, the increase in alpha that has been noted in meditative states is actually less than that found to occur in the normal undisturbed state.

A report by N. N. Das and H. Gastaut[33] indicates that the prime characteristic of deep meditation in yogic samadhi is high frequency waves greater than twenty hertz.[34] In a similar experiment, Goodman tested a well-known Indian teacher of yogic meditation, who first produced beta waves whenever he reported being in meditation.[35] This approach of identifying a meditative state from a simple wave recorded in the output in one area of nerves may give us a lot of data, but it alone will probably not give an adequate understanding of characterization of meditation.

Goodman also tested a kundalini yoga student who was asked to enter several different meditative states at will. The student showed definite changes in the dominant frequencies and in the areas of the brain that produced each state. We also noticed that the kirlian photos of the same student in a previous study showed large structural changes in each of these states. This result was intriguing since the Indian yogi previously tested was also asked to change his state, but no change was seen on his EEG. This may be because he practiced a very limited range of techniques compared to the kundalini yoga student, or because he was much older. It is also possible that he did change his state, but the EEG was not sensitive enough within the appropriate wave range.[36]

P. Copeland did a comparative study of TM, yoga meditation as taught by Paramahansa Yogananda, and a mental breathing exercise in raja yoga as taught by Krishnamacharya.[37] After a careful analysis of the spectral EEG of subjects he reports no significant changes were produced by Yogananda's meditation, or by the raja technique. TM showed a greater tendency for alpha production, but the shift to lower frequency (theta) was later related to the fact that the meditator had fallen asleep. He found there was no unique or generalizable state associated with TM except those also related to sleep. He further suggested that if changes are produced it may be greater in a field of bioenergy not recorded well by EEG.

At this point, our studies with EEG must remain inconclusive, although it does seem to be possible to use EEG in looking at the degree of flexibility a practitioner has in altering the overall brain wave pattern of specific areas.

Another area of research in which the EEG can be helpful

at the present state of technology is in the study of sleep patterns. A considerable amount of research has been conducted on sleep during the 1970s, giving us norms for the various stages of sleep and the periodicity of dreams.

In 1957 Kleitman first described the rest-activity cycle of sleep. This "basic rest-activity cycle" completes itself every ninety minutes in the average human being.[38] Dement and Kleitman found that the time between the onset of one REM (rapid eye movement) period and the next also varies between eighty and ninety minutes. These REM periods are most often correlated with dream activity, and for this reason the cycles are also referred to as sleep-dream cycles. In addition to REM activity, four distinct stages of sleep have been defined and can easily be observed and scored from EEG recordings. Stage one is the lightest sleep, while stage four is the deepest sleep.[39]

Practitioners of kundalini yoga report less need for long hours of sleep than before the beginning of regular yoga exercise. They also claim to sleep more deeply when the yoga has been faithfully practiced. If these claims are true, then we should be able to observe significant changes in the sleep patterns of a regular yogi who is healthy and normal in every other respect. To test this hypothesis, S. Khalsa and M. Raynor selected a kundalini yoga student known to be very regular in his morning exercise and evening meditation for a period of about four years. The student was medically normal and was actively involved in work and society. He was observed with EEG for three nights. The analyzed EEG-EOG recordings showed that he slept four and a half to five hours, which is less than normal. He also spent significantly less time in stage two sleep than the norm and significantly increased time in stage three. He spent 26–30 per cent of his sleep time in stage three which would be expected for less than .1 per cent of the population. On the other hand, he showed as much time in REM near the end of his sleep period as the average person.[40]

Since there was only one subject in this experiment the results are certainly not conclusive. Our findings do suggest, however, that kundalini yoga may influence sleeping patterns. In the study of kundalini kriyas we have found several techniques that are claimed to deal with insomnia, narcolepsy, and other sleep disorders by "reintegrating the brain and the glandular system." We are actively pursuing some well controlled studies in this area. Changes in the EEG measures of well-identified states such as sleep stages, may give us an indirect way of seeing the psychophysiological effects of meditation and yoga on the individual. If the claims test positively, training in the use of these kriyas could help deal with the night disturbances that are so common in our culture.

The study of the glandular system, particularly the endocrine system, is another area of central concern to yogic therapy and to the more esoteric theories of kundalini yoga. Each endocrine gland is associated with a chakra, or energy transducing structure in the aura. The chakras represent different frequencies of energy as well as different psychological states. The balance of these chakras is intimately related to the balance of the corresponding endocrine glands. This link is a basis for understanding the relations between mental and physiological states.

To examine whether there is sufficient reason to suspect that measurable changes are induced in the endocrine system by meditation, G. S. Khalsa and Jaga Nath S. Khalsa selected two kundalini meditations to test.[41] One meditation, "kirtan kriya," was observed in yogic therapy to re-establish regular menstruation in women who had taken contraceptive pills. The disruption of the menstrual cycle in these women is sometimes attributed to a depression of the pituitary function induced by the hormones in the birth control pill. The kriya is claimed to effect thyroid and pituitary secretions as well as "balance the brain" and open the ajna chakra—the center of energy associated with the mystic eye at the brow point. The second kriya was a breathing pranayam that used four, eight, and sixteen-part breaths in left and right nostrils as well as a four-part breath through the mouth. It was claimed to "heal the body by balancing the brain areas." Three male meditators were used to test the pranayam. All subjects were in good health and did not eat the morning of the experiment. Blood samples were drawn from a catheter every fifteen minutes during the experiments. These were analyzed by radio-immune assay for leutinizing hormone (LH), prolactin (Prl), and growth hormone (GH) by an endocrinology laboratory at a VA hospital. These three hormones are measures of pituitary secretion. EKG and EEG were also recorded. Blood drawing and instrumentation was done from outside the meditation room. The cognitive set established before the experiment was that we wanted to examine blood chemistry during meditation. A pretest baseline of about two hours was taken. Each meditation period lasted for about one hour. During these periods, none of the subjects showed any evidence of sleeping by EEG or by subjective report. Finally, the meditation periods were followed by a post-test baseline of another hour.

With both kriyas, increases in leutinizing hormone and prolactin were observed. The first kriya produced the largest changes: 117 per cent in LH and 53 per cent in Prl. (Hormone values may be considered to have an accuracy of 10 per cent.) Growth hormone increased in the first kriya but not in the second. The results suggest that changes in the pituitary secretions can be induced by the kundalini meditation kriyas. This is in contradiction to reports of studies on TM[42] but is given some support by a study on yogic practitioners.[43] In any case, it is not wise to lump all meditations together as if they produced a single physiological and psychological state. As we have suggested earlier, each kriya must be studied by itself. The data, though strongly suggestive, is not conclusive. We intend to repeat the pilot with extensive controls, including a three-day baseline in a fixed environment so that we can record the normal cyclic shifts of the hormones and their relationships to each individual's eating and sleeping habits. We have reason to believe that the increases observed in this preliminary experiment are not due to the cyclic variations in the individuals, since all the subjects showed sharp increases during the same fifteen minute period. If the kriyas do allow selective stimulation of various endocrine hormones as claimed by the practitioners, the implications for use in clinical settings are far-reaching.

PERFORMANCE STUDIES

Kundalini yoga is now being used to improve ability in sports performance by an increasing number of athletes. This has begun to stimulate interest in testing the effects of kundalini yoga on standard measures of physical performance.

R. Moses of the University of Oregon did a study using students selected from physical education classes. In his study, he compares students who attended ten weekly sessions of kundalini yoga with control groups that were involved with body building, judo, wrestling, basketball, tennis, volleyball, and badminton for the same amount of time. He noticed significant increases in flexibility of several body joints, lung capacity, breath retention, and muscle strength for all groups, although the increases were larger in the yogic group than in any of the control groups.[44]

Jaga Nath Singh Glassman at California State College, San Bernardino measured changes in heart rate, respiration, and blood pressure for three different kriyas practiced by the same subject and compared them to the effects of moderate exercise.[45]

The first kriya was breath of fire (described above). The second involved concentration on the pulse, breath, and brow while sitting in a standard cross-legged position. The third kriya was a four-part breath: four short inhalations in which the lungs are completely emptied. There was also a particular hand position (*mudra*) associated with this kriya.

Comparing the effects of these meditative kriyas with the effects of moderate running exercises proved to be very interesting. Blood pressure increased as much during breath of fire as during moderate exercise, yet the heart rate increased only slightly. Breath of fire seems to increase blood pressure while putting very little strain on the heart. The second kriya showed a slower respiration rate and higher blood pressure than in the heavy exercise. The four-part breath increased the heart rate slightly and decreased the diastolic pressure to a very low level (a drop of over fifteen points).

These results tend to show that each kriya produces different physiological changes in the same person. Second, although they do not look as physically active as an exercise such as running, kundalini kriyas can produce comparable physiological changes particularly in relation to changes in blood pressure. Further research into the effects of kundalini yoga on performance is certainly warranted.

PSYCHOLOGICAL STUDIES

A well-controlled study by S. Johnson at the University of Southern California examined the effects of weekly sessions of kundalini yoga on conflict resolution, self-concept, and emotional adjustment.[46] He randomly divided a paid group of eighty volunteers into experimental and control groups. All were tested before and after the twelve-week period. He used extensive statistical analysis to determine any significant changes. He found changes in the experimental group that indicated greater ability to resolve conflict and control their behavior in stress situations. Similar increases were recorded in self-esteem, sense of positive identity, self-satisfaction, personal worth, moral-ethical self, physical self, and positive behavior as recorded by the Tennessee Self-Concept Test. As a result of their participation in the weekly kundalini yoga sessions, the subjects tended to like themselves more, have more confidence, and have more positive feelings about their physical attributes and behavior. The experimental group also showed an increased capacity for realistic positive self-description, and a reduction in the level of general maladjustment, personality disorder, and neuroses. Similar results have also been observed by other researchers.[47] The conclusion derived by Johnson in his study is that "kundalini yoga has benefit as a psychotherapeutic instrument."

H. Stone at Smith College measured the effects of a kundalini yoga class using the Personal Orientation Inventory and the State Trait Anxiety Inventory.[48] The study showed a significant increase in self-acceptance, improved self-image, and reduction in state and trait anxiety after ten weeks of kundalini yoga. This supports Johnson's conclusion that kundalini yoga is conducive to positive psychological change.

Since kundalini kriyas apparently produce changes that are considered to be significant for personality growth and counseling effectiveness, their use as an adjunct to regular therapies may be valuable. KRI is actively involved in developing meditational therapies that can be used effectively in professional settings. The use of kundalini yoga in high-stress environments, such as prisons or detention homes may prove to be of great psychological benefit although careful testing must first be done before viable applications can be made.

CONCLUSION

Keeping in mind that most of these experiments were preliminary studies, our initial data seem very promising. The general indication has been that kundalini yoga is capable of producing significant changes in all major areas of investigation, including psychological, physiological, and bioenergetic systems. The tests show that kundalini yoga can be related to positive changes in self-esteem, openness to experience, cognitive perception, and attitude. Other findings show that yogic practice also influences body rhythms such as the sleep dream cycle, hormone secretion and the nasal cycle, as well as overall fitness. Finally, there is some evidence that kundalini kriyas may be able to stimulate healing or psychic capacities.

Further avenues of inquiry are suggested when these studies and the current experimental literature are compared with claims made in the kundalini yoga teachings. For example, breath of fire is claimed to "cleanse the blood." What this may mean physiologically or in terms of individual health patterns can only be specified at present in a yogic language which lacks sufficient definition for Western scientific mentalities. To promote further discussion of the claim in scientific circles, we can measure changes in physiological correlates that relate to the blood and immunological systems in people that practice the breath of fire. Breath of fire is also said to build the supply of prana in the body and strengthen the aura. To test these claims in our future studies of breath of fire, we will look at its effects on the rate of bacterial phagocytosis by white blood cells, on high frequency EEG, and on the magnetic and electric fields around the body.

Another area of continuing interest is sleep. According to the yogic teachings, a master of kundalini yoga needs little sleep and does not dream. Instead, he sleeps for two to three hours in a deep "awakened" sleep called *turiya,* and deals with all his subconscious pressures during his early morning meditation. This meditation is a conscious mental cleaning process that involves the use of mantra and pranayam. Through this meditation, the subconscious material that would normally enter the mind in the dream state is eliminated or reduced to a minimum via activity during a conscious state. If these claims are true, observable changes in the sleep cycle should be verifiable. The relationship of sadhana, sleep, and dreaming should, in fact, eventually constitute a major departure from mainstream psychology. One of the main processes of psychotherapy is to "make subconscious material conscious through dreams." Analysis dealing with the presence of psychic material usually associated with sleep in an altered state of consciousness produced by meditation, and de-emphasizing the need for dreaming sleep could lead to the development of meditational therapies that bypass the traditional pathways of energy transformation or accomplish the same desired changes by appealing to now-unemployed dimensions of the self.

Future research project areas that have been stimulated by this work and speculation include

1. Investigation of meditative states in band areas of high frequency EEG (20 hertz);

2. Changes in blood chemistry, including ion, hormone, and hormone variations that are induced by the practice of kundalini kriyas;

3. The study of the bioenergetic field surrounding the body by the use of kirlian photography, radiant energy detectors, and electromagnetic field monitoring devices;

4. Development of profile tests to measure personality effects of long term practice of kundalini kriyas, as well as short term effects that result from the practice of different meditations;

5. Testing of cognition, memory, and learning capacity in altered states of consciousness induced by various kriyas;

6. Sleep studies of yogis on the use of kriyas to correct sleep disturbances;

7. Development of new instrumentation relating to EEG, spinal measurements, and imaging of biological tissue;

8. Development of teaching systems abstracted from the kundalini kriyas that clarify the process of altering conscious states in general, and applications of these techniques to social programs dealing with addiction and behavior modification;

9. Discovery of new characterizations of the kundalini energy in its mind/body/spirit manifestations;

10. Long term cultural-anthropological studies of the populations that practice kundalini yoga;

11. Tests of non-local field phenomena such as information transfer over distance (telepathy, out of the body experiences, etc.);

12. The further development of a complete classification system that selects kriyas to use in tests of various yogic therapy claims;

13. A study of the effects of long distance mental healing on lesion tissues and the growth rate of cancerous tissue;

14. Further performance tests that study the yoga kriyas as prime building blocks in the "new athletics."

These and other research projects will be undertaken mostly in co-operation with other institutes, universities, or laboratories. We encourage these co-operative efforts and invite communication about project ideas from a wide variety of sources. At the same time we are securing funds to establish the institute's own laboratory within the coming year.

Besides these practical experimental ventures, researchers at KRI are also actively working toward producing theoretical models to organize and explore kundalini, altered states of consciousness, and the energy fields of the human being. The study of the finite and infinite aspects of energy in relation to human personality and potential is called "Humanology." It was well-developed both in theory and practice by the ancient kundalini yogis. Translating this knowledge and experience into more modern language and paradigms is one of our primary tasks. As we pointed out in the introduction, one of the great difficulties in serious experimentation with altered states of consciousness is the lack of a solid theoretical language and conceptual framework in which we can pose questions and identify the variables relevant to consciousness phenomena.

The attempts by theorist E. H. Walker to relate the quantum mechanical model to states of consciousness is an admirable step in the right direction.[49] In his work, he looks at consciousness as an information processing system that selects the various states operative within the human system. He believes that consciousness can exist without physiological parameters, but that if it is strongly "bound" by a physiological system, it will be influenced by, or even effectively blocked by, the parameters of that system. Relating this physical quantum approach to the psychological-linguistic approach of C. Tart should prove to be very fruitful. Undoubtedly these initial attempts will look as odd to the future sciences as the "fluxions" and "fluids" of Newton do to the modern theorists now. But right now, these are the types of models we need.

R. Grisell, KRI associate senior researcher, for example, has recently constructed a mathematical model called "Hierarchical Field Theory" that postulates a possible field structure to explain ESP and many consciousness phenomena.[50] By looking at the geometrical dynamics of time and space, and introducing the concept of partially interacting fields with greatly different characteristics, he constructs a non-local field theory that provides a terminology for discussing ESP, kundalini, etc., and leads to further speculations about elementary particles and consciousness.

The crucial factors in developing and testing these theories are the kundalini kriyas mentioned earlier. Each kriya alters the consciousness either within the realm of a single state of consciousness or to a discretely different stable state of consciousness. The availability of over a thousand specific kriyas that can be taught to large populations opens the way to a widespread exploration of these altered states. This approach, when combined with the testing of one subject in many techniques, can help isolate the variables related to consciousness change as well as those related to the stabilization of discrete states of consciousness. Understanding how and why various kriyas produce their effects will raise basic questions about the reflex systems of the body, the relationship of various areas of the brain to psychological functioning, and the natural representation of information in different energy modalities.

Ultimately, we hope that all of these experiments and theories increase our understanding as well as our appreciation of the beauty and vastness of this cosmos and the interconnectedness of consciousness in all of its infinite potential.

NOTES

1. Tart, C. *States of Consciousness.* New York: E. P. Dutton, 1975.
2. Davidson, J. "The Physiology of Meditation and Mystical States of Consciousness," *Perspectives in Biology and Medicine.* Spring, 1976.
3. Schacter, S., and Singer, J. E. *Psychol. Rev.* 69:379, 1962.
4. Tart, op. cit.

5. Govinda, L. A. *Foundations of Tibetan Mysticism*. New York: E. P. Dutton, 1960.
6. Penfield, W. *The Mystery of the Mind*. Princeton University Press, 1975.
7. Heisenberg, W. *Physics and Philosophy*. London: Allen & Unwin, 1963.
8. Evans, C. "Parapsychology–What the Questionnaire Revealed," *New Scientist*. January 25, 1973.
9. Puthoff, H. E., and Targ, R. "A Perceptual Channel for Information Transfer over Kilometer Distances," *Proceedings of the IEEE*, March, 1976, 64:3, p. 349.
10. Yogiji, Harbhajan S. K. "Rhythm of the Breath," *Kundalini Lectures*. Claremont, California: Kundalini Research Institute, Winter, 1976, February 18, 1976.
11. Smith, M. J. "Paranormal Effect of Enzyme Activity Through Laying-on-of-Hands," *Human Dimensions*, Summer, 1972.
12. Grad, B. "A Telekinetic Effect on Plant Growth," *International Journal of Parapsychology*, 1973.
13. Yaeger, R. *The Effects of Kundalini Yoga on Onion Root Cell Mitosis*. Unpublished paper. California State College, San Bernardino, 1974.
14. Dean, D. "The Effects of 'Healers' on Biologically Significant Molecules," *New Horizons*, 1975, I, 215–19.
15. Dean, D., and Brame, E. "Physical Changes in Water by Laying-on-of-Hands," *Proceedings, Second International Congress on Psychotronic Research*. Paris: Institut Métaphysique International, 1975.
16. Tiller, W. A. *Kirlian Photography: Its Scientific Foundations and Future Potentials*. Stanford, California: Stanford University, 1975.
17. Kirlian, S. D., and Kirlian, V. Kh. "Photography and Visual Observations by Means of High-Frequency Currents," *Journal of Scientific and Applied Photography*, 1961, 6, 397–403.
18. Ibid.
19. Burr, H. S. *The Fields of Life*. New York: Ballantine, 1973.
20. Singh, R. K. *The Effects of Kundalini Yoga on Kirlian Photography*. Unpublished paper. California State College, Sonoma, 1974.
21. Singh, R. K., Singh, S. K., and Fowlis, G. S. "Kirlian Photography of Meditative States," *Journal of Science and Consciousness for Living in the Aquarian Age*. No. 6, June, 1974.
22. Khalsa, G. S., and Hubacher, J. *Comparative Study of Seven Meditation Techniques Using Kirlian Photography*. Unpublished paper, Kundalini Research Institute, 1975.
23. Connell, J. T. "Reciprocal Nasal Congestion-Decongestion Reflex," *Trans. Amer. Academ. Opth. and Otol.* 1968, 72:422.

24. Khalsa, S. S., and Raynor, M. *Kundalini Yoga and Psychophysiological Correlates: A Pilot Study*. Unpublished paper, University of California, Riverside, 1975.
25. Ibid.
26. Ibid.
27. Ibid.
28. Goodman, G. S. *The Effects of Three Yoga Exercises on the Electroencephalogram in Man*. Dissertation, University of California, Davis, 1972.
29. Khalsa, G. S., and Khalsa, S. K. S. *Breath of Fire, Blood pH, and Hyperventilation*. Unpublished research, Kundalini Research Institute, 1974.
30. Bagchi, B., and Wenger, M. *Electroencephalogr. Clin. Neurophysiol.* 1957, 7:132.
31. Goodman, op. cit.
32. Lynch, J. J., Paskewitz, A., and Orne, M. T. *Psychosomatic Medicine*. 36:399, 1974.
33. Das, N. N., and Gastaut, H. *Electroencephalogr. Clin. Neurophysiol.*, 1955, 6 (suppl.): 211.
34. Dement, W. C., and Kleitman, N. "The Relation of Eye Movements During Sleep to Dream Activity—An Objective Method for the Study of Dreaming," *Journal of Exp. Psych.* 1957, 53, 339–46.
35. Goodman, op. cit.
36. Ibid.
37. Copeland, P. "Meditation and EEG Studies," *Yoga Journal.* July–August 1976.
38. Dement and Kleitman, op. cit.
39. Dement, W. C. *Some Must Watch While Some Must Sleep.* New York: Charles Scribner's Sons, 1974.
40. Khalsa, S. S., and Raynor, M., op. cit.
41. Khalsa, G. S., and Khalsa, J. N. S. *Study of Hormonal Changes (Prl, GH, LH) in Two Kundalini Meditations.* Unpublished paper, Kundalini Research Institute, 1976.
42. Shapiro, D., et al. (ed.) *Biofeedback and Self-Control.* Chicago: Aldine Publishing Company, 1972.
43. Gode, J. D., Singh, R. H., Settiwar, R. M., Gode, K. D., and Udupa, K. N. "Increased Urinary Excretion of Testosterone Following a Course of Yoga in Normal Young Volunteers," Indian J. Med. Sci. 28 (4–5): 212–15, April–May, 1974.
44. Moses, R. *Effect of Yoga on Flexibility and Respiratory Measures of Vital and Breath Holding Time.* Dissertation, University of Oregon, 1972.
45. Glassman, J. S. *Physiology of Yogic Techniques.* Unpublished paper, California State College, San Bernardino, 1975.
46. Johnson, S. *Effects of Yoga Therapy on Conflict Resolution,*

Self-Concept, and Emotional Adjustment. Dissertation, University of Southern California, 1974.
47. Datey, K. K., Deshmukh, S. N., Dalvi, C. P., and Vinekar, S. L. "Shavasan: A Yogic Exercise in the Management of Hypertension," *Angiology*. 1969, 20:325.
48. Stone, H. Unpublished thesis, Smith College, 1975.
49. Walker, E. H. "The Nature of Consciousness," *Mathematical Biosciences*. 7, 131–78, 1970.
50. Grisell, R. *Hierarchical Field Theory: A Theoretical Framework for Extrasensory Phenomena.* Unpublished paper. University of Texas Medical Branch, 1976.

REFERENCES AND SUGGESTED READINGS

Banquet, J. P. *Electroencephalogr. Clin. Neurophysiol.* 1973, 35:143.

Grad, B. "The 'Laying-on-of-Hands': Implications for Psychotherapy, Gentling, and the Placebo Effect," *Journal of the American Society for Psychical Research,* 1967, 61, 286–305.

James, W. *The Varieties of Religious Experience.* New York: Modern Library, 1929.

Leadbetter, C. W. *The Chakras.* Adyar, India: Theosophical Publishing House, 1968.

Muses, C., and Young, A. M. *Consciousness and Reality.* New York: Avon, 1972.

Ornstein, R. E. *The Psychology of Consciousness.* New York: Viking Press, Inc., 1972.

Randall, J. *Parapsychology and the Nature of Life.* New York: Harper and Row Publishers Inc., 1975.

Wenger, M., Bagchi, B., and Anand, H. *Circulation.* 24:1319, 1961.

Yogiji, Harbhajan S. K. "Rhythm of the Breath," *Kundalini Lectures.* Claremont, California: Kundalini Research Institute, Winter, 1976, Feb. 18, 1976.

THE BIOLOGICAL BASIS OF KUNDALINI

Erik Floor

Any person who has felt the illumination of kundalini, or who has appreciated accounts of its effects by others, knows of the vital power of this phenomenon. It is a release of a unique "body chemistry."

Man has long sought a bodily source for his deepest feelings. An early attempt, perhaps successful, to identify a chemical embodiment of exalted spiritual consciousness was the belief in a miraculous substance, soma, described in the Vedas. Three centuries ago Descartes proposed the pineal gland as the seat of the soul. And even today it is not uncommon to refer to the heart as the source of love and compassion.

Today, moreover, because of the very recent successes of physiology in understanding so many bodily processes, scientific metaphors for emotional and spiritual experiences have increasing popular appeal. The squiggly recordings of the electroencephalograph, especially, seem to hold the potential to measure a person's innermost thoughts mechanically.

The phenomena attending arousal of kundalini shakti or energy are particularly amenable to a physiological interpretation. For a definite, often sudden transformation in consciousness occurs which may be preceded by sensations starting in the region of the base of the spine and progressing up the body and into the head. If we inquire a little deeper into the biological basis of this phenomenon, can we find out in terms of modern physiological science what is actually happening in these body regions?

Unfortunately for our curiosity, we can't. There is no apparent reason why it should not be possible eventually to discover what the biological mechanism of kundalini is. All that seems needed is to analyze the phenomenon according to established biochemical and physiological procedures that have proven so effective in other contexts. But at the present time such an analysis has barely begun. Virtually nothing is known about the biology of this amazing process.

One ancient theory of kundalini physiology held that a "coiled energy" lay dormant in the region of the base of the spine. When released, this energy rose in the body, opening consciousness potentials (chakras) along the spine and ultimately the highest center in the brain. What is the "energy"? Probably the most concrete version of this theory conceived of it as normal "reproductive fluids" which were thought actually to enter the spinal cord at its base and travel up into the brain. This idea is quite unnecessary by current concepts in physiology though, and is almost surely wrong. At some more abstract level the notion of an "energy" ascending the spinal region parallels the subjective phenomena observed during the awakening of the kundalini and is probably true.

However that may be, the body has a much more direct and efficient means to connect the reproductive organs, or other structures at the base of the spine, with the brain—nerves. Nerves work electrically. In a fraction of a second nerve pathways carry messages from the tip of the spine to the brain. At its destination in the brain a message can be decoded either to impart information to other nerves or to signal the release of a chemical into the brain that affects both brain and consciousness. The awakening of kundalini often occurs in a flash, a time scale indicative of a process related to nerve activity rather than to fluid flow.

Because of the speed of electrical impulse conduction in nerve tracts, modern theories of kundalini physiology must consider a more likely source of the kundalini shakti. The actual site of the biological trigger for kundalini energy could be in the brain. According to this theory, the sensations felt in the spine and internal organs during arousal of kundalini are the secondary reverberations of a primary activity in the brain that projects outward into the body via the peripheral nerves. The further question of why particular body parts resonate more than others to the fundamental activity in the brain may suggest clues to the nature of the basic brain mechanism itself.

But, one may object, the awakening of kundalini does not feel as though it begins in the brain, or even in the head. Instead it seems to begin at a location quite far removed from the head, that is, in the base of the spine. However, it is crucial to realize that one can't feel any of the brain's activities directly in the same sense that one can feel, say, a finger moving. Thus a person cannot know whether a sensation that seems *subjectively* to originate in the pelvic region actually does arise there or whether, on the other hand, it is a consequence of a process that began in the brain outside of awareness and was subsequently transmitted to the lower body by way of nerve connections.

This is a question that can be approached experimentally, in principle, at least. The answer should begin to tell us where soma is first released in the body at the awakening of kundalini. A hypothetical kundalini researcher who was simultaneously monitoring nerve activity in the brain and lower spinal cord with electronic instruments would be able to tell *objectively* where the initial activation took place. Contemporary neuroscientists (myself included) share a prejudice about how this and similar experiments will turn out.

The cosmically complex human brain, which contains almost as many nerve cells as there are stars in our galaxy, is probably where much of the biological basis of kundalini energy will be found. This viewpoint leads to the prediction that in the experiment described in the preceding paragraph, nerve activity in the brain would precede nerve activity at the base of the spine and the *perception of "energy"* in that area, by a fraction of a second. Of course, the experiment would be difficult to do with the technology available today. And it would be hard to interpret because nerve pathways are so extremely complex. It might not be evident that the right pathways had been measured. But once kundalini's point of origin has been localized to the brain, as it very likely will be, the next question will be what the brain mechanisms of kundalini arousal might be. Some recent advances in brain research afford glimpses into this elusive, so deeply interesting physiology.

NEUROCHEMISTRY AND THE AWAKENING OF KUNDALINI

Philip Lansky

The actual process of Shakti rising up the spine to meet her lord Shiva in the brain is often characterized as a transmutation of sexual to psychic energy. According to this view, one hundred drops of *bindu* (semen) are sublimated and distilled to one drop of highly purified *ojas* (psychic energy).

The subjective experience of the kundalini rising is always described as both sudden and intense. The following is an excerpt from Gopi Krishna's autobiography, *Kundalini:*

> During one such spell of intense concentration I suddenly felt a strange sensation at the base of the spine, at the place of touching the seat, while I sat cross-legged on a folded blanket spread on the floor. The sensation was so extraordinary and so pleasing that my attention was forcibly drawn towards it. The moment my attention was thus unexpectedly withdrawn from the point on which it was focused, the sensation ceased. . . . When completely immersed I again experienced the sensation, but this time, instead of allowing my mind to leave the point where I had fixed it, I maintained a rigidity of attention throughout. The sensation again extended upwards, growing in intensity, and I felt myself wavering; but with a great effort I kept my attention centered round the lotus. Suddenly, with a roar like that of a waterfall, I felt a stream of liquid light entering my brain through the spinal cord.

At this point, we will attempt to consider a possible neurochemical explanation for the phenomenon of the ascending kundalini. From the traditional concepts we know that there is supposedly an interaction between sexual centers in the lower chakras and with psychic centers at the upper chakras around the brain. From Gopi Krishna's account we know that the experience involves the subjective perception of light, and mental phenomena which might be called "hallucinatory." Finally, we have already stated that the uppermost chakra is frequently suggested as being associated with the pineal gland.

The pineal gland is extremely rich in an indolic derivative of serotonin called melatonin. The precise function of melatonin is unknown; however, considerable evidence suggests that the pineal gland and melatonin exert an inhibitory effect upon both the female and male gonads in mammals. Furthermore, the sexual hormones testosterone, estrogen, and progesterone have been shown to in turn inhibit the biosynthesis of melatonin. It would thus seem reasonable that some type of relationship exists between the pineal gland and sexual function. Furthermore, it is well established that the pineal, at least in the lower mammals, contains photoreceptors and might thus be involved in the perception of light.

It is also of interest to note here that melatonin can readily cyclize to a three-ringed compound, 10-methoxyharmalan, which is potently hallucinogenic. (Melatonin itself is not a hallucinogen.) The conversion of melatonin to 10-methoxyharmalan is shown on the next page.

It has been suggested that the endogenous formation of 10-methoxyharmalan may be a cause of hallucination in mental disorder.

Though I will not attempt to define a neurochemical basis for the possible phenomenon of a rising kundalini, it would appear that the pineal may be a reasonable place for the future researchers to begin looking. The pineal is involved in sexual function (relationship of sexual to psychic chakras),

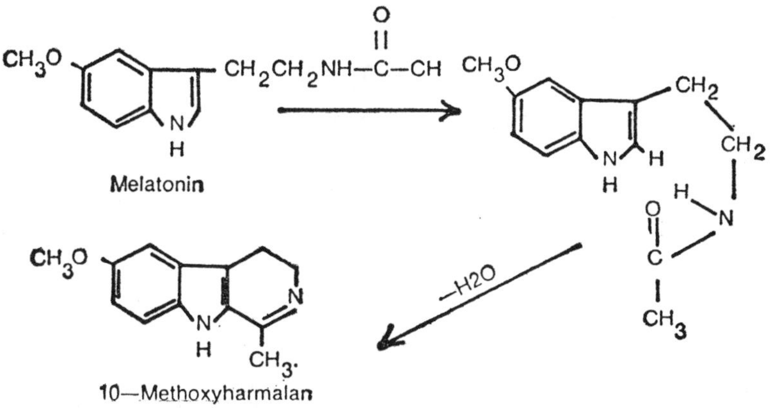

Figure 1. Conversion of melatonin to 10-methoxyharmalan.

contains photoreceptors (reported perception of "liquid light" during kundalini experience), and contains melatonin, which may cyclize to a potent hallucinogen, 10-methoxyharmalan.

KINDLING AND KUNDALINI EFFECTS

Marilyn Ferguson

Laboratory research into the kundalini phenomenon is under way in various parts of the world. The University of Bangalore, India, will investigate kundalini in "Project Consciousness," a government-supported study.

Earlier, the famed Max Planck Institute in Germany undertook a biochemical search for kundalini—subjectively reported to involve electrical sensations, tingling, inner lights, even convulsions, usually followed over a period of time by a moderation of "symptoms" and apparent alterations in the central nervous system.

Those investigating the effects have sometimes looked for parallel effects in electrical stimulation of the brain because of similar anecdotal reports. Now an unexpected finding in epilepsy research may prove relevant.

Kundalini may be analogous in its origin to a lab-induced effect in animals called "kindling." The kindling effect was originally heralded as a model of epilepsy—but now John Gaito of York University reports (*Psychological Bulletin* 83:1,097–1,109) that different mechanisms probably are involved, at least in some cases. The amino acid taurine, which suppresses epileptic seizures in laboratory animals, does not prevent phenomena caused by kindling.

In addition, the kindling effect apparently causes permanent changes in the neural circuitry.

First reported by G. V. Goddard and his associates in 1969, "kindling" refers to the effects of repeated, periodic, low-intensity stimulation of the limbic region of the brain. At first a rat being kindled continues to explore its environment normally.

"However, after a number of trials with the same intensity of stimulation," Gaito said, "the rat will rear up on its hind paws, and the forelimbs will begin to convulse." Over a period of time the bursts of electrical activity kindle similar patterns in adjacent brain regions. Also, the threshold is progressively lowered so that a smaller dose of electricity triggers convulsions.

When the amygdala is stimulated, the afterdischarge spreads to the amygdala on the other side of the brain, then in an orderly sequence to the hippocampus, occipital cortex, and finally to the frontal cortex.

Kindling can start only in the limbic structures. There is essentially no triggering effect in the cortex, brainstem, or thalamus.

Analogies of the kindling effect and meditation effects—especially of the dramatic kundalini phenomena—are interesting. Obviously, most human subjects don't perceive their experiences as pathological, although they may be somewhat unnerving. The effects typically occur after a history of regular meditation and in an unthreatening setting. There is no onset of seizures in the classic sense, and the nervous system effects appear to be positive over the long run.

But the animal research on kindling suggests a possible crude model for the period of latency from the beginning of regular periods of stimulation to the first conspicuous effects.

The kindling studies also may help illuminate the role of the limbic brain structures. The effects vary in strength and onset according to which of these regions is stimulated in the animals, with the amygdala being the most amenable to kindling.

In regard to human subjects, Bernard Glueck of the Hartford (Connecticut) Institute of Living has speculated that the sounds used in mantra meditation might set off a resonance effect in the limbic brain. The "invariant stimulus" of mantra yoga is a repeated sound. Some subjects report the eventual onset of sensations of an electrical nature spreading throughout the head and becoming rhythmic, sometimes almost convulsive or orgasmic in nature. Several of the kundalini cases described by psychiatrist Lee Sannella [in *Kundalini: Psychosis or Transcendence?*] occurred after a period of Transcendental Meditation, which uses a mantra technique.

A RESEARCH NOTE ON KUNDALINI ENERGY

Robert L. Peck

In writing about kundalini thousands of years after its earlier description and effects, I find that I differ from the early descriptions in one area. The early writings read as if it's an either/or situation. Kundalini is either raised or it isn't. Part of this either/or model is based on the use of a snake representing the energy. The snake is either aroused and slides up the backbone, or it is resting coiled around the lower energy center. One cannot have a snake partially in two or more places at once!

My experiences suggest that the flow of energy along or through the nervous system can vary in magnitude. One time the effects can be very strong while at other times the effects appear minimal. With beginning students, the first experiences are very weak; as they progress the effects become more and more pronounced. One could argue that one's awareness of the kundalini is varying, and that the energy is actually the same. The exception is that other effects associated with the rise in energy also seem to develop slowly, such as depth of meditation, God-awareness, ESP phenomena, drop in body metabolism, time sense, etc. Further, one would have to have another model or source of energy for those who have had God-awareness or ESP experiences without yoga training. If we accept that kundalini is the energy source for supranormal occurrences, and that these vary in magnitude and duration, then kundalini must also be variable in magnitude and in time duration.

As a research physicist having worked with electrical conduction in ionic media, my hypothesis of kundalini is that the electrical flow characteristics of the nervous system undergo a change with certain stimuli, causing an increase in efficiency, sensitivity, and control of the nervous system. One possibility is that the normally large potassium or sodium ions are replaced with much, much smaller hydrogen ions for the conduction of electrical impulses. Some researchers, including myself, have demonstrated that hydrogen ions can and do carry electricity in certain materials and under certain conditions. The human body has certainly the right materials. We then have to assume that the conditions are variable. We mentioned earlier the formation of clathrates in the blood which reduce mental awareness. It's quite possible that as hydrogen ions are substituted for larger ions, the clathrates would diminish along with other negative blood chemistry reactions.

KUNDALINI AS PREVENTION AND THERAPY FOR DRUG ABUSE

John R. M. Goyeche

The conclusion that yoga practices allow learned control of the sympathetic nervous system is not a new one. Dr. Vasant Rele of Bombay came to the same conclusion in 1926. In his book *The Mysterious Kundalini* he outlines in great detail how through the practice of yoga, the right vagus nerve, the major nerve of the parasympathetic system, is brought under voluntary control. "The stimulation of the right vagus nerve at its central connection (in the medulla) can control the activities of all the six plexes of the sympathetic system." The vagal center is said to be stimulated by reflex through the spinal cord, primarily through the control of the afferent and efferent impulses of respiration during the process of pranayama, especially. Normally, respiration is controlled automatically by one of the plexes of the sympathetic system and is unconscious. When attention is paid to breathing, however, the impulses become conscious and "are made to pass through the vagus and other nerves of the parasympathetic portion which have their nuclei in the midbrain and bulb."

A word should be said on the "kundalini." This refers to a blissful, ineffable experience which is said to result from the regular practice of yoga and which in most schools of yoga is said to contribute to the continual experience of samadhi. In August of 1972, at the University of Manitoba, I was fortunate enough to record some psychophysical data during the kundalini experience. At that time I was sitting in vajrasana (on my knees) and was merely concentrating on my breathing for fifteen to twenty minutes. After about fifteen minutes I had three kundalini experiences within several minutes. The first two lasted about one minute each, the last only a few seconds. The polygraph record shows that at the onset of each of the three experiences a number of interesting things happened. The most noticeable change is the large localized skin potential response which occurs in the EEG channel, indicative of a sudden sympathetic response. Throughout the entire experience, respiration rate and heart rate accelerate and show little variability. The change in respiration is experienced as a reflex which is not under voluntary control, which occurs automatically and subsides in the same way. Also of interest is the pattern of breathing before the onset of each of these experiences. From a very slow and regular rhythm, the breathing changes for a few seconds to a very shallow, irregular pattern in which it is difficult to ascertain whether inspiration or expiration is occurring. Following this pattern, the other changes begin within a second or so.

What does this psychophysiological pattern mean? It could be hypothesized that the kundalini reflex is a sympathetic reflex elicited to compensate for a critical drop in metabolic level with an accompanying increased level of carbon dioxide. This metabolic drop is in accord with the findings of Wallace and Benson who reported declines in both oxygen consumption and carbon dioxide elimination. The data would seem to fit this interpretation, but obviously much more data is needed. In any case, the kundalini is experienced as an "electrical bliss" vibrating throughout the body. There may be a possible similarity between the kundalini experience and the experience which occurs when amphetamines are injected intravenously. Users have been described as having "rushes" or "flashes" which are experienced as orgasmic in nature. Amphetamine causes a biochemical arousal of the RAS [reticular activating system] in the absence of sensory input and has potent effects on the medial forebrain bundle, the reward system of the brain. . . . In its general manifestations it mimics the stimulation of the sympathetic nervous system. Thus, the kundalini experience may closely parallel the amphetamine experience and indeed may be a good substitute for it.

KUNDALINI: CLASSICAL AND CLINICAL

Lee Sannella

Every spiritual tradition that is concerned with the rebirth process has its own model. Most of these are descriptions that stress the subjective side of the experience, either treating the objective signs as incidental or ignoring them. Thus, these accounts, however valid they may be on their own terms, are not helpful in making objective comparisons of different traditions. When it comes to physiological interpretations, most of these models have little relevance.

An exception is the kundalini model from yoga. Kundalini is seen as an "energy" that usually resides "asleep" at the base of the spine. When this energy is "awakened" it rises slowly up the spinal canal to the top of the head. This may mark the beginning of a process of enlightenment.

In its rise, kundalini causes the central nervous system to throw off stress. The stress points will usually cause pain during meditation. When kundalini encounters these stress points or blocks, it begins to act "on its own volition," engaging in a self-directed, self-limited process of spreading out through the entire physiopsychological system to remove these blocks.

Once a block is removed, kundalini flows freely through that point and continues its upward journey until the next stress area is encountered. Further, the kundalini energy diffuses in this journey, so that it may be operating on several levels at once, removing several different blocks. When the course is completed, the energy all becomes focused again at the top of the head.

The difference between this final state and the initial state is not simply that kundalini is focused in a different place, but that in the meantime it has passed through every part of the organism, removing blocks and awakening consciousness there. Thus, the entire process of kundalini action can be seen as one of *purification* or balancing.

Just as an electric current produces light when it passes through a thin tungsten filament, but not when it passes through a thick copper wire, because the filament offers appreciable resistance while the wire does not, so also does the kundalini cause the most sensation when it enters an area of mind or body that is "blocked." But the "heat" generated by the "friction" of kundalini against this "resistance" soon "burns out" the block, and then the sensation ceases.

Similarly, just as an intense flow of water through a thick rubber hose will cause the hose to whip about violently, while the same flow through a firehose would scarcely be noticed, so also does the flow of kundalini through obstructed "channels" within the body or mind cause motions of those areas until the obstructions have been "washed out" and the channels "widened." (The terms "channel," "widen," "blocks," and so on must be taken metaphorically. They may not refer to actual physical structures, dimensions, and processes, but be only useful analogies for understanding this model of kundalini action. The actual process is undoubtedly much more subtle and complex.)

The spontaneous movements, shifting body sensations and other phenomena reported in our cross-cultural survey . . . and in our own cases, can easily be interpreted as manifestations of kundalini action. Furthermore, Bentov has recently proposed a physiological model for kundalini that accounts for much of what we have reported and observed.* His study is evaluated in terms of our results later. Because of the objective orientation of his kundalini model, its universal appli-

* See "Micromotion of the Body as a Factor in the Development of the Nervous System," by Itzhak Bentov (Appendix A to Sannella's book), which follows. *Editor.*

cability, and its susceptibility to physiological interpretation, we shall adopt it as the basis for our discussions.

However, there are differences between our own observations and the classical kundalini concept. Most notably, we observe, and several traditions report, that the energy or sensation rises up the feet and legs, the body, back and spine to the head, but then passes *down* over the face, and through the throat, finally terminating in the abdomen. This is entirely in accord with predictions from Bentov's model, but somewhat at variance with the reports of Muktananda, Gopi Krishna, and classic yoga scriptures.

Therefore we propose the term *physio-kundalini* to refer to those aspects of kundalini awakening, both physiological and psychological, which can be accounted for by a purely physiological mechanism. We shall refer to the physio-kundalini process, the physio-kundalini cycle, the physio-kundalini mechanism, and the physio-kundalini complex. Bentov's model describes such physiological changes that require no supernormal forces.

The slow progression of "energy-sensation" up through the body, then down the throat, accompanied by a variety of movements, sensations, and mental disturbances that terminate when this traveling stimulus reaches its culmination in the abdomen is so characteristic that we shall call it the *physio-kundalini cycle.*

When the energy encounters a resistance, then overcomes it and purifies the system of that block, we shall say that the location of that block has been "opened." The "throat-opening" is one typical example. This gives us a terminology linked to the kundalini concept, suited to the level of our observations and amenable to physiological interpretation. At the same time, it preserves the full integrity of the classical meaning of kundalini without committing us to a belief that this mythical concept is accurate to anything objectively real. . . .

* * * *

We now have two models of kundalini: the classical yogic description and Bentov's physiological model, plus our own clinical observations. Those aspects of the process which *could* have a purely physiological basis, either that which Bentov proposes or some other, we have designated physio-kundalini. The majority of our clinical observations fall within the physio-kundalini category, and we have just examined to what extent they might be accounted for by Bentov's model. But the physio-kundalini process, as we have observed it, differs from the classical yogic description in certain important respects.

Most notable of these is the pathway taken by the kundalini "energy" or body sensation as it travels through the system. Classically, the energy "awakens" at the base of the spine, travels straight up the spinal canal, and has completed its journey when it reaches the top of the head. Along this route, however, there are said to be several "chakras" or psychic energy centers which the kundalini must pass through to reach its goal. These chakras contain "impurities" that kundalini must remove before it can continue its upward course.

On the other hand, in the usual clinical picture, the energy sensation travels up the legs and back to the top of the head, then down the face, through the throat, to a terminal point in the abdomen. What is the relationship between these two descriptions?

We must be aware that yogic descriptions, in addition to being dogmatic, are often very subtle. Western scientists say that the actual location of sensory perception is in the sensory cortex, even though the sensation is *felt* to be in the periphery. Similarly, the yogis might mean that the sensations, blocks, and openings (such as the throat opening) which are *felt* to be in various body parts, are in some subtle way *represented* in the spinal chakras.

Still another possibility is suggested by the experience of one of Muktananda's students (in a personal communication) who says he feels energy spreading throughout his body, but especially descending from his forehead over his face to his throat, then to his chest and abdomen, *then* to the base of his spine, and *only then* into and up the center of the spine itself. He says the sensation in the spine is more subtle and difficult to perceive than that of the peripheral areas—perhaps because most of the energy has not yet entered his spine.

The time factor is also different in the classical and clinical pictures. All the characteristic elements of the physio-kundalini complex are included in the classic description. And yet we find quite "ordinary" people who complete the physio-kundalini cycle in a matter of months, whereas yogic scriptures assign a *minimum* of three years for culmination of full kundalini awakening in the case of the *most advanced* initiates. Here we have the suggestion that full kundalini awakening includes a larger complex of which the physio-kundalini process is only a part.

It is too early to say exactly what the relationships are, except that perhaps the physio-kundalini mechanism is a separate entity which may be activated as part of a full kundalini awakening. Much of the problem stems from the difficulty of comparing different stages when many processes are happening concurrently. Individual differences complicate the picture. But it would be possible to clarify things by remembering the theoretical definition of kundalini action as a *purificatory* or balancing process.

If the "impurities" or imbalances have any objective reality, it should be possible to demonstrate them with physiological and psychological tests, and to correlate their removal with specific signs and symptoms observed clinically. Since we now know that the process may be triggered and how it may be recognized in its initial stages, long-term case studies, covering the entire course of the process, are a logical next step in these investigations. They would be invaluable in documenting *specific* objective ways in which the kundalini process is beneficial.

Diagnostic Considerations

Our results indicate a clear distinction between the physio-kundalini complex and psychosis, and provide a number of criteria for distinguishing between these two states. We have seen, in some of our cases, that a schizophrenic-like condition can result when the person undergoing the kundalini experience receives negative feedback, either from social pressure or from the resistances of his own earlier conditioning.

Evidence that these states are distinct and separate comes from two of our cases who became "psychotic" after being confined to a mental institution for inappropriate behavior. Each of them reported that during their stay in their respective mental institutions they were quite sure that they (and several of the other patients) could tell which of their number were "crazy" and which just "far out and turned on."

Possibly this is a situation where "it takes one to know one," and a person whose own kundalini has been awakened can intuitively sense the "kundalini state" of another. This is of special interest, as it may point to a use of such people in assisting to decide which way the balance lies between the two processes in any particular patient.

Clinicians usually have a finely tuned sense of what is psychotic. Mainly, it is this sense for the smell of psychosis that tells us if the patient is unbalanced in this way, or is, instead, inundated with more positive psychic forces. Also, there is a feeling for whether the person is dangerous to himself and others. Persons in the early phases of kundalini awakening, if hostile or angry, are, in our experience, rarely inclined to act out.

Also, those in whom the kundalini elements predominate are usually much more objective about themselves, and have an interest in sharing what is going on in them. Those on the psychotic side tend to be very oblique, secretive and totally preoccupied with ruminations about some vague but "significant" subjective aspect of their experience which they can never quite communicate to others.

With our own results and Bentov's model, we have several more distinguishing features. Sensations of heat are common in these "high" states, but are rare in psychosis. Also very typical are feelings of "vibrations" or flutterings, tinglings, and itchings that move in definite patterns over the body, usually in the sequence described earlier. But these patterns may be irregular in atypical cases or in those who have preconceived ideas of how the energies "should" circulate.

With all this, bright lights may be seen internally. There may be pains, especially in the head, which suddenly arise or cease during critical phases in the process. Unusual breathing patterns are common, as well as other spontaneous movements of the body. Noises such as chirping and whistling sounds are heard, but seldom do voices intrude in a negative way as in psychosis. When voices *are* heard, they are perceived to come from within and are not mistaken for outer realities.

Recommendations and Discussion

Our results support the view that this force is positive and creative. Each one of our own cases is now successful on his or her own terms. They all report they handle stress more easily, and are more fulfilled than ever before in relationships with others. The classical cases indicate that special powers, as well as deep inner peace, may result from the culmination of the full kundalini process. But in the initial stages, stress of the experience itself, coupled with a negative attitude from oneself or others, may be overwhelming and cause severe imbalance.

Experience suggests an approach of understanding, strength, and gentle support. The spontaneous trances which disturbed one individual ceased when we encouraged him to enter a trance state voluntarily. By recognizing a distinction between "psychotic" and "psychically active," we had communicated to him an attitude that the trances were valid and meaningful. Because of our own acceptance of the condition, the patient was able to accept it.

The trances themselves ceased to "control" him as soon as he gave up his own resistance to them and the forces behind them. Similarly, another case had severe headaches, but these stopped as soon as she ceased trying to control the process and simply "went with it." The pain, in other words, resulted not from the process itself but from her resistance to it. We suspect that is true of all the negative effects of the physio-kundalini process.

Symptoms, when caused by this process, will disappear spontaneously in time. Because it is essentially a "purificatory" or balancing process, and each person has only a finite amount of "impurities" of the sort removed by kundalini, the process is self-limiting. Disturbances seen are therefore not pathological, but rather therapeutic, constituting a removal of potentially pathological elements. The kundalini force arises spontaneously from deep within the mind, and is apparently self-directing. Tension and imbalance thus result, not from the process itself, but from conscious or subconscious interference with it. Helping the person to understand and accept what is happening to him may be the best that we can do.

Usually the process, left to itself, will find its own natural pace and balance. But if it has already become too rapid and violent, our experience suggests it may be advisable to take steps such as heavier diet, suspension of meditations, and vigorous physical activity to moderate its course.

The people in whom the physio-kundalini process is most easily activated, and in whom it is most likely to be violent and disturbing, are those with especially sensitive nervous systems—the natural psychics. Many of our cases had some psychic experience prior to their arousal. Natural psychics often find the physio-kundalini experience so intense that they will not engage in the regular classical meditation methods that usually further the kundalini process; instead, they either refrain from meditation or adopt some mild form of their own devising. But much of their anxiety may be due to misunderstanding and ignorance of the physio-kundalini process. Rather than increasing their fear, we should be giving them the knowledge and confidence to allow the process to progress at the maximum comfortable natural rate.

Much could be accomplished by changing attitudes, first

around people experiencing the kundalini, but ultimately in society as a whole. This is not just for the person's benefit, but for all of us who need models in our own spiritual search. Some other cultures are more advanced than our own in terms of their recognition of the positive value of spiritually or psychically developed people.

The trance state in Bali serves an important adaptive function for the children. In parts of Africa, trance is a social and religious necessity, required for kundalini arousal.

In South Africa a state which Western psychiatry would probably call acute schizophrenia is a prerequisite for initiation into the priesthood by one Kalahari tribe.

Here, we must speak of the many creative people who are now suffering because of mistakes that we in the [psychiatric] profession have made in the past. We have a special obligation to make every effort to correct those mistakes. At this time in our society it could be that such charismatic and strangely acting people as shamans, trance mediums, and *masts* (the God-intoxicated) might find themselves in custodial care.

Possibly there are many now so situated who could be found and released to more positive uses among us. The problem is to recognize them among the other inmates of our institutions. Here Meher Baba's work with masts would be a useful precedent to study. If it is true that, to a certain extent, "it takes one to know one," a special and invaluable use for people who have already experienced the physio-kundalini process would be to assist us in such a project.

There are many undergoing this process who at times feel quite insane. When they behave well and keep silent they may avoid being called schizophrenic, or being hospitalized or sedated. Nevertheless their isolation and sense of separation from others may cause them much suffering. We must reach such people, their families, and society with information to help them recognize their condition as a blessing, not a curse.

Certainly we must no longer subject people, who might be in the midst of this rebirth process, to drugs or shock therapies, approaches which are at opposite poles to creative self-development.

These people, though confused, fearful, and disoriented, are already undergoing a therapy from within, far superior to any that we yet know how to administer from without.

MICROMOTION OF THE BODY AS A FACTOR IN THE DEVELOPMENT OF THE NERVOUS SYSTEM

Itzhak Bentov

Introduction

In the last few years, both young and old people in the United States and in Europe have taken up the practice of meditation. Regular practice of meditation has a calming and stabilizing effect on its practitioners.[1,2,3] With prolonged practice, many physiological changes occur in the body. Among them is a change in the mode of functioning of the nervous system. These changes can be monitored by the application of a modified ballistocardiograph to a seated upright subject.

Theoretically, when meditation is practiced properly, a sequence of strong and unusual bodily reactions and unusual psychological states is eventually triggered.* Most meditators realize that these reactions are caused by meditation and don't become alarmed. However, sometimes this mechanism

* The "rising of kundalini," as described in classical yoga literature, is a stimulus or "energy" activating a "center" (chakra) at the base of the spine and working its way up the spine. The stimulus stops at several centers along the spine, as it rises. These centers are located opposite the major nerve plexes in the abdomen and in the thorax, which are also stimulated in the process. Eventually the stimulus ends up in the head. Along its path, it often causes violent motion in some parts of the body, signifying that there is "resistance" to its passage. The rising of the kundalini may happen suddenly or over a period of several years. After entering the head, the stimulus continues down the face into the larynx and the abdominal cavity.

can be triggered in nonmeditators. Our observations indicate that exposure to certain mechanical vibrations, electromagnetic waves, or sounds may trigger this mechanism. It is the purpose of this article to bring to the attention of the medical profession this mechanism and some of its symptoms.

Summary

The ballistocardiogram of a sitting subject, who is capable of altering his or her state of consciousness at will, shows a rhythmic sine wave pattern when the subject is in a deep meditative state. This is attributed to the development of a standing wave in the aorta, which is reflected in the rhythmic motion of the body. This resonating oscillator (the heart-aorta system) will rhythm-entrain four additional oscillators, eventually resulting in a fluctuating magnetic field around the head.

Our initial experiments indicate that the five resonating systems are:

1. Heart-aorta system producing an oscillation of about 7 Hz in the skeleton, including the skull. The upper part of the body also has a resonant frequency of about 7 Hz.
2. The skull accelerates the brain up and down, producing acoustical plane waves reverberating through the brain at KHz frequencies.
3. These acoustical plane waves are focused by the skull onto the ventricles, thus activating and driving standing waves within the third and lateral ventricles.
4. Standing waves within the cerebral ventricles in the audio and supersonic ranges stimulate the sensory cortex mechanically, resulting eventually in a stimulus traveling in a closed loop around each hemisphere. Such a traveling stimulus may be viewed as a "current."
5. As a result of these circular "currents," each hemisphere produces a pulsating magnetic field. These fields are of opposing polarities.

This magnetic field–radiated by the head acting as an antenna–interacts with the electric and magnetic fields already in the environment. We may consider the head as simultaneously a transmitting and receiving antenna, tuned to a particular one of the several resonant frequencies of the brain. Environmental fields may thus be fed back to the brain, thus modulating that resonant frequency. The brain will interpret this modulation as useful information.

This paper presents a preliminary report on the possible mechanism of the so-called "kundalini." The kundalini effect is viewed by the author as part of the development of the nervous system. This development can be elicited by the practice of any of several different types of meditative techniques, or it may develop spontaneously. Research into this area is continuing and investigation of the kundalini effect by different methods is in progress.

Micromotion Measurement with the Capacitive Probe

Small body motions accompanying the motion of blood through the circulatory system may be measured with a capacitive probe apparatus. A subject sits on a chair between two metal plates, one above the head, and one under the seat, five to ten cm from the body.

The two plates of the capacitor are part of a tuned circuit. The movement of the subject will modulate the field between the two plates. This signal is processed and fed into a single channel recorder, which registers both the motion of the chest due to respiration and the movement of the body reacting to the motion of the blood in the heart-aorta system. The resulting recording trace (Figure 2) is very similar to that of a ballistocardiogram,[4] in which the subject lies on a platform, to which are attached three mutually perpendicular accelerometers or strain gauges, to measure the body's motion in response to blood flow. But in the capacitive probe measurements, gravitational forces and the elasticity of the skeleton and the general body build play important roles.

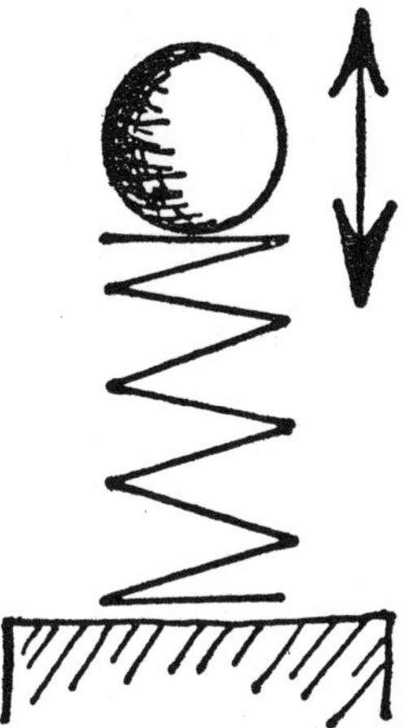

Figure 1. Mass on a spring.

As an analogy, a seated subject can be represented by a mass on a spring (Figure 1): the spring is the spinal column and the mass is the weight of the upper part of the body. Upon the ejection of blood from the heart, this mass is set into motion and starts oscillating at its natural frequency when the person is in a deep meditative state.

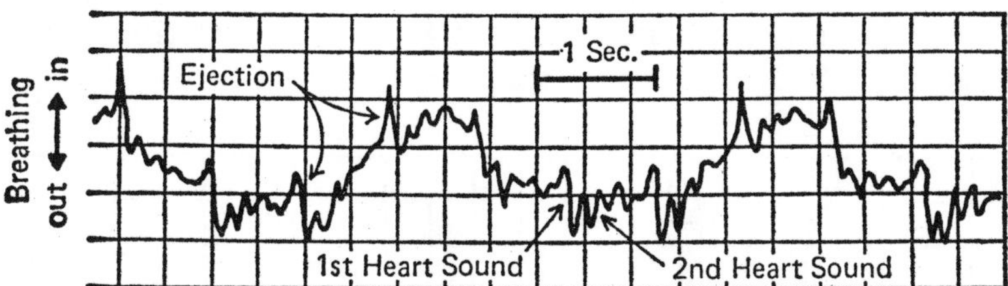

Figure 2. Baseline resting state record.

Figure 2 shows a baseline resting state record, in which the micromotion of the body is superimposed over the motion of the chest, caused by breathing. These are the large slow waves of about a three-second period, or twenty breaths/minute. The first 7 Hz wave is caused by the ejection of blood from the left ventricle, which makes the body recoil downward and sets the body oscillating. The second wave corresponds closely to the action of the blood flowing through the aortic arch, lifting the body up. The third wave occurs at about the same time as the closing of the aortic valve and the slight backflow of the blood, called the dichrotic notch. The first and third waves correspond closely to the first and second heart sounds.

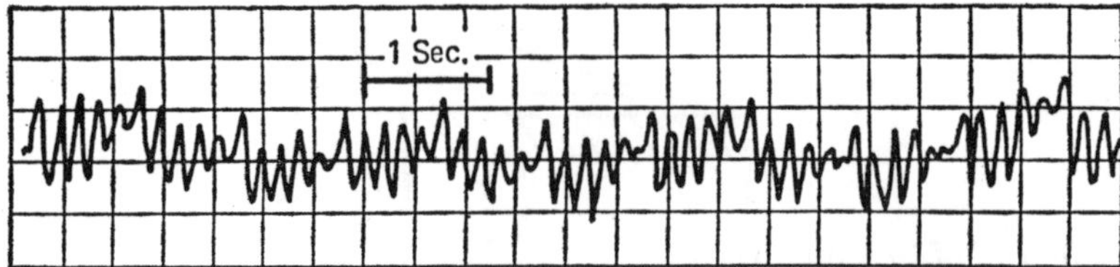

Figure 3. Deep meditative state record.

Figure 3 shows a recording, in which the subject is in a deep meditative state, a few minutes after the baseline reading. Breathing is very shallow, as shown by the practically even level of the 7.5 Hz waves. The irregularity, which characterized the baseline behavior (Figure 2) is gone. Large amplitude regular waves–practically pure sine waves–are present. An almost pure sine wave is what characterizes this state. The body moves in a simple harmonic motion.

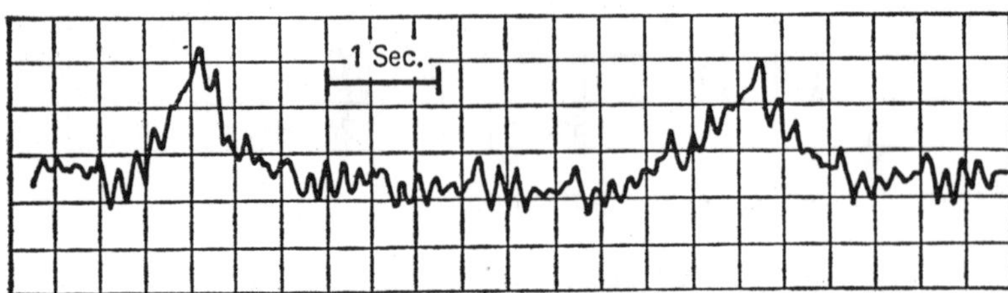

Figure 4. Return to baseline resting state record.

Figure 4 shows the return to baseline of the same subject. Breathing is deeper again, the irregularity of the wave pattern is back, but is not as irregular as before. Total elapsed time for the recording was about 20 minutes.

We have noticed that the regularity in rhythm is obtained at the expense of breathing. The subject can stay in the shallow breathing state for a long time without having to compensate later by deep rapid breathing. This is a state in which the demand for oxygen by the body seems to be lowered. If one stops breathing for a while without being in a deep meditative state,[5] the same regular pattern will be achieved. However, oxygen deficiency builds up quickly and overbreathing will be necessary to restore balance, while in the meditative state this overbreathing does not occur.

The Development of a Standing Wave in the Aorta

The regular movement of the body indicates that a standing wave is set up in the vascular system, specifically, in the aorta.[6,7] This is the only feasible explanation of the regular sine wavelike behavior of the body. This standing wave, as will be shown later, has far-reaching consequences and affects several other resonant systems in the body, which are all driven by this large signal.

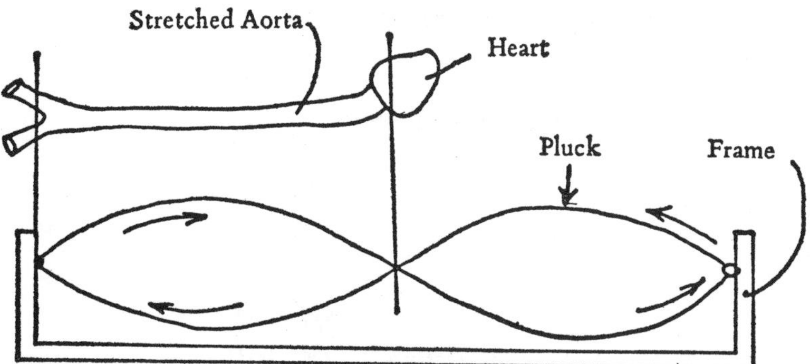

Figure 5a. Comparison of the aorta to a stretched vibrating string. The length of the stretched aorta is equal to one half the wavelength of the string.

The aorta is the major artery of the body. When the left ventricle of the heart ejects blood, the aorta, being elastic, balloons out just distal to the ventricle. Under these conditions, a pressure pulse travels down along the aorta. When the pressure pulse reaches the iliac bifurcation, part of it rebounds and starts traveling up the aorta (Figures 5a, 5b). When the timing of the pressure pulses traveling down the aorta coincides or is in phase with the reflected pressure pulses, a standing wave is achieved. This standing wave of approximately 7 Hz will cause the body to move in a rhythmic fashion, provided the aorta is properly tuned. Presumably, a feedback loop is set up between the bifurcation and the heart, which then regulates the breathing so as to make the lungs and the diaphragm contact the aorta and regulate its impedance. This allows the pressure pulse to be in phase with both the ejection and the dichrotic notch. This is an entirely automatic process during deep meditation.

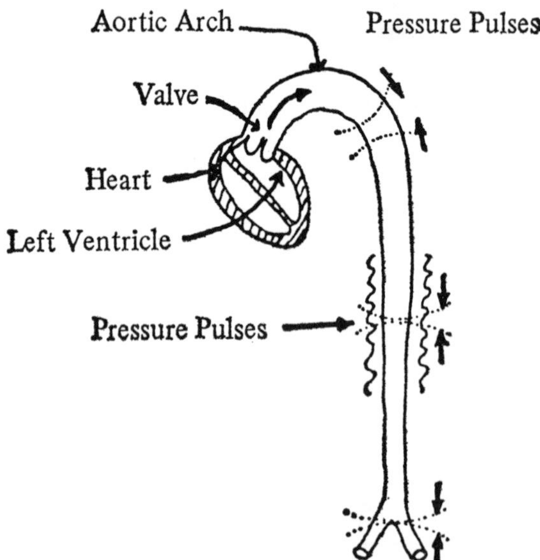

Figure 5b. Collision of the oppositely traveling pressure pulses causes a destructive interference pattern and vibration of aortic walls.

Acoustical Plane Waves in the Body

The movement of the body is relatively small, 0.003 to 0.009 mm, but the body and particularly the head are very dense, tight structures. By moving up and down, the skull accelerates the brain with a mild impact in both directions (Figure 6). This sets up acoustical and possible electrical plane waves reverberating within the skull. The brain may be considered as a piezoelectric gel, converting mechanical vibrations into electrical vibrations, and conversely.

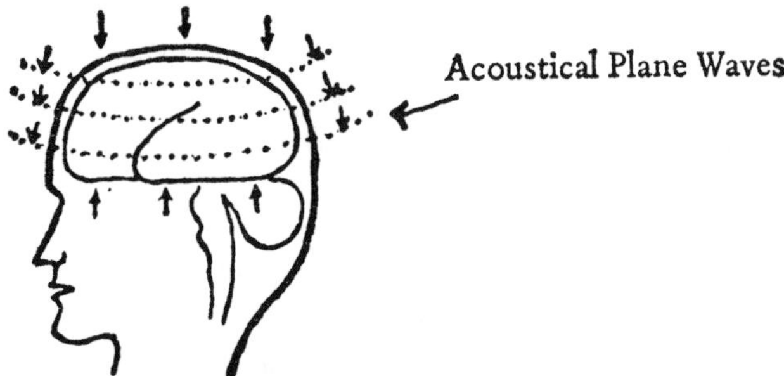

Figure 6. Acoustical plane waves moving through the brain.

The acoustical plane waves reflected from the cranial vault are focused upon the third and the lateral ventricles, as shown in Figures 7 and 8.[8] High-frequency acoustical waves generated by the heart are reflected from the cranial vault and are focused upon the third and lateral ventricles of the brain.

Acoustical Standing Waves in the Ventricles

A hierarchy of frequencies couples the 7 Hz body movement to the higher frequencies in the ventricles.

The body can be considered as a bag of elastic skin containing stiff gel and supported by a rigid armature. The motion

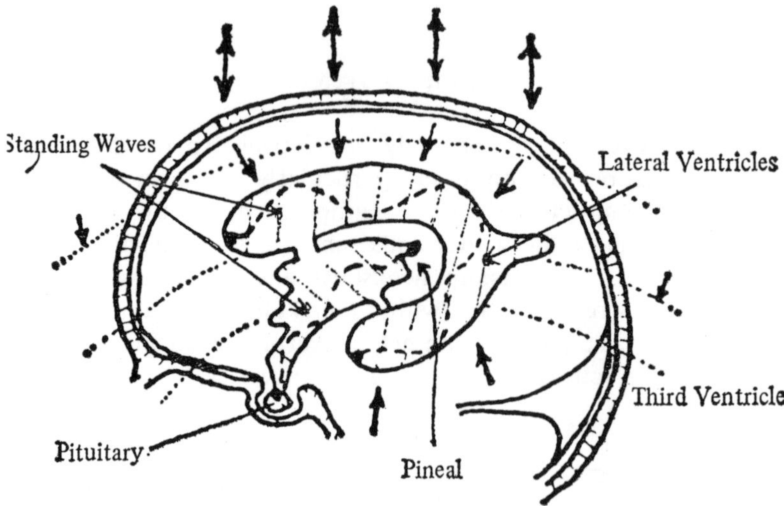

Figure 7. Lateral cross section of brain, showing acoustical standing waves.

of the heart-aorta system sets this gel vibrating in different modes. Assuming the velocity of signal propagation to be 1,200m/sec. the fundamental frequencies for the different parts of the body would be along the vertical axis of the body: (1) brain, 4,000 Hz; (2) circumference of skull, 2,250 Hz; (3) whole body length, 375 Hz; (4) trunk and head, 750 Hz; (5) heart sounds, 35 to 2,000 Hz.[9]†

Part of the energy of the acoustical waves coming from the cranial vault is reflected from the interface of the ventricles and sets the cerebrospinal fluid vibrating. The calculated fundamental frequency of the lateral ventricles is 4,000 Hz and that of the third ventricle, 12,000 Hz. These are the basic standing waves within the ventricles. Again, as long as the

† The high-frequency component of the heart sounds, although very low in intensity, may be able to drive the ventricles directly. The stimulus will be conducted by the left side of the neck, up into the skull, and reflected back from the cranial vault to the ventricles.

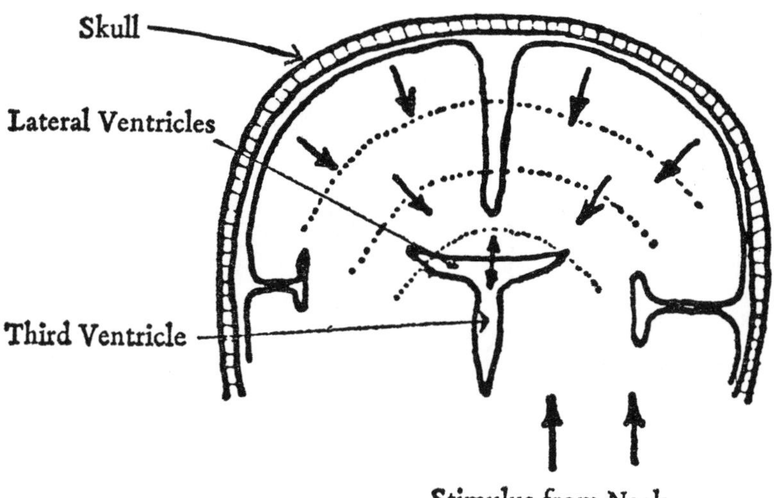

Figure 8. Frontal cross section of brain.

body is in a deep meditative state, it is assumed that these two oscillators stay locked in step with the heart sounds. This phase-locking may occur with the high-frequency end of the heart sounds, i.e. above the 2,000 Hz range. The vibrations produced in the brain tissue by the standing waves in the ventricles are conducted to the middle ear and converted into sound. This is the sound that will be recognized by the meditator as an "inner sound" (Figure 9). These sounds may start abruptly, last for a few seconds or minutes, and die out.

Frequency distribution measurements of "inner sounds" reported by 156 meditators are made by asking each meditator to compare the sounds heard during meditation with sounds produced by an audio-frequency oscillator through an earphone in one ear. The subject rotates the oscillator frequency control to match oscillator tones with those heard or remembered as the "inner sound." The frequency distribution is not smooth, but shows several sharp peaks, harmonics of the fundamental frequency, and possibly beat frequencies produced between the third and lateral ventricles of the brain, which

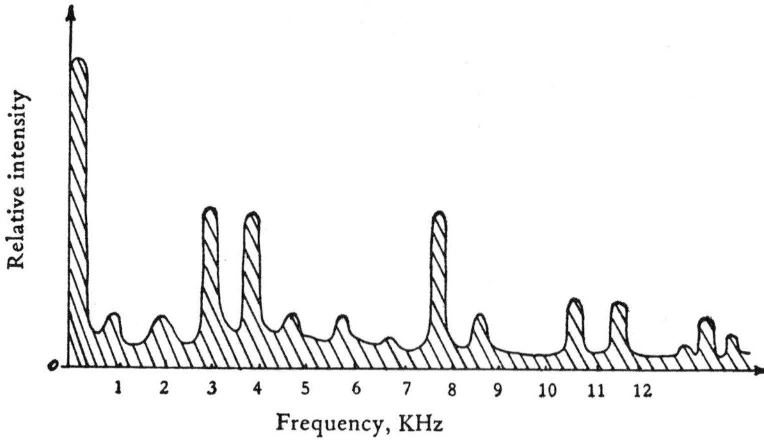

Figure 9. Frequency distribution of "inner sounds" heard by meditators.

are connected by a fluid bridge. In the frequency range below 1 KHz, acoustical standing waves running through the entire body, and the higher harmonics of the heart beat and the heart sounds appear.

The Circular Sensory Cortex "Current"

Figure 10 shows a lateral or side view of the brain. A cross section of the left hemisphere, along line AB through the sensory cortex, is shown as Figure 11.[10] The labels in Figure 11 show sensory cortex areas corresponding to specific sensory functions, and to three pleasure centers, which elicit pleasurable sensations when stimulated. These are: (1) cingulate gyrus; (2) lateral hypothalamus; (3) hippocampus and amygdala areas.

Just above the roof of the lateral ventricle starts the medial fissure, the cleft which separates the two hemispheres.

When a standing wave is present in the ventricles, the roof of the lateral ventricles acts as a taut skin on a drum that moves rapidly up and down, as shown in the sketch (Figure 8).

The roof of the lateral ventricles is the corpus callosum, a bundle of nerve fibers connecting the two hemispheres.[11] The vibration of the corpus callosum and of the brain mass in general may serve as a pace-setter in the phase synchronization which occurs between the two hemispheres during meditation.[12]

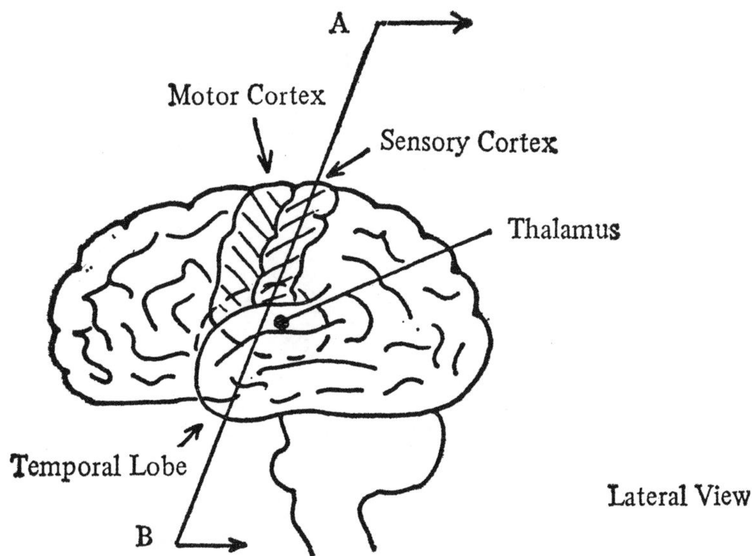

Figure 10. Lateral view of the brain, with section line AB.

When the sensory cortex is stimulated electrically or mechanically, paresthesias occur in the area of the body corresponding to certain points on the cortex. These points are mapped out on the surface of the cortex as shown in Figure 11. As the roof of the lateral ventricles vibrates, it stimulates first the toes, then the ankles, then the calves, thighs, and as the stimulus rounds the corner of the hemisphere, the pelvis is stimulated. As the stimulus spreads along the cortex, it will affect the trunk, moving along the spine toward the head.

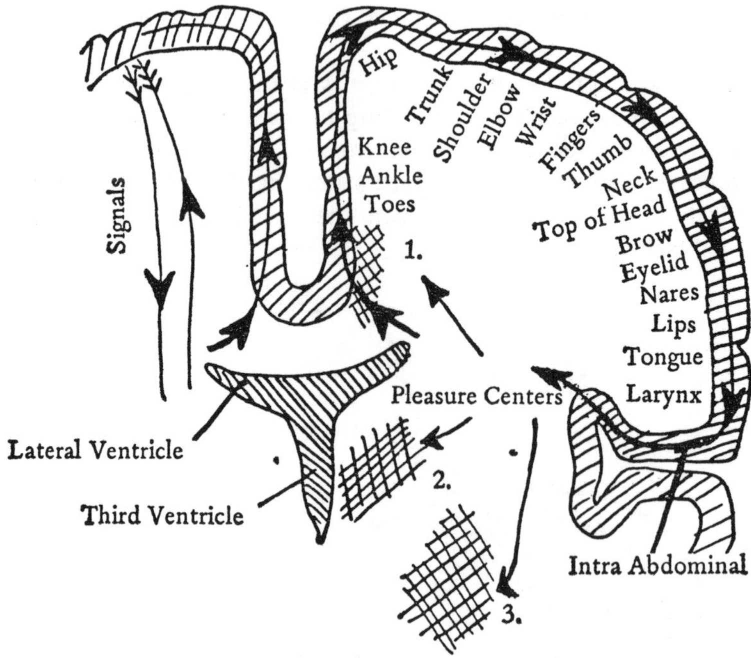

Figure 11. Cross section of the left hemisphere of the brain, through section line AB of Figure 10.

The cortex has different acoustical properties from the white matter and the cerebrospinal fluid. The white matter is made up mostly of myelinated fibers, a fatty substance which will tend to damp out an acoustical signal. The cortex may be viewed as a water-based gel that conducts vibration well.

Thus, an acoustical interface exists between the white matter, the cortex, and the cerebrospinal fluid. The cortex will therefore preferentially tunnel the acoustical signal.

This mechanical vibratory action is assumed to cause electrical polarization of the tissue of the cortex, to allow enhanced conductivity of the tissue to the stimulus moving along the cortex. This moving stimulus may be viewed as a current. According to our hypothesis, this current is responsible for the effects of the "awakened kundalini" on the body.[13,14]

Sensory signals usually come to the cortex through the thalamus and go back the same way (Figures 10, 11). It is interesting to note that those parts of the body, which are represented on the surface of the cortex facing the cranium, are felt more strongly by a person experiencing the kundalini stimulus. Those chakras, or energy centers, are most actively felt, while portions of the cortex, which are cushioned and are located inside the folds of the brain, are less noticeable to the individual. This may well occur because the arch between the tops of the two hemispheres and the temporal areas are exposed to a double stimulus—one coming up from the ventricles and one coming down from the cranial vault, accelerating the brain downward. The larynx is the last point on the cortex facing the skull, and it is also the last chakra to be activated and strongly felt. Presumably, the stimulus continues inside the fold of the temporal lobe and closes the circuit, as shown in Figure 12. This is shown by EEG measurements, indicating that during meditation there are currents of opposing polarity, relative to the midline, flowing along the sensory

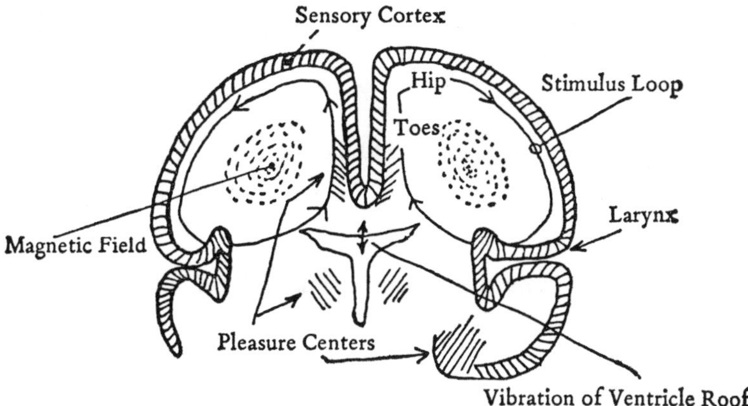

Figure 12. Frontal cross section of brain.

cortex of both hemispheres. These occur in both the alpha and theta range of brain wave frequencies.

As the stimulus travels through, it crosses an area which contains a pleasure center. When the pleasure center is thus stimulated, the meditator experiences a state of ecstasy. To reach that state it may take years of systematic meditation, or again, in certain people it may happen spontaneously.

As long as the four oscillators (1) the aorta, (2) the heart sounds, (3) the standing waves in the ventricles, (4) the circulating sensory stimulus or kundalini current are in phase and resonating, all parts of the body move in harmony. The fifth oscillating circuit is activated when the senory cortex tissue has been finally polarized to the point where there is a circulation of electrical current in the hemispheres and a magnetic field develops inside the core of each current ring, as shown in Figures 13 and 14.[15]

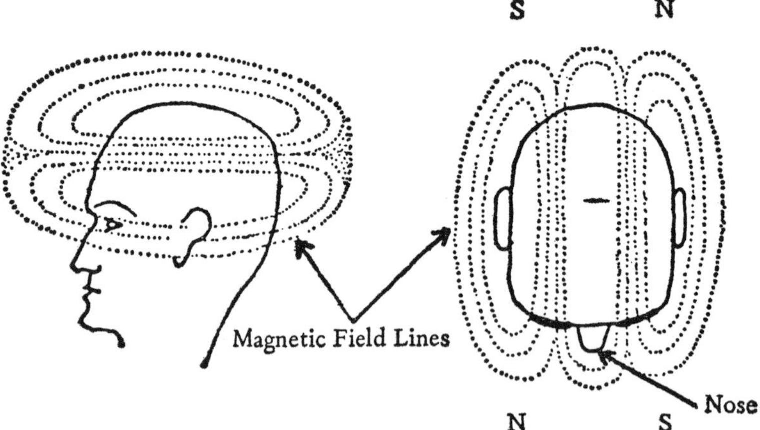

Figures 13–14. Lateral and top views of head, showing magnetic field lines.

This magnetic field pulsates in harmony with the other oscillators. The observed "normal" rate of the circulation of the sensory current is about 7 cycles/sec.

Pulsating magnetic fields of the order of 10^{-9} gauss are produced by the currents circulating in the brain. These currents may be detected by an electroencephalograph electrode on the skin surface of the head. However, they are quite variable.[16] The sensory cortex currents will produce fields of symmetrical shape but with polarities associated with the two brain hemispheres opposing each other, as shown in Figures 13 and 14.

Thus by meditating in a quiet sitting position, we slowly activate five tuned oscillators. One by one these oscillators are locked into rhythm. This results eventually in the development of a pulsating magnetic field around the head. When this occurs, one may simultaneously observe other characteristic and automatic changes in the functioning of the nervous and circulatory systems. It is the purpose of meditation to bring about these changes in order to increase the ability of the nervous system to handle stress and overcome it more easily. The noise level in the nervous system is thus reduced, and the system becomes more efficient and permits a fuller development of the person's latent physical and mental capacities.

Any of the five tuned oscillators can be triggered individually after a short period of stimulation. Any one of them will get the sensory cortex current circulating and will soon lock the heart's and the body's motion into an artificial state of meditation. This is a dangerous practice, which may be traumatic to an inexperienced meditator.

Magnetic Feedback

Fifteen subjects sitting upright were subjected to hemispheric stimulation by an externally applied varying unipolar magnetic field of 0.5 gauss maximum intensity measured at the skin surface. The field was produced by a C-shaped electromagnet, with thirty-cm pole gap spacing, activated by a voltage-offset sine wave power source, with frequency 3.75 Hz, and stimulus duration two minutes for each subject. The apparatus formed a closed magnetic circuit with lines of force going through the brain. The polarity of the applied field could be reversed. The responses of the subjects in a blind experiment were collected in tabular form. (See Table 1.)

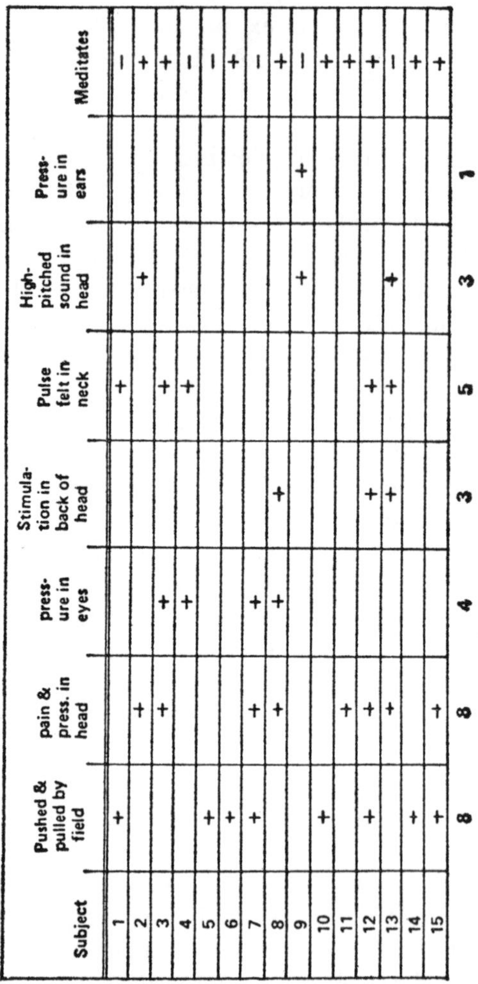

Subject	Pushed & pulled by field	pain & press. in head	press-ure in eyes	Stimula-tion in back of head	Pulse felt in neck	High-pitched sound in head	Press-ure in ears	Meditates
1	+				+			−
2		+				+		+
3		+	+		+			+
4			+		+			−
5	+							−
6	+							+
7	+	+	+					−
8		+	+	+				+
9						+	+	−
10	+							+
11		+						+
12	+	+		+	+			+
13		+		+	+	+		−
14	+							+
15	+	+						+
	8	8	4	3	5	3	1	

Table 1. Summary of responses of fifteen subjects to unipolar 3.75-Hz, 0.5-gauss maximum intensity, two-minute-duration magnetic-field stimulation applied to one hemisphere of the brain.

Micromotion of the Body

More than 50 per cent of the subjects tested described sensations of pain or pressure in the head, also a sensation of being pushed and pulled by the applied magnetic field. These results suggest an interaction of the field around the head with the externally applied field.

Discussion

The symptom-sign of this "sensory-motor cortex syndrome," or what has been characterized as the kundalini process in ancient literature, can be quite variable and sporadic. Its complete presentation usually begins as a transient paresthesia of the toes or ankle with numbness and tingling. Occasionally, there is diminished sensitivity to touch or pain, or even partial paralysis of the foot or leg. The process most frequently begins on the left side and ascends in a sequential manner from foot, leg, hip, to involve completely the left side of the body, including the face. Once the hip is involved, it is not uncommon to experience an intermittent throbbing or rhythmic rumbling-like sensation in the lower lumbar and sacral spine. This is followed by an ascending sensation which rises along the spine to the cervical and occipital regions of the head.

At these latter areas, severe pressure-caused occipital headaches and cervical neck aches may be experienced at times. These pressures, usually transient but occasionally persistent, may also be felt anywhere along the spine, right or left side of chest, different parts of the head and the eyes. Some individuals will notice tingling sensations descending along the face to the laryngeal areas. The tracheolaryngeal region may also be felt as a sudden rushing of air to and fro. Respiration may become spasmodic with involuntarily occurring maximum expirations. Various auditory tones have been noted, from constant low-pitched hums to high-pitched ringing. Visual aberrations and temporary decrease or loss of vision has been observed. The sequence of symptoms continues later down into the lower abdominal region.

Because a particular symptom or sign of the altered sensory and motor systems may occur or persist for months or years, the sequence of symptoms may not be obvious, nor appear casually connected. Also, only in a few of the known cases will all of the symptoms in this sequence become vividly apparent to each person. Normally, physical and laboratory examination reveals either little or no pathology and therefore, except in rare cases, many of the complaints are probably dismissed as psychosomatic or neurotic symptoms.

Meditation has been considered, here and elsewhere, as a stress removal process.[17,18] The symptoms noted above are indications that release of stress is taking place. Stress, as defined by H. Selye, is "a state manifested by a specific syndrome which consists of all the nonspecifically induced changes within a biological system."[19] The intensity of the symptoms is an index of the severity of the stress being released. On the whole, these symptoms should be looked upon as a positive sign of normalization of the body. The unusual aspect of this mechanism is that the release of stress is experienced as a localized stimulation of a particular part of the body, as opposed to the accepted notion that stress is a diffuse general state.

A large percentage of individuals who meditate and who have previously used psychedelic drugs for extended periods of time, or are experiencing unusual stress, are more likely to show these symptoms. These will eventually subside by themselves, without the need for any medical intervention.

It is the spontaneously triggered cases that present a problem, since the individual does not know the cause of these symptoms, and tends to panic. The psychological problems may mimic schizophrenia, and be diagnosed as such by the physician. As a consequence, drastic procedures may be used to alleviate the problem.

An awareness of the existence of the above-noted symptoms and the mechanism which triggers them is important, in view of the constantly increasing number of persons practicing meditation, and therefore likely to experience these effects of stress release.

Possible Rhythm Entrainment Effects

Our experiments show that when a person in deep meditation is suddenly called to come out and stop meditating, the normal response is reluctance to abandon that state and a lapsing back into deep meditation repeatedly. This seems to suggest that a "locking in" situation is present. It is well-known that the larger the number of frequency-locked oscillators in a system, the more stable the system and the more difficult it is to disturb.

When a situation exists, where there are two oscillators vibrating at frequencies close to each other, the oscillator which is operating at a higher frequency will usually lock into step the slower oscillator. This is rhythm entrainment. When in the state of deep meditation, a person goes into sine wave oscillation at approximately seven cycles/sec, there is a tendency for him or her to be locked into the frequency of the planet (Figure 15).

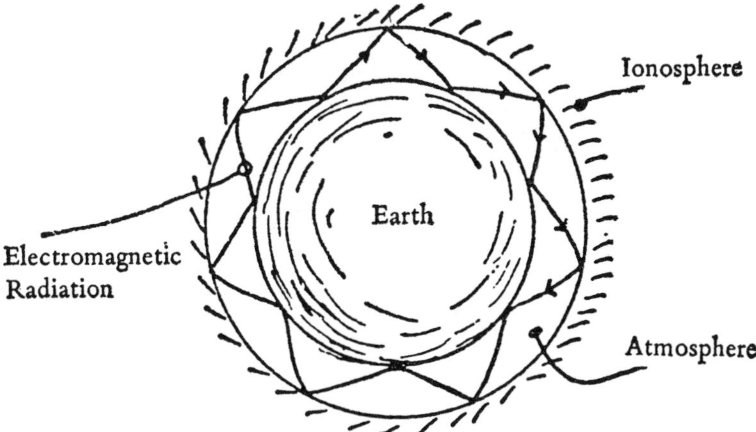

Figure 15. The Earth's atmosphere is shown as a resonant cavity.

We have talked about resonant cavities and how a stimulus can set such a cavity vibrating at its own resonant frequency. Our planet has a conductive layer around it called ionosphere, which starts about eighty km from the earth's surface. The cavity between the earth and the ionosphere (the atmosphere) is also a resonant cavity. Certain types of electromagnetic radiation travel through this cavity, being reflected alternately between the Earth's surface and the ionosphere, and vibrate at characteristic resonant frequencies.

In 1957, W. O. Schumann[20,21] calculated the earth-ionosphere cavity resonance frequencies at 10.6, 18.3, and 25.9 Hz. More recent work by J. Toomey and C. Polk (1970)[22] gave the values 7.8, 14.1, 20.3, 26.4, and 32.5 Hz. The lowest frequency, 7.8 Hz, is approximately equal to the velocity of electromagnetic radiation divided by the earth's circumference:

$$\frac{2.998 \times 10^8 \text{ m/sec}}{4.003 \times 10^7 \text{ m}} = 7.489 \text{ or } 7.5 \text{ Hz}$$

This is the reciprocal of the time required for a beam of electromagnetic radiation to go around the earth.

The planet is very much affected and quite closely coupled by its plasma fields with the sun. These two bodies and their interacting fields form our immediate environment. The sun produces energy in a wide spectrum, from powerful X rays to acoustical signals.[23,24] The solar wind shapes the magnetosphere and the plasmaspheres of our planet. All these layers contain charged particles produced by the sun. In the Van Allen belts, these particles oscillate back and forth along the magnetic lines of the earth between the north and the south poles. Much of this vibration occurs in the frequency range 1 to 40 Hz, well within physiological frequencies.[25]

There is a strong coupling between these oscillations and the changes in the magnetic field of the earth. These microfluctuations of the magnetic field are on the order of 10^{-5} gauss, about 10,000 times stronger than the fields around our heads. We live within this constantly active natural electromagnetic environment, with the added perturbations of broadcasting TV and radio stations.[26]

Given these conditions, it would be reasonable to assume that the fluctuations in these planetary environmental fields have affected human evolution in subtle ways over the ages—in ways which are not quite clear to us yet.[27]

Our knowledge of physiology considers the present state of the human nervous system as being at the peak of its development. However, this article suggests a mechanism which may cause changes in the cerebrospinal system. When a fetus develops in the womb, it undergoes changes which mirror human evolution from a fish through the amphibian to the mammal. But our findings suggest that this evolution very probably has not come to a halt with the way our present nervous system is presently functioning. The hidden potential of our nervous system may be vast.

The mechanism outlined above describes a possible next step in the evolution of the nervous system, which can be accelerated by the use of certain techniques. We can speculate that this development will have the effect of an increased awareness of the self as a part of a much larger system. We can postulate that our magnetic "antennae" will bring in information about our extended system—the planet and the sun—and will allow us to interpret geophysical phenomena and signals to better advantage.[28]‡

†† Note 28 shows that one of the orientation mechanisms of the homing pigeon depends on the magnetic fields of the earth. Indications are that the pigeon's built-in magnetic field is interacting with the earth's magnetic field. The pigeon's field would be analogous to the magnetic field around our head, when intensified by the sensory cortex "current."

NOTES

1. Wallace, K., and Benson, H. "The Physiology of Meditation," *Scientific American,* February 1972.

2. Banquet, J. "Electroencephalography and Clinical Neurophysiology," *EEG and Meditation,* vol. 33, p. 454, 1972.
3. Benson, H. *The Relaxation Response,* William Morrow & Co., New York, 1975.
4. Weissler, A. *Non-Invasive Cardiology,* chapter on ballistocardiography, Grune and Stratton, New York, 1974.
5. Wallace and Benson, op. cit.
6. Bergel, D. *Cardio-Vascular Fluid Dynamics,* chapter 10, Academic Press, New York, 1972.
7. New, P. "Arterial Stationary Waves," *American Journal of Roentgenology,* vol. 97, no. 2, pp. 488–99.
8. Ruch, T., Patton, H., Woodbury, J., and Towe, A. *Neurophysiology,* 1st edition, p. 262, Saunders Publishing Co., Philadelphia, 1962.
9. Luisada, A. *The Sounds of the Normal Heart,* Warren H. Green Publishing Co., St. Louis, 1972.
10. Ruch, Patton, Woodbury, and Towe, op. cit.
11. Ibid.
12. Banquet, op. cit.
13. Bucke, R. *Cosmic Consciousness,* E. P. Dutton & Co., New York, 1970.
14. Krishna, G. *Higher Consciousness,* Julian Press, Inc., New York, 1974.
15. Cohen, D. "Magnetoencephalograph: Detection of the Brain's Electrical Activity with a Superconducting Magnetometer," *Science,* vol. 175, no. 4022, February 11, 1972.
16. Ibid.
17. Benson, op. cit.
18. Selye, H. *The Stress of Life,* McGraw-Hill, New York, 1956.
19. Ibid.
20. Schumann, W. "Electrische Eigenshwingungen des Hohlraumes Erde-Luft-Ionosphere," *Zeitschrift für Angewandte Physik,* vol. 9, pp. 373–78, 1957.
21. Persinger, M., ed. *ELF and VLF Electromagnetic Field Effects,* Plenum Press, New York, 1974.
22. Ibid.
23. Thomsen, D. "On the Edge of Space," *Science News,* vol. 94, no. 9, p. 216, August 31, 1968.
24. Ewing, A. "The Noisy Sun," "Ion Signals Across Space," *Science News,* vol. 92, no. 11, p. 250, September 9, 1967.
25. Konig, H. "Biological Effects of Low Frequency Electrical Phenomena," *Interdisciplinary Cycle Research,* vol. 2, no. 3, 1971.
26. Becker, R. "Electromagnetic Forces and Life Processes," *MIT Technology Review,* vol. 75, no. 2, p. 32, December 1972.
27. Ibid.

28. Walcott, C., and Green, R. "Orientation of Homing Pigeons Altered by a Change in the Direction of an Applied Magnetic Field," *Science,* vol. 184, no. 4133, April 12, 1974.

REFERENCES AND SUGGESTED READINGS

Gauquelin, M. *The Cosmic Clocks,* Avon Books, New York, 1974.

Stapp, Col. J. P. "The 'G' Spectrum in Space Flight Dynamics," *Lectures in Aerospace Medicine,* January 16–20, 1961.

Tart, C. *Altered States of Consciousness,* John Wiley & Sons, New York, 1969.

SYMBOLIC EXPRESSIONS OF KUNDALINI THROUGH THE UNCONSCIOUS

Tontyn Hopman

It is only natural that people in whom kundalini begins to be active should have manifestations of the process in their unconscious. These will most likely take the form of vivid dreams, fantasies, and visions of light, heat, dryness, and such symbols of transformation as snakes, butterflies, frogs, certain forms of fire, death, and resurrection. The unicorn may appear signifying sublimated sexual power, or the thunderbolt as supreme creative potency in the form of transcendental energy acting on the mundane.

Of all these, the very ambivalent symbol of the snake is likely to appear most frequently. An actual encounter with a snake is always unexpected and startling. Similarly, a person to whom a snake appears in a dream often sees in it something extraordinary or even threatening. It is of some importance whether the dream snake is poisonous. If so the dreamer is probably facing some ominous situation, the peril or negativity of which he has not yet recognized, but which he is likely to experience—with a startle—in the days following the dream. Jung pointed out that the Gnostics related the serpent to the spinal cord and the spinal marrow, and that it is an excellent image of the way the unconscious expresses itself suddenly and unexpectedly with its peremptory and terrible incursions. A snake dream indicates that an important, probably transforming event is about to occur. If the snake is nonpoisonous, its appearance, apart from signifying metamorphosis, may mean that somewhere in the dreamer a process of healing is going on. Since the time of the ancient Greeks, who depicted their great mythic healer Aesculapius with a snake around his staff, there has always been one symbol or another in which the snake winds around a staff as an emblem of medical doctors or pharmacies all over the world.

Extraordinary potency and psychic energy are always suggested by the appearance of the snake, and the idea of transformation or resurrection obviously derives from the fact that snakes shed their skins. The snake with special attributes may occur as the crowned one, symbolizing his superior value, or as the snake with crystal in its head, suggesting it brings priceless spiritual realizations. There is also the feathered or winged snake, denoting a spiritualization through an integration of matter and spirit.

Example of a Kundalini Dream

Wings and feathers suggest the element of air, the realm of the Spirit. This is shown clearly in the following remarkable dream of a young woman who passed through an awakening:

> She dreamt that she and her father were lying lazily in the grass of a hillside, enjoying the sunny summery atmosphere. Presently they both became aware of a soft mechanical noise like "put . . . put . . . put . . ." as two beds, one after another, came floating along from left to right, as if driven by unseen little motors. The beds came to halt so close to them that she and her father could each recline on one of them as they continued their leisurely journey in the calm summer air of the sunbathed landscape.
>
> The dream picture changes. The young woman finds herself in the farmer's house, high up in the Alps, where she spent part of her youth. Suddenly she is startled by a sharp noise of rapidly increasing intensity coming from outside. She runs to the window and to her intense consternation sees a squadron of jet planes diving straight

> down in her direction. With a crashing noise the squadron tears down straight at her, seeming in the next few seconds certain to crash into the farmhouse. Then, with a split-second maneuver they skim over the house's rooftop, missing it by inches. A moment later the door of the room in which the young woman finds herself opens and the uniformed chief pilot of the squadron enters and with authority explains to her that this is how kundalini (he actually uses that word in the dream) works. It has these two aspects: the one in which one drifts into a serene calm, the other laden with a violently threatening crisis that is averted only at the very last moment.

It is extremely important to understand that these seemingly unavoidable crises have a meaning. They are part of the transforming and cleansing process that always accompanies both the awakening and the years that follow. The ultimate catastrophe so often is avoided by the realization that in some department of life one is pursuing a wrong course. A last-minute turnabout, at the height of a crisis, can then bring a change that may well affect one's entire destiny. Or the crisis may have the quality of a creative destruction of that which is false or obstructive to our unfoldment. Such crises, either in the mind or in relation to the outer world, are part of the highly concentrated experience that the process makes one go through. The knife-edge path is by no means illusory. Everything may really be at stake. Each time they occur there is a total challenge affecting our whole being. The Spirit knows no half measures or lukewarm adjustments. How else could a person really be transformed except through the most intense experiences?

And here lie the real dangers to those who want to awaken kundalini by artificial means or under the guidance of commercial gurus. They really risk madness and death. But to those in whom the awakening happens spontaneously, the right inner or outer teacher will appear at the right time. It is to the great credit of Gopi Krishna that he went the whole length of this perilous path entirely on his own. But just because of that he is able to present the world with a live and entirely new perspective about the phenomenon that is bound to have an inconceivable impact on a time that seems just ripe for it.

The ambivalent quality of the process is presented beautifully to the young woman in this dream. It is explained that the awakening encompasses both the state of being in harmony with Tao and the knife-edged path with its violent purifications and sudden, catastrophic perils. It is significant that in the first part of her dream she is accompanied by her father. Gopi Krishna has pointed out that the activated process runs in families. Awakening is primarily possible through favorable hereditary conditions. In this connection, remarkably, the dreamer's father had a partial awakening, and her own daughter, at the age of seven, illustrated her own dream in which a large snake protected a bowlful of precious stones.

Of course, dreaming of snakes, butterflies, fire, etc., by no means indicates that an awakening is going on. Everybody has periods in his life when inner changes are going on. On the other hand, it is not at all advisable for those in whom the awakening is going on to pay much attention to their probably vivid dreams and visions. The participation of the unconscious in the process may produce an avalanche of such material, but unless one understands the symbolic language of the psyche very well, one may be drawn into a labyrinth from which it is very hard to get out. And where is the analyst who has reliable knowledge of the workings of kundalini? Of course, if one has been deeply upset by it, a psychologist may bring relief. But caution should be exercised in interfering with the process. The better attitude toward the unconscious would be one of positive acceptance. Through rejection of its expressions, the unconscious can become negative. If we maintain an attitude of openness and willingness to cooperate, the Guiding Principle in us can bring about significant changes without any great effort on our part.

Example of a Snake Dream

> A man dreamt that he was standing among empty shelves. Suddenly a large green snake appeared and, before he knew it, had coiled itself around him several times, putting its head on his. Obviously he finds himself completely at the mercy of this formidable creature.

Neither in the visionary world nor in reality is it good to be in such a position, in which one's freedom of action is so completely frustrated. On awakening from the dream this man realized his precarious situation. However, he had developed a good relationship with his own psyche and decided to paint his dream as one does in art therapy. Such a course can render perilous dream content harmless by transferring much of it to the outer world. Then it is there, right in front of one, fixed but still reflecting its potency on the observer–but in a much less threatening manner. The result was astonishing. Within a week the same man painted a spontaneous vision in which the snake was clearly contained within a mandala. It was no longer a snake about to strangle or bite him but rather one that was an integral part of an archetypal order, contained in that order. While painting this second picture this man experienced an influx of strength and a sense of exultation.

Example of a Sex Dream

How the unconscious takes part in the process is clearly illustrated in one of the sex dreams that so often accompany the awakening:

> A middle-aged man dreamt he was bending forward to such an extent that his head came level with his genitals.

Next day, preoccupied with the intense atmosphere of that dream, he got the idea to take up the same position as he had in his dream. The result was startling. For the first time he saw that his testicles were making very visible spastic contractions. Gopi Krishna has explained this phenomenon, whereby the organs act as pumps to rush the sublimated sexual fluids to those parts of the brain and body that are in dire need of this fuel at the height of our transformation. Clearly this man's unconscious wanted to make him aware that the process had started in him. It is important to become conscious of the process because we must not only begin to realize what is happening but also we must want to cooperate with it. Then we may no longer live to excess. We must avoid all great strains and pay attention to our diet and sleep. Sexual contact during the first six to twelve months after the awakening should probably be avoided because otherwise the process may go out of control. It becomes necessary to find the suitable middle way.

Some Reactions to the Awakening

During and for a period of time after the awakening, it may be quite hard to accept the reality of kundalini. One is aware of going through a turmoil of both beatific and upsetting visionary or synchronistic experiences. One wants nothing more than to return to the old, uncomplicated state and have nothing more to do with the new situation. Perhaps we already intuit the discipline acceptance of it implies. It means living with the Unknown. Most people tend to avoid transformation. They would rather do anything to change the environment and the circumstances instead of changing themselves. And so they are inclined to put it all aside as a nightmare that they can laugh about when the normal waking state is fully there again. But the serpent power has its own very unmistakable means to make itself known and respected. And so in the end they cannot help but admit that a new energy is active in them.

Another dangerous possibility is to take the opposite standpoint and believe that one has been chosen by divinity to become someone very special endowed with superhuman powers. Such a person may even interfere with and try to direct the process. The results are very much more painful than in the former case. One who does this is in danger of self-inflation. That means unconsciously he identifies his small ego with the higher self in him that is the sole originator and director of the process. In his immediate surroundings he may become a laughingstock and in his own mind this situation creates an imbalance with which he upsets himself in a painful way and loses his contact with outer reality. It is not for nothing that the world's great faiths rank humility as one of the prerequisites on the spiritual path.

It seems that most people in whom the awakening occurs appear for some period of time to be upset by it, unless it has been with them from birth. The turbulent changes that may occur in the unconscious may be presented to them as dreams or visions of momentous forces of nature, as great storms threatening to tear down trees and houses, or as agitated oceans throwing up perilous waves. Earthquakes or landslides may shatter the dreamer's abode or fires may destroy it. These represent elements of the psyche in the process of transformation. Dreams as well as fantasties can have a strong impact on the conscious mood and depress or uplift us all day long. Faced with such apparent threats, the most helpful attitude one can take may well be what Gopi Krishna calls the "prayerful mood," that state of mind in which it is recognized that the ego does not have an answer to the immediate problem or threat and can do nothing about it but remain in a state of humble, unarticulated prayer to the Unknown. This, he says, puts us in a direct contact with our larger self.

The Conscious Attitude

Consciously we can assist in the process of remaining or returning to normal by evening out the unbalancing effect on the nervous system and the mind. This can be done by the very simple means of regulating food, sleep, and calm, possibly by being with persons with whom we have a harmonious and loving relationship and by humbly trying to live with, even for, the new energy in us. We have to find out for ourselves whether, and how much, we can go on with entertainment, parties, smoking, and drinking, what kind of sexual life is in harmony with our new state, and what environment furthers it. It may be that some of the noise of the day has to give way to stillness. We have to find out to whom we can speak about our problems, if we speak of them at all. So the real art of living, for those in whom the process is activated, would be to continue, as much as possible, to behave as before and at the same time to keep clean and fueled the lantern that they themselves are so the flame may burn brightly in it.

SOME POSSIBILITIES FOR FURTHER KUNDALINI RESEARCH

John White

The ramifications of the kundalini concept extend into many areas of science and the humanities—indeed, all of life. The preceding articles in this section, drawn from diverse sources, clearly are only initial investigations into a vast field. This brief article is intended to gather together other such preliminary probes that came to my attention during my research, or that I conceived, and to offer them for consideration.

Literary Criticism

It was suggested in the commentary to Part II that Poe's life and works ought to be re-examined in terms of kundalini. Such an examination could well be extended to other writers and other aspects of literature. For example, it has been pointed out by various critics that fairy tales often have hidden psychological meaning. The story of Sleeping Beauty can be seen as a dramatization of the awakening of kundalini. So can "Snow White and the Seven Dwarfs." In the latter story—once it is stripped of its Hollywood veneer—the dwarfs appear to represent the chakras and Snow White represents the higher self, the human potential for growth to a state of infinite bliss. The prince can be seen as grace, the guru giving shaktipat, divine love, the vehicle that awakens the higher self.

One of the pioneering researchers in this field was the eminent psychologist Carl Jung. This is a little-known aspect of his career. In 1932, at his headquarters in Zurich, Jung held a seminar on kundalini. The transcript is nearly fifty pages long and was unavailable for inclusion here. It was published in *Spring* (see Appendix) as "Psychological Commentary on Kundalini Yoga." Here is an example of Jung's insightful approach to kundalini in the field of literary criticism, taken from the commentary.

> I will give you an example from a medieval book, the famous *Hypnerotomachia,* or *Le Songe de Poliphile.* . . . It was written in the fifteenth century by a Christian monk of a famous Roman family. He got into the unconscious, as we say. It is like the beginning of Dante's *Inferno,* but expressed in entirely different terms. He depicts himself as traveling in the Black Forest, which in those days, especially to Italians, was the *ultima Thule* where the unicorn still lived, as wild and unknown as the forests of central Africa to us. And there he loses his way, and then a wolf appears. At first he is afraid, but afterward he follows it to a spring where he drinks the water. That is an allusion to baptism. Then he comes to the statues and peculiar symbolic inscriptions, which he quotes, and which are most interesting from a psychological point of view. Then suddenly it becomes uncanny and he is frightened. He wants to go back, and he turns to go out of the cave again. But there a dragon is now crouching that bars the way and he cannot go back; he simply has to go forward. The dragon is kundalini. You see, the kundalini in psychological terms is that which makes you go on the greatest adventures. I say: "Oh, damn, why ever did I try such a thing?" But if I turn back, then the spirit of adventure goes out of my life and my life is nothing any longer; it has lost its flavor. It is this quest which makes life livable, and this is kundalini, this is the divine urge. For instance, when a knight in the Middle Ages performed marvelous deeds, like the great labors of Hercules, when he fought drag-

ons and liberated virgins, it was all for his lady—then she was kundalini. And when Leo and Holly [in H. Rider Haggard's novel *She*] go to Africa to seek She, and She urges them on to the most incredible adventures, She is kundalini.

Yes, the anima is the kundalini.

Quantum Physics

The renowned German physicist C. F. von Weizsäcker, director of the Max Planck Institute for the Life Sciences in Starnberg, Germany, wrote a long Introduction to one of Gopi Krishna's books, *The Biological Basis of Religion and Genius* (see Appendix). In it he pointed out the functional near-equivalency between the ancient concept of prana and the modern formulation of quantum mechanics regarding the nature of space.

"At the center of his entire argument," von Weizsäcker remarks, "Krishna places an evolution of the organ of consciousness, which can be described in physiological terms. Our sciences know nothing whatever of such an evolution. This is the field of contest. . . ." He adds that this view of sexuality serving evolution either in reproduction or in the heightening of consciousness is dependent on the esoteric concept of prana. But "prana is not necessarily incompatible with our physics. Prana is spatially extended and vitalizing. Hence above all it is moving potency. The quantum theory designates something not entirely remote from this. . . ."

In my *Future Science,* an Appendix entitled "The X Energy: A Universal Phenomenon" lists more than a hundred terms, from cultures around the world throughout history, for a fifth force in nature that is functionally equivalent to prana. There is, as one physics researcher, Dr. Charles Musès, puts it, a protobiological character revealed by quantum physics in the subatomic world. This is a subject in which the so-called mind-matter problem can be fundamentally investigated, with a rich harvest of data on the physics of paranormal phenomena likely to be gained.

Sleep and Dream Research

In correspondence with me several years ago, a psychiatrist speculated that REM (*r*apid *e*ye *m*ovement) sleep—the stage of sleep during which dreaming occurs—may be a nightly form of mild kundalini experience.

This proposition is developed as follows. First, the penis-serpent equivalency is routinely accepted in psychological thought. Second, during REM sleep, males experience penile erection while females experience some engorgement of the clitoris. So REM sleep is a stage of our unconscious life that is profoundly connected with our sexual nature. Even if the content of the dream is not explicitly sexual, these physiological effects are generally present. Moreover, analysis of dreams usually reveals latent sexual meaning, well disguised by fantasy.

The possibility of a REM sleep-kundalini relationship is further suggested by the fact that a person deprived of dream time during sleep will eventually show signs of psychotic behavior. He will go insane. Kundalini tradition likewise holds that *mastanas,* a Persian word denoting "God-intoxicated" people whose behavior is nevertheless deranged, have "stumbled" on the kundalini path. *Mastanas* are distinguished from *farzanas,* those pursuing disciplines of higher consciousness who have not taken a misstep into madness.

If kundalini is the link between sexuality and madness, it would seem to be obvious in the case of schizophrenics. My correspondent pointed out that Bleuler and other psychiatric pioneers observed that schizophrenic men often had erections. He asked, "Might kundalini cause an erection by the same mechanism that REM sleep causes them, and might REM sleep therefore be considered an aspect of kundalini?" He suggested that since the value of REM sleep for mental health is clearly established, kundalini yoga may in part be a technique for obtaining the benefits of REM at will.

This is not implausible when one considers that both dreams and the forms of meditation using visualization have in common the generation of internal bioluminescence. If, as Lansky suggests, the light experienced during the awakening of kundalini has a neurochemical basis, then kundalini yoga and meditation in general may be methods of "bringing dreams into waking life"—that is, integrating states of consciousness into a greater, more harmonious mode of living. Indeed, kundalini tradition holds that the demarcation between the unconscious and the conscious is reduced, even eliminated, in kundalini masters. Their state of samadhi is continuous, even when they are asleep, so their dream life takes on a markedly different quality. Dream studies of such people might yield surprising new data.

Medical Literature Search

In *Nuclear Evolution,* page 130, Christopher Hills remarks that kundalini "has already been studied objectively by several doctors for many years (to my knowledge at least seventeen years) in yogic hospitals and ashrams such as the Kaivalyadhama laboratory at Lonalva near Poona. A friend of mine, Dr. S. Vinekar, the Director of Research, demonstrated a map tracing of the kundalini path by using EEG and GSR equipment to record its electrical effects in 1961 at a conference of renowned yogis in Patna. . . . The opening of the chakras and the path of the kundalini is described in many ancient texts and Dr. Vinekar merely checked these documented statements from an objective medical and biophysical point of view."

These data, if still available, ought to be collected as part of a large and well coordinated search through the international medical literature for information on kundalini. One wonders what similarities and differences there might be, for example, between Vinekar's mapping and Bentov's.

In any case, one person cannot do it all, nor can he be expected to be familiar with all the literature that exists on a subject as vast as kundalini. Therefore a systematization of knowledge from the physical, biological, and social sciences is strongly needed in this field. Then a content and pattern analysis can be made to extract the profiles of kundalini phenomena in order to conduct controlled experiments. What might be found, for example, if the medical condition commonly called "brain fever" were examined in terms of kundalini? Would the bouts of brain fever that occurred to an inventive genius such as Nicola Tesla take on new significance? I suspect so.

That is a matter to be investigated. However, the standard procedure for scientific investigation in general, before beginning an experiment, is to make a search of the literature in order to avoid "reinventing the wheel." That certainly is appropriate in the case of kundalini research because there have been very few attempts to collect, collate, and catalog such literature. Here is an area for scholarly effort.

Biology and Molecular Genetics

Gopi Krishna has given specific indications for scientifically demonstrating the reality of kundalini. I will summarize them here.

First, a person in whom kundalini is fully developed will clearly be a genius, no matter what his IQ was before the experience. This position represents a radical departure from the view of intelligence which holds that it is determined once and for all by the condition of the genes at birth. How is genius determined? The standard IQ tests are one obvious measurement. In addition, *new* knowledge will come from such a person. He will be a *creative* genius, not simply an intellectual prodigy.

Second, as kundalini transforms a person, the nervous system and brain undergo microbiological changes that will be observable (although the necessary equipment for observing them may not yet exist).

Third, the "food" that the body uses to nourish the nervous system during the transformation comes from the sex organs —the "essence" of seminal fluid in men and what Gopi Krishna calls "the erotic fluids" in women. Thus the reproductive organs increase their activity dramatically, producing many times more copiously than usual. There may also be unusual involuntary contractions of the penis or vagina-uterus ensemble as the sexual fluids are drawn into the body.

Fourth, the fluid sexual essence, existing at the molecular or even the atomic level, streams from the reproductive organs through neural pathways into the spinal canal and then upward into the brain (*urdhvas retas*—the reversal of the sexual fluids). This can be verified by a spinal tap.

Fifth, the bloodstream also carries nerve food during this organic transformation. Hence the composition of the blood changes due to the awakening of kundalini, and ought to be examined in any research program.

Sixth, heart activity (pulse rate) and other internal organs undergo radical changes in operation. Hormonal balance, for example, can be expected to shift. Likewise, perception, digestion, and elimination change dramatically—still further clues to look for in the full spectrum of physical-mental-behavioral transmutations that necessarily must occur as nature prepares the organism for a higher state of being through a total cellular reorganization.

Finally, since the person in whom kundalini is fully awakened will have high moral character and other traits (such as psychic and literary talents) typically associated with spiritual masters, psychologists and others will be able to compare these factors before and after the awakening of kundalini. His psyche and values should be those of a self-actualized person.

These suggestions by Gopi Krishna can be dealt with straightforwardly. Another possible test along the lines he suggests, which I propose here, is in the field of molecular genetics. Gopi Krishna maintains that enlightenment is an evolutionary process, with heredity playing an important role by stamping the genes of the enlightened so that their biological gains through spiritual disciplines can be passed to their progeny. This prediction can be tested by comparing genetic structure prior to and during the awakening of kundalini. Presumably, the DNA will show some difference before and after.

Clinical Psychology and Psychotherapy

In Swami Narayanananda's *The Primal Power in Man or The Kundalini Shakti* (see Appendix), there is a good example of how the kundalini concept can bring striking new perspectives to the data of orthodox psychology and thereby open new avenues of psychotherapeutic research and application. Narayanananda examines an all too common situation—sorrow—in a way that shows its transformative potential. The usual psychological approach to grief consists in having the grieving person learn to "cope" with his circumstances. He is counseled to "be realistic" and accept the loss "like an adult." This is not an incorrect approach—only incomplete. It is incomplete because it fails to recognize the possibility of using deep sorrow in the service of consciousness expansion. (Alfred Tennyson's poem *In Memoriam* is a beautiful example of how sorrow can lead to transpersonal awareness.) Consider Narayanananda's description of the psychophysiology of sorrow:

> Kundalini shakti awakes and rises up even when one is in deep sorrow. . . . In deep sorrow, the mind constantly lives on one object, viz., the beloved object. This constant thinking of one thing and this constant living on one object, brings about automatic concentration of the mind. This one-pointedness of the mind [activates] the kundalini shakti. For, every [instance of] deep one-pointed thinking is only an unconscious [action] on the kundalini shakti. This [action] heats the kundalini shakti. And the heated shakti tries to rise up, as the sor-

> row-stricken man becomes indifferent, for the time being, to the senses, sense-pleasures and their objects. So the . . . shakti tries to rise up. But in deep sorrow the shakti does not rise up fully, as the man has not gained the purity of body, nadis and the mind. It rises up only partly. Often the heated kundalini shakti sends hot currents to the different parts of the body and more to the brain center. These hot currents that reach the brain center heat the brain, make the mind fickle, bring insomnia, brain disorder, insanity and incurable diseases. For the hot currents keep the mind wide awake and if a person does not know how to check the currents and to bring down the partly risen kundalini shakti to safer centers, one suffers terribly and it may ruin the whole life of a person or lead one to insanity. This is why we see many become insane, many get brain defects, and many others get some incurable diseases after deep sorrow.

From this perspective, "breakdown" is an opportunity for "breakthrough." Psychologists, psychiatrists, psychotherapists, counselors, and others in the helping professions could begin to incorporate into their practices those techniques (such as meditations, visualizations, and breathing exercises) that are designed to direct the grieving person through the grief state into higher awareness and insight. Since concentration, as Narayanananda points out, is automatically but unconsciously present during grief, it needs only to be recognized as such and used consciously. The clinical applications here are vast.

A datum bearing directly on the relationship between deep grief and the potential for awakening kundalini was provided by a correspondent who directed my attention to a passage in Havelock Ellis's 1942 *Studies in the Psychology of Sex* (Volume 1, Part 2). Ellis quotes a man who, at the end of the last century, reported the following:

> When my child died at the age of six months, I had a violent paroxysm of weeping and for some days I could not eat. When I kissed the dead boy for the last time (I had never seen a corpse before), I felt I had reached the

depths of misery and could never smile or have any deep emotions again. Yet that night, though my thoughts had not strayed to sexual subjects since the child's death, I had a violent erection. I felt ashamed to desire carnal things when my dead child was still in the house, and explained to my wife. She was sympathetic, for her idea was that our common grief had intensified my love for her. I feel convinced, however, that my desire was the result of a stimulus propagated to the sexual centers from the centers affected by my grief, the transference of my emotion from one set of nerves to another. I do not perhaps express my meaning clearly.

Headache Research

Swami Muktananda remarks in his autobiography (see the excerpt in Part II) that during his kundalini awakening, "I used to suffer from acute headaches." This symptom has been explored by Bentov and Sannella in their physio-kundalini syndrome research. In *New Age* magazine (March 1978), Bentov gives further details of their findings. One symptom of the physio-kundalini syndrome, he says, is "tremendous headaches, steelband-like headaches" in which the "pressure goes on and off at first, but eventually becomes constant."

This comment prompted a correspondent of mine, Mineda McCleave (see her article in Part IV), to explore speculatively a possible relationship between headache and kundalini. More than forty million Americans suffer some kind of severe periodic headaches, and it is estimated that up to twenty-one million of them are migraine victims. McCleave herself has a history of migraine, and feels on the basis of personal experience that Western medicine is treating kundalini symptoms, especially headache, without recognizing the true nature of the process. Some of the points of correspondence she sees between headache research and kundalini research are:

—Tension headache often begins with a pressure that builds until it becomes constant. At that point it is called a "hatband" headache because it seems to fit around the head like a hatband. This matches Bentov's description of "steelband-like headaches."

–In classical migraine (as distinguished from common migraine) there is an "aura" or warning signal preceding the pain. Sufferers describing the aura mention subjective phenomena such as spangles of light, flashing lights, streaks and dots of light, fireworks, exploding stars, a halo or rainbow surrounding people they see, weird images of animal and human forms, visual distortion, hallucinations and other mental aberrations. This may be functionally related to the hallucinatory experiences often reported upon the awakening of kundalini.

–Most migraine sufferers are above average intelligence, and some have been geniuses. These include Lincoln, Jefferson, Grant, Darwin, Tolstoy, Nietzsche, Tchaikovsky, Virginia Woolf, Alfred Nobel, Karl Marx, George Bernard Shaw, Lewis Carroll, and Edgar Allan Poe. This may be evidence of Gopi Krishna's claim that kundalini activity produces genius.

–Just as Bentov noted that the kundalini-induced headache may become extremely active about 2:30 A.M., the first headache of a cluster headache–a form of particularly severe headache that generally strikes males–often hits its victim between 2 and 5 A.M.

–It has been reported that migraine may be connected to the menstrual cycle in women. Many migraine patients have their first headaches in their teen years and twenties. In women the migraines usually vanish after menopause, and seldom do they occur for the first time after menopause. This appears related to the sexual aspect of kundalini's awakening.

–Studies have shown that many people have an increase in sexual urge when the barometer falls to 29.9 or lower. The Migraine Foundation of Toronto, Canada, reports that about one third of migraine patients, including children, have their attacks triggered when barometric pressure drops to 29.9 or lower. The further the drop in pressure, the more severe the migraine.

–There seems to be an inherited predisposition toward migraine. Gopi Krishna claims there is a hereditary factor involved in the awakening of kundalini.

McCleave concludes that classical migraine, tension, and cluster headaches may be unrecognized symptoms of a degree of kundalini awakening. She suggests that the information gathered by the medical profession and consolidated by the American Association for the Study of Headache (5252 North Western Ave., Chicago, Ill. 60625) be studied by kundalini researchers.

IV

Kundalini and the Occult

The following articles deal with various aspects of kundalini as expressed in occult forms. The word occult is not a pejorative term, although certain degenerate occult practices clearly warrant condemnation. Here we are simply observing a relationship between little-understood phenomena and the dynamics of the kundalini concept.

In its most general sense, occult means secret, hidden, beyond the bounds of ordinary knowledge, unknown to the general public. At the center of all occultism is the attempt to gain higher knowledge and control of the forces of nature, especially the life energy that is the basis of true magic and paranormal phenomena. In its highest form, occult science merges indistinguishably with true mysticism.

This is illustrated by a passage from Robert Anton Wilson's recent book *Cosmic Trigger,* which is an account of his extensive investigations into occult pathways in search of "the final secret of the illuminati." In discussing Aleister Crowley, an occultist par excellence who evolved a magical-meditative system called Scientific Illuminism, Wilson writes:

> I remembered Crowley's discussion of Jesus, Buddha, Mohammed, St. Paul, and Moses in Book One of *Magick.* Jesus, Crowley points out, says nothing about the source of his Illumination; Buddha speaks of being tempted by various demons and then seeing the Clear Light; St. Paul tells us he had been "caught up into Heaven and seen and heard things of which it is not law-

ful to speak"; Mohammed claims he was visited by the Archangel Gabriel; and Moses simply says he "beheld God." Crowley comments: "Diverse as these statements are at first sight, all agree in announcing an experience of the class which fifty years ago would have been called supernatural, today may be called spiritual, and fifty years hence will have a proper name based on an understanding of the phenomenon which occurred."

Crowley's statement shows that mysticism and genuine occultism are closely allied. It also shows Crowley's belief, paralleling Gopi Krishna's view of kundalini, that courageous, clear-minded research and the systematization of knowledge will yield understanding of the basic laws governing "supernatural" phenomena and higher consciousness. Might the "proper name" Crowley expected be kundalini research? I suggest that it is.

Not all mystics and occultists are on a par, of course, or motivated by the same values and purposes. Clearly, there is a negative side to occultism. But the heart of genuine occult practices appears to be synonymous with aspects of the kundalini concept. In my book *Everything You Want to Know About TM,* I provide an example of the profound importance that kundalini-based studies of the occult can have. I offer the example here, beginning with this identification test:

"Who is this man? He was a vegetarian who studied yoga, freethought, and various occult arts. He contemplated entering the priesthood. He consulted astrologers, used psychedelic drugs, and read widely in the wisdom literature of the Near East and Orient, including Tibetan Buddhism, Gnosticism, and various mystics. He believed in the reincarnation of souls into animal bodies, and wept when his canaries died. He exercised every day in front of an open window. He attended seances and was himself mediumistic. He loved playing with children."

This apparently gentle soul, this Flower Child, this Friend of the New Age was none other than—Adolf Hitler. Several recent studies of Hitler have given us this new and radically revised portrait. They show that Hitler was an occultist of a high order, with distinct mystical traits. (They also make clear the difference between a mystic and a saint.) In *The Occult Reich, the Occult and the Third Reich* and, most important of all, *The Spear of Destiny,* clear, strong documentation of the occult foundations of the Nazi movement is presented. These books convincingly propose that Hitler was a mystic of sorts whose inner circle of supporters were occultists practicing black magic who had considerable knowledge about altered states of consciousness. Hitler's high native intelligence and active kundalini were raised to near-genius level through personal experience of transcendent consciousness, gained primarily through use of psychedelic drugs such as peyote and through initiation into occult practices for expanding awareness.

The mind-expanding experiences Hitler had as a young man gave him sporadic access to an illumined state that later led him to say to one of his generals, "The purpose of human life is to gain a mystic view of the universe." This is a surprising statement, far out of keeping with the stereotyped, one-dimensional image of Hitler that historians have thus far given us. It shows his deep affinity with the thought of evolutionists such as Gopi Krishna, Teilhard de Chardin, Sri Aurobindo, R. M. Bucke, and others.

Hitler's evolutionary notion of a super race was formed not so much through reading philosophers such as Nietzsche as it was from direct experience of higher consciousness. But if der Führer had a significant degree of mystical understanding, he failed woefully to develop it in a balanced, integrated way, and thus—quite obviously!—failed to develop saintly character traits necessary for the full awakening of kundalini. Lacking the guidance of spiritual values and ethical restrictions, his inner vision and high intelligence became distorted by malignant internal and external influences. Psychopathology developed, leading to the holocaust of World War II. If further Hitlers are to be avoided, kundalini research appears to be essential.

Alchemy provides another useful example of the links between kundalini and the occult. Alchemy's true purpose is not the chemical manipulation of gross matter, as is commonly thought, but rather the transmutation of unrefined elements of the human psyche. These elements are symbolized by various substances that have a precise meaning assigned to them. In the "laboratory" of the achemist's own body, the "lead" of ordinary awareness becomes the "gold" of higher consciousness, just as the yogi seeks to transform his being through specific practices. The term kundalini does not occur in the alchemical tradition, but the alchemical processes, encoded in cryptic language, have been decoded by modern commentators such as Dr. Israel Regardie in *The Philosophers' Stone* and shown to be, in part at least, tantric practices. As mentioned earlier, tantra's aim is to awaken the kundalini energy and bring about a state of heightened awareness.

Studies in occult subjects provide uncounted instances of kundalini's generally unrecognized centrality to even the most respected fields of orthodox thought. Medicine, for example, is symbolized by the caduceus, the staff of Hermes* around which are entwined two serpents. The serpents can be equated with ida and pingala coiling around the central channel of life, the spinal sushumna. Health, therefore, from the original hermetic perspective, is symbolized by properly balanced physiological activity that harmonizes the life force throughout the body, and the medical practitioner is one who has intimate knowledge of how to modify and correct any imbalances.

The serpent, as an occult symbol of higher knowledge, immortality, and the human potential to become godlike, permeates ancient cultures around the world and survives into the modern age in many forms. Most obvious is the Genesis myth, where the serpent, "more subtle than any other wild creature," leads Adam and Eve to understand that the fruit of the tree of knowledge of good and evil can enable them to "be as gods." If we put aside the philosophical question of

* The staff of Aesculapius, entwined by a single serpent, is also often used as the symbol of medicine.

why the Lord originally forbade such knowledge to humans, it is clear that the serpent is kundalini and that Genesis is a myth concerning states of consciousness. By eating the fruit of our own tree-shaped cerebrospinal system—the spinal trunk and its exfoliation into the many-leaved (or thousand-petaled) brain—man can gain knowledge that may indeed kill him. "For in the day that thou eatest thereof thou shalt surely die," the Lord tells Adam. There are two senses in which a person can die—figuratively and literally. Regarding literal or biological death, we have seen indications that kundalini, improperly raised, can cause it. When properly raised, however, kundalini can result in a figurative death, an ego-death, involving transformation of the nervous system and the experience of divinity. In this experience, the "old Adam" dies, to use St. Paul's phrase, and a new person is born, reborn, as a child of the cosmos, no longer self-centered or even Earth-centered but rather universally centered and cosmically conscious. This, I suggest, is the meaning of the Star Child floating in space at the end of that occult cinematic experience, *2001,* a saga of the evolution of the human race from an apelike condition to a beckoning new stage of transhuman development.

Professor Weston La Barre, in his book *They Shall Take Up Serpents,* demonstrates that the phallus and the serpent were symbolically identical in the higher thought of the ancient Mediterranean world of Africa and Asia Minor, centering in Egypt. The serpent, for example, appears on the Pharaoh's diadem at the site of the mystical "third eye," indicating the relationship between sexual and supersensory experience. Gopi Krishna supplements this by pointing out that the kundalini concept is the only sensible explanation of an otherwise mysterious piece of Egyptology: paintings and statuary depicting men—even a Pharaoh and a male god—in meditation with an erect phallus. This is not meant by the artist to be erotic at all, Gopi Krishna says, but rather is a frank and literal depiction of a biological fact about kundalini. Swami Muktananda's story in Part II is a modern confirmation of this.

Going beyond La Barre's research, Gopi Krishna has

found evidence for kundalini experience in the ancient records of Tibet, Sumer, the Indus Valley civilization, China (where the serpent appears as the dragon), Greece (for example, the python-oracle at Delphi), and in the feathered serpent of Mexico and South America.

The functional relation among the phallus, the serpent, and higher states of consciousness is demonstrated well in Gopi Krishna's description of his own initial kundalini experience. A few pages after the excerpt from his autobiography presented here, he describes an orgasmic-like kundalini experience he had: "There was a sound like a nerve thread snapping and instantaneously a silvery streak passed through the spinal cord, exactly like the sinuous movement of a white serpent in rapid flight, pouring an effulgent, cascading shower of brilliant vital energy into my brain, filling my head with a blissful luster. . . ."

The relation between sexual climax and spiritual ecstasy so often encountered in occultism and mysticism suggests the general outline of a still-further stage of evolution toward which the human race is slowly tending. The details of this biological advance are dim–occulted, if you will. Nevertheless, I offer the following in a speculative way.

In sexual climax, the pranic life energy rushes upward through the spinal cord into the brain. (Ejaculation of semen in males is *not* the primary characteristic of climax. Rather, it is the brain stimulation through the nervous system that is sought through sexual activity–a characteristic that applies equally to females.) The kundalini concept postulates that this life energy can be focused and directed in such a way that the bliss of orgasm is heightened manyfold and made permanent as *ananda.* Gene Kieffer, president of the Kundalini Research Foundation (see Appendix), elaborates on this aspect:

> The most powerful motivating force of life, as Freud has shown, is sex and the pleasure drawn from the sexual act. Similarly, the most powerful motivating force to draw man onto the evolutionary path, according to the

> traditional concept of kundalini, is ananda. This highly extended state of consciousness, permeated with an extreme form of rapture, is said to be possible only when the consumption of prana is greatly enhanced.

The new state of consciousness—characterized by ananda, heightened mental faculties, and the development of new supersensory channels of perception—begins to impose itself upon the exterior world through loving and wise action in society, thereby helping to bring about a transformation of the human condition. And it is noteworthy that the word climax comes from the Greek *klimax,* meaning ladder (to heaven—that is, to a paradisal state).

Recent data from parapsychology and thanatology give us new insight into the condition of a person in higher consciousness at the end of physical life. The yogic tradition, which designates the death process as *mahasamadhi* ("casting off the body" or the ultimate enlightenment), apparently named it so for an important reason. The yogi brings to bear all his yogic training and power by choosing the time of his death and exiting consciously from the body in nonphysical form through the fontanelle at the top of the skull, just as, phenomenologically speaking, semen is ejaculated through the penis and just as kundalini energy passes rapidly up the spinal column. (Interestingly, a French term for orgasm is *petit mort,* little death—the momentary extinction of ego consciousness.)

The yogic death-experience is literally ecstatic. The word ecstasy is derived from the roots *ex,* out of, and *stasis,* a fixed or static condition. Ecstasy is the ancient term for out-of-the-body experience or astral projection, the "flight of the soul." It is the experience in which one finds his consciousness, his center of self-awareness, floating in space exterior to the physical body.

This experience is the objective of many occult paths and mystery school initiations. It is part of their training to remove fear of death and the limitations of a physical body. In the past few years, a number of investigators have given accounts and analyses of this experience in books such as *Life*

After Life, The Astral Journey, Ekstasy, and *At the Hour of Death.* The interesting point here is that those who have undergone the experience almost uniformly reported loss of fear of death, while a sense of blissful, serene well-being flooded their awareness. Death, they said, is seen to be simply a change of state. From a condition of being fixed in a body of gross, static substance, one is freed into a realm where consciousness is contained in a body of much finer substance, more subtle and rarefied, and capable of much greater mobility and freedom.

Yogic training, therefore, is in part a systematic process in which one deliberately conquers fear of death and learns to exit consciously and painlessly from the body at the end of a life of service to humanity. This is stated explicitly in some of the ancient yogic texts, and more recently by Swami Rama in *Living with the Himalayan Masters.* In a chapter on techniques of casting off the body, he writes, "It is not like committing suicide, but is an exact process or way of leaving that body which is no longer an instrument for enlightenment. Such a body is considered to be a burden—an obstacle which might obstruct the journey of the dying man. . . ."

A journey to where? From the yogic perspective, the goal is to explore the nature of the nonphysical postmortem condition, recognizing that consciousness is ultimate reality and that it tends to be structured in levels of existence traditionally called the astral plane, the etheric plane, the causal plane, etc. These other space-time frameworks have entities indigenous to them, among which are the "beings of light" described by many people who have voluntarily or spontaneously experienced the ecsomatic condition. *These beings are probably an evolutionarily advanced form toward which human life is tending, and psychological enlightenment is therefore a prefiguration of that distant condition in which the entire body is enlightened or of luminous substance.* The beings of light, it is said in many occult and spiritual traditions, are in turn assisting the birth process by which *Homo sapiens* is emerging into the new world of higher consciousness. I propose that the higher humanity be named. *Homo noeticus.*

Knowledge of the higher worlds: This is the thrust of all spiritual disciplines, ceremonial magic, occult practices, shamanic training, and religious ritual–to employ it with precision for the evolution of the race to a greater state of existence, eventually freed from the bonds of flesh.

It was precisely this condition that Hitler, via the Third Reich, was seeking. His understanding was woefully incomplete, however. The purpose of life, the greatest sages say, is not simply to gain a mystic view of the universe; rather it is to gain that view *and then lovingly share it with others.* Hitler's violent, coercive tactics resulted in a horrible caricature of the evolutionary process.

Aleister Crowley's occultism was fundamentally an attempt to control and direct evolution. D. Brian Hanlon states in a *Gnostica* magazine (October–November 1977) review of Israel Regardie's biography of Crowley, *The Eye in the Triangle,* that Scientific Illuminism was aimed at producing Adepts, evolutionary mutants–fully enlightened individuals who had attained realization of their own divine genius. Crowley came to believe that this was the "next step" in human evolution, "an awakening to the meaning of the man of the future," as Regardie describes it.

In the following selections, we examine a wide variety of possible relationships between occult phenomena and kundalini. The brief excerpt from Kenneth Grant's *Cults of the Shadow* shows the widespread influence of kundalini in cults of Africa and Asia. It also gives evidence of the evolutionary impulse taking focus in practices designed to develop the body of light, the subtle vehicle for consciousness that is deathless and refined of gross matter. Grant notes that this is the great mystery motivating the cults.

By far the most difficult and controversial article is the excerpt from J. M. Pryse's *The Restored New Testament.* Pryse maintains that the Book of Revelation is a coded text detailing the awakening of kundalini through occult practices and that the core truth of the Christian tradition is development of the solar body of light, the immortal vehicle for consciousness that Jesus demonstrated through the crucifixion and resurrection. Such a message will not be welcomed in certain quarters of Christendom. It is included here, however, because Pryse's argument is logically tenable and because it is an elaboration on the preceding article by Mineda J. McCleave, "Christian Mysticism and Kundalini."

In an article in *Astrologia* (Vol. 1, No. 2) in 1974, Dr. Charles Musès discusses "The Most Ancient Resurrection Doctrine of Egypt Reconstructed"–a subject that relates directly to the cultic mysteries. Musès writes that the central purpose of ancient Egyptian metaphysics was to gain the "hatching" of the higher energy-substance body, able to function with greatly enhanced senses in a higher objective world. I will quote the article at length because of its importance for this section.

> Without that higher body in such released form, the transition of death would find the person still imprisoned in the cocoon or egg protecting the as yet not fully developed higher body. Hence in such cases all that death can bring by way of new experiences is veridical-seeming, very vivid dreams, pleasant, unpleasant, or mixed according to the degree of development of love and release from fears that prior earth-body experience had afforded the particular person. It is important to note, however, that the highest use of the *bardo* (to use the convenient Tibetan term) state is continued development of the higher body, leading to increased powers in the next incarnation, and in some cases proceeding to such a degree that the necessity for future earth-lives is greatly curtailed or even, in exceptional cases, wholly eliminated. In these last cases there is a direct entrance into the immortal state of higher objectivity from the antiworld or bardo plane.
>
> *With* the "hatching" or birth of the higher body, however, there is no longer any necessity to return to an earth-type existence in a carbon-based, fragile and comparatively imprisoning body or vehicle of entity-expression.

> The most ancient Egyptian teachings were concerned with an occult science—now lost and as yet far beyond the reach of our technology—whereby while *still in this life,* the carbon-based body, by suitable extradimensional radiation, could be transformed into the new type of energy-substance and form the imperishable, radiant body. In this manner, the initiate so treated could enter into a higher dimensional *objective* world, without the necessity of the *bardo* states and without the trauma of physical death.
>
> The cosmic beings, more advanced than the human stage, that could administer such a process were symbolized primarily by the great Hawk Deity Horus, flanked by Isis, the Goddess of Immortal Life, and Nephthys, the lady of the Palace of Resurrection or House of Horus. The person undergoing the transformation was assimilated to Osiris, the god-who-died, overcome by Set, the ruler of the inevitable mortality of earth-life conditions. Set's power, however, is the inverse of Horus'. By proper administrations and techniques one can be transformed into the other, thus substituting unalloyed, felicitous immortality as an ongoing, ever-developing individuality† rather than the traumatic, constantly death-interrupted immortality, with its disruptions of memory and personality that attend the ordinary experience of earth-life.

If we accept this assertion, it gives us still greater insight into the "mystery" that unites kundalini and Christianity. It implies that the process by which the yogi transmutes his psychophysical being is the same as that by which Jesus the man, presumably trained in one or more occult traditions originating in Egypt or the East, developed the higher transfigured body that allowed him to undergo physical death and yet "rise again" as proof that he was truly Christed, begotten of the immortal Creative Force—as an example for others to follow on the evolutionary path to eternal life.

† *Not* in the ordinary human body, however. C. Musès.

Kundalini, Evolution and Enlightenment

The grand theme of human history is the evolution of consciousness and growth to a godlike condition. This theme has taken a wide variety of spiritual, occult, and scientific forms. Occult studies, this section will demonstrate, can contribute much to elucidating the underlying unity of science, occultism, and religion. An open-minded approach to the occult will undoubtedly bring to light important new data for kundalini research—data that bear on human growth to higher states of being, including the possibility of controlling and accelerating that growth. It is an awesome prospect.

STIGMATA AND KUNDALINI

Geoffrey Nicoletti

In 1974 and 1975 I had the good fortune to work on behalf of Padre Pio, the world-famous Italian mystic priest, at the American office of his official Cause for Beatification in Norristown, Pennsylvania. When Padre Pio died in 1968, he had been a stigmatic continuously for fifty years. My reflections on this unusual man have led me to see a functional relation between stigmatic wounds and the kundalini experience.

Stigmatization, or religious wounds, is not unique to Christianity, although the best-known cases are those in imitation of Jesus's wounds. Moslems, for example, have experienced stigmata while contemplating an image of Mohammed in battle. However, I shall confine illustrative material in this brief article to Christians who have demonstrated stigmatization.

Stigmata are not necessarily bleedings. Many of those 321 cases listed by Dr. Imbert-Gourbeyre in his 1894 book *La Stigmatasion* suffered invisible stigmatization. Others, however, did bleed. Some bled on religious days only; some bled continuously, stopped completely for years, and then bled again. Some stigmatics had only one wound while others had the five major wounds of Jesus—hands, feet, and side. According to René Biot, author of *The Enigma of the Stigmata,* from which most of these facts are derived, some stigmatics began to bleed after age sixty. There is even one individual who gave off boiling water from the "lance wound"!

Even the concept of "Christian stigmatization" is not quite

accurate, since the historical record is mainly composed of Catholics. Further, most of these were in religious orders. Only 12 cases are from the laity. Of 321 stigmatics which Imbert-Gorbeyre lists, 280 were women. And most of the 321 were Italians–10 from Sicily alone. Even the "lance wound" has been located on different sides of the body with different stigmatics. A most striking fact is that 16 stigmatics belonged to the same convent.

The historical record of stigmatization begins with St. Francis of Assisi, who received the visible wounds two years before his death in 1226. Unlike any other stigmatic, St. Francis not only had wounds, but also his blood, in these locations, formed nails that were visible–as were the wounds –after his death when he was laid out for veneration. The possible nature of the wounds is discussed in *Mystical Phenomena* by Albert Farges and also by Rev. Herbert Thurston in *The Physical Phenomena of Mysticism,* among others. The Catholic Church holds that there are three possible sources: God, the Devil, and one's self. One stigmatic, Louise Lateau, was studied by the French Academy in the nineteenth century. Some stigmatics, like Therese Neumann and Therese Higginson, appear to have been quite neurotic. But others like Padre Pio, in spite of his self-flagellations, appear to have had quite stable minds.

It is the history of this Capuchin priest that I will draw upon in this examination of the kundalini force. There are many reasons for choosing Padre Pio. He is the only stigmatic I know whose bleedings continued for a great length of time. He reports in his diary that as early as 1910 he felt, invisibly, the stigmatization. In 1915, he had sporadic bleedings that persisted for the next three years. Then, from 11 A.M. on September 20, 1918, till his death on September 23, 1968, Padre Pio bled–slowly but continuously–day and night without interruption.

Professor Bignami, Dr. Georgio Fiesta of Rome, and Dr. Romanell of Barletta conducted independent examinations of the wounds during the visible stigmatization period. They would not determine the cause of the wounds, nor could they treat them successfully. They did not understand why there was no festering, no loss of weight, no shock, no coagulation, and, of course, no death. At the same time, when Padre Pio had gashed his head, he responded to normal treatment. This was true of his hernia operation also. Not only had the doctors never heard of localized bleedings of a permanent nature—there are short-lived sweats of blood—they also had to consider the strange fact that Padre Pio's blood acted normally in the rest of his body.

A possible connection between the wounds and the kundalini experience is found in the concept that there exists a multitude of chakras in the body, including the hands. Because of the nature of the wounds, because the blood gave off a perfume—many eyewitnesses reported this, including chemists required to study the blood—and because healings were associated with the stigmata of Padre Pio, we should ask what force or energy was manifesting itself through this phenomenon. I conjecture here that the force sustaining the bleedings, imparting the perfume, and promoting the healings could be kundalini manifesting through minor chakras.

The literature on kundalini suggests that it can be dangerous when aroused. If stigmatics, not knowing of this dormant force, awakened it, I suspect that many would suffer the ills of kundalini improperly aroused. The description of the ill effects of kundalini match the descriptions of the ills of the stigmatics of whom we have biographies. Catherine Emmerich is a classic example. So is Rose Ferron, who was bedridden for four years, and Therese Neumann, who was declared hysterical by doctors before a visible manifestation of stigmatization. Neumann had suffered an awful back injury while attempting to put a barn fire out for her employer. As part of a bucket brigade, she collapsed from exhaustion, injuring her spine. We can also note more generally that stigmatics were given to flagellations, and above all, many were given to celibacy. The latter characteristic is a primary connecting link to the dynamics of the kundalini experience.

Even Padre Pio, in his private diary of 1910–22, the years during which he developed stigmatization, tells his spiritual director in letter after letter of severe headaches that the doctors could not alleviate. Padre Pio speaks continuously during those years of a spiritual fire within him. And he was released by the Italian Army during World War I because of outrageous fevers that broke thermometers at 125° F! They were sudden, not continuous, but nonetheless accurately recorded. A horse thermometer was needed to get a true reading. The doctors released Padre Pio to go home to die; he was incapable of keeping any food down.

Kundalini is said to bring the awakening of psychic faculties. In Padre Pio we find a lifelong ability for bilocation (out-of-body projection with full materialization of the astral body at a location away from the physical body), levitation (this was reported to me by the chaplain of Chestnut Hill College, who witnessed one instance), and other gifts such as drawing out the astral sight through the pupilless eyes of Gemma di Giorgi (who is still alive) and thus enabling her to see.

It seems that Padre Pio was not spared the physical torments of kundalini but was spared from neurosis or psychosis. From 1931 to 1933, the Vatican ordered him isolated. His behavior at that time proves his sanity as he did not "confess," crack, or grow bitter. He also did not rebel against requirements placed on him at various times in his life to cover his wounds (the hands by gloves), preach no sermons, write no books or letters, nor pose for photographs.

It should be noted, in fairness, that one of every ten photographs of Padre Pio are posed shots; these are of him with groups of soldiers, children, nuns, etc., where charity and courtesy would have been violated if he refused. One of the most photographed men in the world, Padre Pio is seen with a serious look in his eyes and an occasional smile, but no neurotic, sweet-faced gaze toward a never-never land. His mysticism pointed him toward people; his religious context has created a reverse prejudice against him where those interested in psychic phenomena ignore this giant for lesser psychics. Because he heard confessions for fourteen hours daily as a young priest, because he ate one meal a day and slept four hours a night, and because of his virtuous character, can we say he was neurotic? Psychotic? He was even known to whip his Franciscan cord in rage at people—fanatics—who tore at his clothes as if he were a living statue rather than a person.

Carl Jung, in *Religion and Psychology, East and West,* sees the Buddhi factor, the sixth body of which Theosophy speaks, as what we now call the collective unconscious. Is it so farfetched to reread the mystics of the Church—and here, especially, the stigmatics—that their "spiritual fires" are descriptions of a force they didn't consciously recognize but nevertheless awoke—the kundalini force? Even the moment of permanent visible stigmatization of Padre Pio on the morning of September 20, 1918, is described by him, in his diary, as the result of a "fiery tool." Could the inner light that Hesychasts see when meditating on Mount Athos be the awakened kundalini? If the Catholic Church would prefer seeing the mystic relating to people rather than merely in a nice one-to-one relationship with God, is it inappropriate to use kundalini as part of the awakening of charismatic powers? When I read the reports by eyewitnesses of Padre Pio's sudden explosion of the aura, am I reading of a manifestation of the kundalini?

I recognize that from the viewpoint of Catholic mystics, this force, described differently by them, is not a central part of their lives, either psychologically or theologically. But from the viewpoint of kundalini research, can we posit the existence of two parallel phenomena—stigmatization and kundalini—and say there is no functional relationship between them in psychophysical terms? It seems reasonable to presume that the stigmatics experienced the kundalini force, even though Jesus was central to their spiritual lives.

UFOs AND KUNDALINI

Gene Kieffer

It seems truly fantastic how consciousness communicates with itself through the marvelous mechanism of the human organism. Those who have awakened kundalini in themselves tell us how they must grope for words to convey even the barest details of what has happened to them. Though each has his unique story to tell, there is a consistency among them all that I believe is genuinely convincing.

From what I have learned in talking to these people, and to a somewhat lesser degree from my own studies and experience, I have come to the conclusion that kundalini is responsible for many of the UFOs that abound in our times. This theory, not original with me, can only gain credence after science begins its research on kundalini.

To get a rudimentary picture of kundalini, one can think about trying to give a chimpanzee a transfusion of consciousness from a human mind. New concepts would suddenly begin to well up in a shallow pool of consciousness, like a sun just appearing on the horizon.

Now imagine what the case would be if the recipient really were an intelligent chimpanzee and the donor an intellectual. The rush of new knowledge would literally blow its mind. This is similar to what happens when kundalini is awakened, especially if one is totally unprepared for the experience. Even when one has spent years preparing by refining the body and mind through rigorous mental, physical, and spiritual disciplines, a sudden burst of this extremely potent psychic energy into the brain can be fatal. The burned-out transformer furnishes an apt comparison.

I have a friend who awakened kundalini some twelve years ago. At first he hovered on the edge of insanity. He knew something extraordinary was taking place both within as well as outside the body. He could not begin to comprehend what was happening to him, however. Finally he began to converse with an entity in the form of a serpent. Though frightening, it was better than no sure communication at all.

Later another entity appeared in no definite form, but as an inner voice. It explained that what was really going on was the building of a transmitter that could be used to communicate with people from another planet. There can be little doubt that this news came as a welcome relief. My friend was far more kindly disposed to the astronaut than the hideous serpent. He had always been a devout Christian. Had a truer explanation been given to him by "his inner voice," even then, it would have been rejected because it would have been incomprehensible. His sanity would have been swept away.

Today, though the renovation of his brain and nervous system continues apace, he no longer requires the same symbolism. The terror he had experienced in the beginning gave way to a bond of affection between himself and the "foreign invader." He told me that should this Presence leave him now, he would surely rather die than go through life alone. What first impressed itself upon his consciousness as a cloud of death, in the form of a serpent as real as life, has revealed itself as his own Self or soul.

Along with this new understanding has come a vastly expanded view of the universe, my friend says. His consciousness is expanding, and as it does, it requires an expanded circuitry throughout his entire body—especially his brain and nervous system. The obsolete design that had served him so adequately before is hardly any better suited for his new personality than the brain of a chimpanzee can be for the mind of a man.

One who has awakened kundalini can sometimes observe the internal operation as though he were a bystander watching an army of expert technicians at work on a giant computer.

There was a television special, *The Incredible Machine,* in which the circulation of the blood was shown in X-ray microcinemaphotography. The narrator intimated that the white cells display an independence that could only be explained on the basis of their having an intelligence of their own. One film sequence showed the cells working their way up the narrow tributaries, and finally into the tiniest capillaries, in single file. Each one would squeeze its way through as though it were a microscopic glob of intelligence.

The way consciousness operates in the human nervous system, I am told, is almost the same, only much more awe-inspiring. There are amazing photographs taken by a laser beam of liquid droplets of electricity. Consciousness also takes the same spherical shape, like subatomic globes of luminosity. Once kundalini has been successfully aroused, each of these, glowing with intelligent life, performs a specific task in refurbishing the nervous system.

The culmination of The Great Work is a new personality, completely different from the one that formerly occupied the mind and body. It is as though the person had been reborn. The old personality merges with another, much larger, personality. Whatever the explanation may be, the personality that finally emerges sees the world in a way that is entirely different from the way an ordinary person does.

UFOs can take on a different meaning, also. They need not be visitors from another planet, but can be phenomena originating in another universe. This other universe may exist side-by-side with our own. They need not be a part of our three-dimensional world at all. My belief is that UFOs of the type that would come from another planet, either in our galaxy or some other, will not be encountered by man until a great deal more spiritual progress has been made here on Earth. Otherwise, the UFOs would interfere with the orderly, natural evolution of the race by introducing foreign influences. Guidance, at this stage, is meant to come from within ourselves.

But UFOs do manifest themselves through individual consciousness, and as such, they do require a rational explanation. The best way to tackle this problem, therefore, would be for scientists to investigate kundalini. This would be comparatively easy and would involve a modest investment, considering the magnitude of the undertaking.

It is possible for scientists to gather together a group of two or three hundred dedicated individuals who would make it their soul objective to awaken kundalini. A spontaneous arousal of kundalini under the observation of competent investigators would be a scientific "first." The phenomenon could be studied as never before in modern times.

If UFOs are indeed a part of the broad spectrum of psychic phenomena, kundalini research should give scientists a front-row seat at some of the most spectacular displays. An awakening could be studied both objectively and subjectively. It has been said by Gopi Krishna, the Kashmiri yogi-philosopher, that kundalini is responsible for all, or almost all, phenomena of the mind. This, I believe, is true.

In 1968, December 20, at 10:30 P.M., to be exact, I made "contact" with a UFO. I had learned to generate slightly more psychic energy than was normal for me, and I could raise it to the fourth, or heart, chakra quite easily. This is nothing unusual. Many people can do it after only a brief period of training. But at that time I had no knowledge of kundalini and very little of psychic matters, either. On this particular occasion, though, I decided to try an experiment and use the energy to carry a signal or message into space. I wanted to communicate with a UFO.

Within minutes the contact was made, and though I was certain at the time that I saw the object visually, as a luminous green, slightly pulsating, amorphous vehicle, I later came to the conclusion that it was a projection of my own self. Whatever the case, we were soon in "telepathic contact," and I was given instructions to report what I was learning to a certain person employed by NASA in Alabama. This I did, via telephone, at 2:00 A.M. on December 21. The three-and-a-half-hour delay was due to my fear of making a fool of myself. I procrastinated until the subconscious impulse overrode all objections.

Nevertheless, the man at NASA was entirely receptive and accepted my report in all seriousness. He even relayed it to Cape Kennedy, where Apollo 8 was about to be launched on the first mission to the moon. The message I had given NASA was that the astronauts would undergo a "spiritual experience" once they had begun their lunar orbit. Had I known when I made the phone call that the countdown had long begun and that the launch itself was to be made that very morning, at dawn, I would no doubt have refused to go ahead with it. Later, a few hours after the launch, I was told by my contact at NASA that there was even some discussion as to whether the mission ought to be aborted.

I say this only because it shows how seriously the government used to take UFO reports, which were fairly common in those days.

This one, single experience does not make me an expert, certainly. I only believe that my understanding of what happened is more rational when placed in the context of kundalini, which subsumes all other theories dealing with the mind. I believe it is the unified field theory that science has been seeking. Every fresh discovery in the field of high-speed particle physics seems to confirm this view. Even the new findings of astronomers fit very nicely into the concept of kundalini.

As we expand our perception of the physical universe, we also expand the circuitry in our brain. It is a chicken-and-egg proposition. If our understanding of the phenomena we observe through our senses and explain through our intellect is not absolutely true to nature, then the networks constructed by consciousness in our nervous system and brain are distorted. We are, I am afraid, building an unreal world for ourselves that may bring about its own destruction in the not-too-distant future. That is why many hard-nosed scientists will not look at psychic phenomena.

Theoreticians have no broader view of the "real" world than does the ordinary person. Their explanations, no matter how complex and elaborate, soon prove inadequate when applied to the frontiers of science. The intellect has been building a castle of sand for some three hundred years. Unless it is shored up by an explosion of intuitive knowledge quickly, the whole towering edifice could topple at any time.

The answers lie in a more thorough understanding of the evolutionary processes at work in the human organism. For they are always at work, imperceptibly building and remodeling the nervous system, particularly. Kundalini research, which in essence would be an attempt to accelerate the evolutionary processes to an incredible degree, can lead to a whole new dimension of consciousness for the race. And in this new dimension of consciousness, man would stand taller than ever he dreamed possible through all the ages of his laborious ascent.

THE DIVINE FIRE: TUMO AND KUNDALINI

John White

One of the lesser-known but nevertheless spectacular human powers is called by its Tibetan name, *tumo* (or *gTum-mo*, a more precise romanized spelling of the word). Tumo is the production of extraordinary body heat. The phenomenon got its name from lamas (Tibetan Buddhist holy men) and yogis in the Himalayas of Tibet and India who developed the ability to control their body temperature at will. "The yogi is beyond heat and cold," says yogic tradition. Photographs show lamas standing naked in the snows as an act of worship or endurance. They have been known to stand that way for twelve to twenty-four hours.

Madame Alexandra David-Neel brought the phenomenon to the attention of the West when she described it in her book, *Magic and Mystery in Tibet*. In a chapter entitled "Psychic Sports," she writes on "the art of warming oneself without fire up in the snows":

> To spend the winter in a cave amidst the snows, naked, and escape freezing is a somewhat difficult achievement. Yet numbers of Tibetan hermits go safely each year through this ordeal . . . [by generating tumo,] the subtle fire which warms the generative fluid and drives the energy in it, till it runs all over the body along the tiny channels of the *tsas* [veins, arteries and nerves].[1]

Others reporting this have added that the hermits often go entirely without cooking or heating fires in their caves.

Before the Chinese Communists took over Tibet, there was a College of Ritual Magic which offered courses in tumo, telepathy, clairvoyance and other aspects of psychic development. The final exam in the tumo course would make most Western college students blink in amazement. To pass the course, a student was required to sit naked on a frozen Himalayan lake or river in midwinter and then put on wet sheets, one by one, until they were dry from the heat of his body. As David-Neel reported it,

> The neophytes sit on the ground cross-legged and naked. Sheets are dipped in the icy water; each man wraps himself in one of them and must dry it on his body. As soon as the sheet has become dry, it is again dipped in the water and placed on the novice's body to be dried as before. The operation goes on until daybreak. Then he who has dried the largest number of sheets is acknowledged the winner.
>
> It is said that some dry as many as forty sheets in one night.[2]

Another witness, Dr. Erwin J. Dingle, reported in *Borderland of Eternity* that on a frozen lake 16,000 feet above sea level, he saw lamas being wrapped in wet woolen blankets which dried within minutes. One lama, he was told, had been doing this for two days without stop. Looking at the man, Dingle saw that the snow had melted around him to a distance of ten feet.

This strange phenomenon is not limited to the mysterious Orient. Here in the West one can find reports of saints and mystics who have also experienced this "fire of love" as they attempted to become one with God. It was Richard Rolle, the fourteenth century English mystic, who gave the title *Fire of Love* to the record of his tumo-like experiences. George Fox, the Quaker, walked barefoot through the streets of Litchfield, England, even though it was snowy midwinter, because he felt warmed by the love of God.

A Dominican nun, Suora Maria Villani, was described during her lifetime as "continually consumed by an unsupportable flame of love." She drank more than three gallons of water a day to relieve her feeling of intense heat. When she died at 86, surgeons opened her chest and found smoke and heat issuing from her heart.

The heat was so intense that they signed an affadavit describing her fantastic condition.

St. Catherine of Genoa had to dip her hands in water during her last illness because she felt a tremendous inner warmth. After she expired, her body remained warm for more than a day, and attending nuns could warm their hands by placing them near her heart. St. Philip Neri walked about in winter with his clothes open from the waist up, explaining that he had to because of the great internal heat he felt.

Some years ago, a young woman living in Connecticut asked my help in controlling her own involuntary condition of extreme heat—a heat so unbearable that she feared for her sanity. Her skin was so hot that she took icy showers and drove around in a convertible with the top down in winter, while wearing only a halter and shorts. These measures barely gave her relief.

Akin to this young woman's problem, medically termed "hyperthermy," are two other paranormal phenomena. The first is spontaneous human combustion. There are well-documented instances in which people have burned to death, mysteriously but without foul play, leaving only a tiny amount of ash behind yet without setting fire to any of their surroundings or even, at times, their clothing. Medical examiners have admitted their bafflement.

One fairly typical case of spontaneous human combustion is that of Dr. John Bentley, a physician in Coudersport, Pennsylvania. On December 5, 1966, he underwent spontaneous combustion. It completely consumed his body except for a leg and bedroom slipper. It occurred in his house, but there was no fire noted except for the charred edges of a hole in the floor where the body had apparently burned through and fallen into the basement. The coroner pronounced the death accidental. This case, reported by researcher Larry Arnold of Harrisburg, Pennsylvania in *Pursuit* (Fall 1976), is one of more than two hundred documented instances of inexplicable spontaneous human combustion.

In a similar fashion, Radha, a fifteenth-century Hindu saint, apparently cremated herself voluntarily. It is said that she announced the time of her death and then, to the amazement of gathered onlookers, walked away from them and was consumed in a burst of light, leaving only a small heap of ashes.

Such legends are almost impossible to verify and may be embellished by time, but there are more recent accounts of similar events observed by competent witnesses. In one such instance, reported in *Psychic* (May/June 1971) a Sikh holy man, Sadhu Singh, performed intentional self-combustion without benefit of any fuel and died sitting placidly in a yoga position. Mystified police ruled out foul play or accidental fire.

According to the report, the 114-year-old yogi had flames coming from his abdomen which, a retired surgeon said, was "not hot when I felt it." Other witnesses included police, science professors and medical men. What they saw was a "candle-like flame" which completely consumed Sadhu Singh's body over a six-hour period, leaving only a residue of ashes. Further, the report notes, apparently there were none of the other physical symptoms normally associated with burn victims. Even the straw mattress on which he was seated and his clothes burned only with the body, and in the course of hours."

The second-tumo-related phenomenon involves psychic healers who produce strong heat from their hands when they work. I worked with one whose bare hand, held over my arm with at least two inches of space between us, made me feel as if I were that close to a large candle. This same phenomenon is widely experienced by those investigating psychic healing and those receiving treatment.

How is it possible to alter and control what is regarded as an involuntary bodily process? Can people burn themselves to death without an external source of heat or flame? The College of Ritual Magic is no longer around, but its knowledge is still available, and scholars and scientists outside Tibet have been studying the mysterious phenomenon.

David-Neel herself wrote that only those who are qualified to undertake the training may hope to succeed because the secret knowledge is obtainable only from lamas with the power to confer it. The most important qualifications, she said, are: to be already skilled in the various practices connected with breathing; to be capable of a perfect concentration of mind; going as far as the trance in which thoughts become visualized; and to have received the proper *angkur* or initiation rite which confers a secret formula.

D. H. Rawcliffe in *Illusions and Delusions of the Supernatural and Occult* offers this view. Candidates for the study of tumo, he says, are selected only if they have a naturally high resistance to cold. Then follows a long period of gradual acclimatization during which special breathing exercises and self-hypnosis are learned. While in trance, the student fixes his mind on an image of heat such as a fire or the sun. The rest is merely a matter of self-induced anesthesia.

The process for induction of tumo's supernormal heat is described by Perle Epstein, author of the 1975 *Oriental Mystics and Magicians*. Long and arduous training is necessary, she writes:

> First the student must wear nothing but a simple cotton loincloth. Really brave disciples wear nothing. Novices start by sitting outdoors on a straw mat; more advanced students sit on the snow or even on top of an ice mound. No food or drink, especially hot, is permitted before practicing. The man may sit in the lotus posture or with both legs on the ground, if he prefers using a stool. The *mudra* (symbolic hand gesture) consists of an extended forefinger and pinky, with the middle and fourth fingers folded into the palm. Again the yogi practices rhythmic breathing, holding breath and, in exhaling, imagining that all anger, lust, selfishness, etc. are being tossed out of the system. At the other end, with each inhalation, he imagines that all Buddha qualities—love, compassion, purity of heart—are flowing into him.
>
> With a peaceful mind, he visualizes a golden lotus flower at his navel. Within the shining flower, he imagines the syllable *ram*. Above this he sees the syllable *ma* (Rama being an incarnation of God), from which a female deity, Dorgee Naljorma, emerges. Every letter of these syllables must be regarded by the yogi as a living and powerful entity filled with fire. Now he continues the process of identifying himself with the goddess and placing the letter *a* in the navel and the syllable *ha* at the crown of his head. The breathing now becomes like a bellows fanning up a low flame that assumes the shape of a ball within the letter *a*. With each breath taken, the force of the flames seated in the navel grows stronger.

> Holding the breath for longer and longer periods, the yogi concentrates hard on the increasing fire as it moves upward from the navel through the *uma* vein. The uma is visualized first as a thin thread filled with flame and currents of breath. Then it grows, expanding from a finger's width to an arm's width, and at last filling the entire body with a blaze of flame and air. The man now loses all bodily consciousness, seeing himself as nothing more than a flaming vein in a sea of fire. It takes at least an hour to reach this stage.
>
> Working backward now, the yogi reverses the steps of his vision, as his mind drops all sense of observation and merges with the Void. In this trance he no longer has any sense of cold, no sense of being either perceived or perceiver. Suspended beyond the senses, the yogi may now remain in meditative bliss (samadhi) for as long as he wishes. Experienced practitioners of tumo claim that a pleasant level of heat is sustained by the body throughout.

Epstein concludes that the phenomenon is attributable to hypnosis.

Biofeedback offers another insight into the production of tumo. At the Menninger Clinic in Topeka, Kansas, Dr. Elmer Green and his wife Alyce have been exploring voluntary control of internal states for nearly two decades. One of the most spectacular events they recorded there occurred when a yogi, Swami Rama of Rishikesh, India, produced a 10° F. temperature difference between two points on the palm of his hand, above the radial and ulnar arteries. Dilation and constriction of the arteries seem to have been the means by which Swami Rama controlled the blood flow, and thus the temperature, the Greens reported.

Another medical researcher, Dr. Herbert Benson of Harvard Medical School, has a similar view. He and several colleagues obtained the aid of the Dalai Lama in finding three Tibetan Buddhist monks who'd spent more than six years practicing tumo, and in 1981 studied the monks to see what occurred. The team measured skin temperature at various points on the bodies of the monks, taking measurements every five minutes during control, meditation and recovery periods. All three monks showed remarkable temperature changes in their fingers and toes, and lesser changes at the calf, chest, forearm, navel and lumbar areas. Their rectal temperature didn't change at all. The greatest temperature change observed was 8.3° C. in the toe of one monk. Benson and his coworkers reported in *Nature* (January 1982) that the monks "exhibited a greater capacity to warm fingers than has been previously recorded during hypnosis and after biofeedback training." They doubted that the monks increased their metabolism to produce more body heat. Rather, they hypothesized, "The most likely mechanism to account for the increase in finger and toe temperature is vasodilation" or increasing the blood flow through the affected area.

At least one new element of explanation was suggested by Benson in his 1987 book, *Your Maximum Mind*, which describes additional research with Tibetan monks adept at tumo.

In February, 1985, some research scientists in Benson's group took two filmmakers to a monastery in the Kulu Valley in northern India. There the monks performed tumo while the movie cameras recorded it.

The equipment was set up in a small monastery. About 3 A.M., twelve monks proceeded to take off all their clothes except for small loincloths. They sat cross-legged on the floor, dipped cotton sheets measuring three feet by six feet into pails of water whose temperature was about 49° F. Next they wrung out the sheets and wrapped them around their upper bodies. Then they started to perform tumo meditation and, as Benson puts it, an amazing phenomenon began to occur. "Although most people would have begun to shiver violently when exposed to such cold wetness, these monks didn't react at all. Instead, they sat calmly, and within three to five minutes, the sheets wrapped around them began to *steam*! The room filled with water vapor so that the lenses of the cameras became fogged over and had to be wiped off constantly. Within thirty to forty minutes, the sheets draped around the monks were completely dry."

The monks repeated this two more times, and not once did they shiver or shake from the cold. Footage of this was shown on the television program *Discover*, and it is truly extraordinary to see the water vapor rising like mist around the monks.

Even more extraordinary was the night—again in February, 1985—Benson's team observed monks perform tumo outdoors at an altitude of 19,000 feet in near-Arctic climatic conditions. At a frigid, inhospitable spot, with the temperature at 0° F., the monks took off their sandals and squatted down on their haunches. Then, Benson reports, the monks leaned forward, put their heads on the ground and draped light cotton wrappings on themselves. In this position, being essentially naked, they spent the entire night practicing a special type of tumo meditation which seemed to put them into suspended animation. They didn't even react when a light snow fell during the night. They simply remained quietly in their meditative posture for about eight hours, looking as if frozen. Then, at a signal, they stood up, shook off the snow, put on their sandals and calmly walked back down the mountain.

Benson theorizes that the Relaxation Response was involved in the monks' physiological resistance to cold, with the addition of a process called nonshivering thermogenesis. "This involves the ability of the body under some circumstances to burn or metabolize a type of fat called brown fat, which is able to generate very large amounts of heat," he writes. "In the past, scientists thought that only certain types of nonhuman mammals, especially those which hibernate, could burn this type of fat. But now it appears that human beings may also have the capacity to generate heat from this fat. We hypothesize that the monks may have learned to do so through the use of generally unknown powers of the mind."[3]

What is the conventional view of Western physiology regarding this? Dr. Norman Shealy, a holistic physician and author of *Occult Medicine Can Save Your life*, summarized present medical knowledge of this phenomenon in a letter to me. Writing from the Pain Rehabilitation Center in LaCrosse, Wisconsin, Shealy remarked:

> We know that almost anyone can be trained to raise skin temperature to 96° F. In addition, it has been demonstrated that with biofeedback training one can raise the temperature of the scrotum to 104°, almost 6° above normal. This implies either a marked decrease in local circulation or an increased

> general metabolism in that area so that we know that it is possible even without "paranormal abilities" to learn to control body temperature at least up to 104°. It's unlikely that it would be possible or safe for anyone to raise the temperature much above 104° as tissue damage begins to occur at 108°. Especially, of course, the brain is very susceptible to temperatures above 104°.[4]

Is it not surprising, then, that the Italian mystic, Padre Pio, regarded by many Catholics as a saint, went through agonizing periods when his temperature rose as high as 125° F.

Yet even 125° F. is far from the highest recorded human temperature. In personal correspondence, Larry Arnold provided me with a dozen other such cases. These included an 1880 incident reported in *Medical Times and Gazette* in which a woman registered temperatures up to 130.8° F. in her groin and vagina. In 1895 a New York doctor named Jacobi told the Association of American Physicians that a hysteric fireman in profound hyperthermy reached a temperature of 148° F. After a fall, he was unconscious for four days. Thereafter he experienced convulsions and complained of pains and, of course, a high temperature. For five days his temperature was recorded at different areas of the body, using different thermometers. The abnormal heat was always confirmed, and averaged 120-125° F. In what may be the world's hyperthermy record, Arnold noted of the same AAP meeting, a Dr. Welch of Baltimore told of a case involving a temperature of 171° F.

Data such as these take us outside the ordinary medical view of body temperature regulation. They take us to the ancient yogic concept of *kundalini*. If the concept is valid, it would provide a means of explaining a physiological phenomenon—tumo as voluntary regulation of body heat—that one of the foremost authorities on body mechanisms regulating temperature assured me, from his office at Yale University, simply couldn't be done.

Certain ancient Sanskrit texts handed down in yogic and other esoteric traditions concerned with developing higher human abilities state that people have a dormant power called kundalini. This potential power is both consciousness and energy. The energy, it is said, can be activated and controlled through various spiritual disciplines so that a person attains expanded consciousness, psychic powers and other extraordinary faculties. This is done by releasing the kundalini energy from its usual position near the base of the spine and channeling it upward into the brain. Thus, tumo in its voluntary condition could be one of the psychic abilities gained by the awakening of kundalini.

Swami Rama sheds light on this in his *Living with the Himalayan Masters*. In a chapter about yogic techniques of "casting off the body" or dying, he writes: "By meditating on the solar plexus, the actual internal flame of fire burns the body in a fraction of a second, and everything is reduced to ashes. This knowledge was imparted by Yama, the king of death, to his beloved disciple, Nachiketa, in the *Kathopanishad*. All over the world, instances of spontaneous combustion are heard about, and people wonder about such occurrences. But the ancient scriptures such as *Mahakala Nidhi* explain this method systematically."[5]

But what about the involuntary tumo condition? The ancient texts also speak about that, saying that in some cases kundalini can go astray. This might be an accident of birth or it might result from improper living or naive experimentation with powerful occult techniques. In such cases, the kundalini energy streams through the body in wild fashion, producing tremendous body heat which can result in sickness, insanity and even death. Various secret techniques for handling this condition have been handed down in texts and by word of mouth among yogis. One method is to pack the person in wet clay.

In a personal communication to me, the deceased Indian yogi-scientist Gopi Krishna, author of *Kundalini, the Evolutionary Energy in Man* and widely regarded as the world's foremost authority on kundalini research, elaborated on the phenomenon of tumo as a byproduct of kundalini activity. He noted that *pingala*—what yogis call the "solar nerve" along the right side of the spinal cord—is considered to be hot, while *ida*—the "lunar nerve" on the left side—is cold. These nerves, according to his interpretation of yogic physiology, are the right and left sympathetic nerves, respectively. "It is a well-known fact in India," he wrote, "that the arousal of the kundalin power can cause such a heat in the system that the *sadhaka* (spiritual aspirant practicing yoga) has to stay immersed in water for hours at a time or a thick layer of wet earth has to be applied to the body to absorb the heat generated. . . . In the case of a morbid arousal of the power, burning or chilling sensations are felt.''[6] (The chilling would be due to an imbalance of kundalini energy entering ida, the cold lunar nerve, rather than pingala.)

An explanation of tumo compatible with present physiological concepts was given by Mayne R. Coe, a medical researcher with a Ph.D. in biochemistry, who wrote about ''Discovering the Yogis' Secret'' in *Fate* (September 1969). In Coe's investigation of tumo, conducted through personal experimentation in freezing temperatures, he learned he could dry a wet woolen blanket through cold shocks to his naked skin. This forced glycogen, a sugar stored in the liver, into his bloodstream, where it was oxidized, providing body heat. The wool blanket acted as an insulator against the surrounding cold.

''My pores were alternately closing and opening,'' he wrote, ''as I was chilled and then warmed by the flush of my skin and the insulating properties of the wet wool that confined the heat to my body and the air inside the blanket surrounding me. . . . Instead of exposing the body nude to the air for extended periods of time to generate the mystical tumo, you shock the body into heat production. The ice-cold blankets shock the body to a warm glow and don't conduct the heat away as outside air or immersion in water would. It is quite easy to sit this way for an extended time at very low temperatures.'' Coe claimed a record of drying a wet woolen blanket dipped in water eight times over a two-hour period during 18° F. weather.

While Coe's discovery makes good physiological sense and goes a long way toward explaining tumo, it doesn't provide a comprehensive explanation of all the data—for example, the lamas who stand *naked* in the snows. Nor would it be sufficient to explain fully the case of Man Bahadur, as reported by Dr. L. G. Pugh in 1963 in the *Journal of Applied Physiology* (and summarized by Anthony Campbell in his book *TM and the Nature of Enlightenment*).

According to Pugh, who was a member of the British Medical Research Council on an expedition to the Himalayas in 1961, a 35-year-old pilgrim named Man Bahadur appeared one day at the expedition base camp on the Mingbo glacier, which is at an altitude of 15,300 feet. Bahadur was clad only in thin cotton trousers and jacket, a thin woolen vest, a cotton shirt, a thin woolen sleeveless pullover, an old khaki overcoat, and a large turban. He had no shoes or gloves.

Bahadur stayed with the expedition several weeks. During the first four days he was seen on the glacier at heights of between 16,500 and 17,500 feet. "On the fourth night," Campbell writes, "there was a blizzard, and next day a search party was sent to look for him. He was found, alive and well, beside a river, 600 feet below the expedition camp. During the nights Man Bahadur had spent on the glacier the temperature had falled to between −13 and −15 degrees Centigrade. Man Bahadur had had no food during this time, and had slept in the lee of a rock, covered by his overcoat. He had, he said, slept soundly and had not been awakened by shivering."

Man Bahadur's performance cannot be explained solely on the basis of Coe's principle of cold shocks to the skin because wet clothing was not involved in his survival. Had Bahadur learned voluntary control over his pranic currents so that he could, at will, direct greater than normal energy upward through pingala via meditation and/or visualization? And how could he maintain that condition during sleep? To what extent was his ability to withstand cold a result of special conditioning through autosuggestion? Pugh, who studied Bahadur through two weeks of physiological testing, had no answers to these questions. In fact, he had no explanation at all. It was, he declared, a mystery to him.

Perhaps a complete explanation of tumo includes all of the foregoing factors. In any case, the reality of tumo has been unquestionably established by competent observers and by Benson's unique film. Tumo's value for researchers in medicine, physiology, psychology and parapsychology should be obvious. Moreover, burgeoning interest in psychotechnologies, which has brought meditation, visualization, firewalking, psychic healing and other hitherto esoteric aspects of the human potential to public attention, will certainly be eager for more knowledge about tumo. Last of all, the welcome prospect of adapting to the environment through our own natural abilities, and without the burdening interference of technology, is particularly timely. The possibility of energy shortages due to physical limitations may spur humanity at large to discover this little-known psychic resource.

NOTES

1. pp. 216–217, *Magic and Mystery in Tibet*, Alexandra David-Neel. Dover: New York, 1971. The original appeared in French in 1929 and was first translated into English in 1932.
2. *Ibid.*, p. 227.
3. p. 21, *Your Maximum Mind*, Herbert Benson. Times Books: New York, 1987.
4. Personal communication, 1977.
5. p. 452, *Living with the Himalayan Masters*, Swami Rama. Himalayan International Institute: Honesdale, Pennsylvania, 1978.
6. Personal communication, 1982.

CULTS OF THE SHADOW

Kenneth Grant

That the oriental systems of tantra were based upon the Draconian or Typhonian cults of ancient Egypt may be adduced from the deposit of many Egyptian terms in the texts of the tantras, particularly in those of India. For example, shakti, meaning "power"–the central concept of the tantras –was known ages earlier, in Egypt, as *Sekht* or *Sekhmet,* the consort of the gods. She typified the fiery heat of the southern sun that had its biological analogue in the sexual heat of the lioness, a symbol of African origin. *Pasht,* in Sanskrit, means "animal," and in the tantras *pashu* has a specific connotation with reference to bestial modes of congress, i.e. sexual congress not sanctified by orthodox tradition. *Pashu* likewise existed in Egypt as Pasht or Bâst,* the feline goddess who "catted," and whose brood gave its name in later ages to the bast-ards which originally signified children born of the mother alone at a time when the role of the male in the process of procreation was unknown, or when the individualized fatherhood was not recognized. In the tantras, the animal passions were typified by the *pashu,* i.e. one who was disqualified from the performance of tantric rites involving the use of the sexual energies.

The *Khart* in Egypt was the god Horus as a child (Hoor-paar-Kraat); he reappears in the Indian pantheon centuries later as Kartikeya, the son of the sun-god. The god On in Egypt was the Sun, and the name was perpetuated in the

* Cf. the English word, beast.

Vedic religion as *Ong* or *Om,* the primal vibration of the creative spirit.

Yet another striking example is the name of the goddess Sesheta who typified the female period; in Hinduism, Sesha is the serpent with a thousand heads; it is also a name in the tantras for the lunar vibration or "serpent of darkness" that manifests itself periodically in women. Such examples of the Egyptian origin of tantric concepts could be multiplied almost indefinitely.

The Ophidian cults of Africa were purged of their tribal and contingent accretions during their fusion with the Draconian tradition of Egypt. But it is in the Kaula Division of the *vama marg,** or Left Hand Path, that the most perfect form of this tradition was continued in India and the Far East. Of this division the *chandrakala*† or "moonray" recension retained some of the primal characteristics of the Ophidian cults.

The application to the human body of the Ophidian processes was revealed in three principal degrees in which the secrets of sexual magic were demonstrated with the use of *suvasinis* or "sweet smelling women" who represented the primal goddess and who formed the Kaula Circle.‡

The ability to function on the inner, or astral planes, and to travel freely in the realms of light or inner space, derived from a special purification and storage of vital force. This force in its densest form is identical with sexual energy. In order to transform sexual energy into magical energy (*ojas*), the dormant Fire Snake at the base of the spine is awakened. It then purges the vitality of all dross by the purifying virtue of its intense heat. Thus the function of the semen–in the

* *Vama* means "woman." She was typified by the moon, the nether, the bottom, the infernal, as distinct from the ether, the summit, the supernal; the left as distinct from the right. *Marg* means "way" or "path"; hence, the term *vama marg* denotes the way involving the use of woman, the lunar current, the infernal powers, etc.

† *Chandra* = moon; *Kala* = ray, essence, path etc.

‡ I.e. the Circle of the Supreme *Kala* (*Mahakala*): the *Chandrakala* or Moonray Goddess.

tantras–is to build up the body of light,* the inner body of man. As the vital fluid accumulates in the testicles it is consumed by the heat of the Fire Snake, and the subtle fumes or "perfumes" of this molten semen go to strengthen the inner body.

The worship of *shakti* means in effect the exercise of the Fire Snake, which not only fortifies the body of light but gradually burns away all impurities in the physical body and rejuvenates it; for the life processes, unchecked, deposit quantities of ash or waste matter in the system. This is governed by the Fire Snake from her seat in the coccygeal (prostate) gland: the excretory region alluded to in some tantras as the feet of shakti.† The effluvia from this region, when retroverted, have power not only to build up the body of light but also to create new worlds, new dimensions, in which the adept can function as easily as he functions upon the mundane plane. In the non-initiate the waste matter, not being purged and drawn up by the heat of the Fire Snake, remains as the end-products of catabolism and forms semen, urine, feces, and–in women–menstrual fluid. The fire leaks out of the average person in these substances which, solely because they are imbued with a spark even of this fire, are useful adjuncts in magical work. Their abuse, as in the sorcery of later ages–when they were not properly understood and improperly applied–accounts for the monstrous abnormalities of the pseudo witch cults and their demonic sabbaths.

When the subtle essences, the "flowers" of these substances, are drawn off and kept within the human organism they direct their fire within and create the magical bodies that are used in the rituals of the Kaula Circle. Initiates have methods of preventing the deposit of semen in the testicles, and urine has curative properties as well as being a stimulant; the tantras give instructions for its use in the rejuvenation of the physical body. Of far more importance, however, is its value as a bisexualizing agent which, if ingested at certain

* The astral body.

† See *Aleister Crowley and the Hidden God,* Chapter 10, note 24.

times of the month, creates a condition wherein the initiate becomes androgynous and without fear. The feces incinerated (i.e. burned to ashes) likewise are used in tantric rituals, and the siddhas refer often to the god Shiva smeared with ashes. Behind this symbol, repulsive as it may appear to non-Orientals, or, more correctly, to non-initiates, lies the great mystery of rejuvenation, physical and astral, and the creation of new worlds.

CHRISTIAN MYSTICISM AND KUNDALINI

Mineda J. McCleave

In his commentary to Gopi Krishna's autobiography, James Hillman made the following observation: "The failed examinations [for college entrance] cut Gopi Krishna off from a substitute career in which his spiritual aims could have become an intellectual or academic ambition. . . . After the examination failure, there was only one way to go: his own."

At eighteen, I quit high school. At twenty, my outlook on life was summed up in one word: *Weltschmerz!* At twenty-one, I celebrated my birthday in a state mental institution. It was there, while reflecting upon my predicament, that it dawned on me: I was a dynamic failure. When I was discharged, there was only one way to go: my own.

The reason I draw a parallel between Gopi Krishna and myself will, I trust, become clear in this article.

To have entered the practice of psychiatry might have satisfied my intellectual and academic ambitions. Destiny, however, intervened, and my aim in life became a spiritual one. Feeling an aversion to the world, in which I was a misfit, I took refuge in religion. I read many books on comparative religion, mysticism, metaphysics, positive thinking, reincarnation, hypnotism, and yoga philosophy. Through his books, Paul Brunton became my teacher. The Bible became my handbook.

My approach to religion always remained Christian-oriented, but I soon discovered the value of incorporating insights gained from other areas. I had been disillusioned by my

Church, but I could not reject Christ or the Bible. Neither could I reject the common thread of love weaving through all the major religions. I was dissatisfied with theological explanations of the Bible, but not with the Bible itself. The words within spoke to me with a kind of comfort and meaning that did not seem to dim, in spite of all the confusing passages and unsatisfying commentaries about the Bible.

Still, I could not understand the *meaning* of God, Christ, the Holy Spirit, love, good, evil, heaven, and hell, nor could I accept the infallibility of the Scriptures. I had read in the Book of Acts* three separate accounts of Paul's conversion experience on the road to Damascus (Acts 9:7, 22:9, and 26:14). The accounts were all "different" in one or more aspects. When I read the same three accounts in the Revised Standard Version, the same differences were apparent. Fundamentalists may overlook such conflicting accounts, but an inquiring mind questions their authenticity.

Nevertheless, I still sensed that the Bible was inspired literature, and I began to study it earnestly. I could not understand many of the parables, and I noticed that Jesus often explained the parables in greater detail to his disciples than he did to the multitudes. In Luke 8:10, Jesus said, "Unto you it is given to know the mysteries of the kingdom of God: but to others in parables; that seeing they might not see, and hearing they might not understand." It seemed he was holding something back from the masses. St. Paul used the same technique. He told his followers he was feeding them with milk, as they were not yet ready for strong meat. As they grew in understanding, he fed them stronger nutrients. He wrote in I Corinthians 4:1, "Let a man so account of us, as of the ministers of Christ, and stewards of the mysteries of God." Why were there so many references to "a mystery" and "mysteries" in the Bible? These things puzzled me. I wanted desperately to understand the Bible, including the mysteries. I prayed for wisdom and understanding. With my faith firmly anchored in God, and hoping—as St. Peter urged—to add

* All biblical quotations are from the King James Version. *Editor.*

knowledge to my faith, the next inevitable step was that I should be drawn to the study of occult books dealing with Bible mysteries.

Most of the religious books I had read warned me against studying occult literature. They claimed that such material was the work of the devil; it was demonic, satanic, evil, and filled with black magic. However, by the time I had progressed to reading occult books, I had already made a covenant with God. It was simple. I would *trust* him and he would *protect* me. I prayed for guidance in the selection of my reading material. I discovered there were good occult books and bad ones, and trusted God to help me choose the good ones.

Strangely, I found these condemned books to be the opposite of what I had expected. The books were filled with thoughts of love, beauty, forgiveness, mercy, faith, and strong moral injunctions. Many of the writers *recommended* a more thorough reading of Scripture. I learned that the term "occult" does not, intrinsically, mean "evil." It simply means hidden, secret, concealed, and/or esoteric. The more I read in the forbidden books, the more I began to understand the Bible. Knowing, by this time, that the occult teachings were filled with "hidden wisdom," I realized that St. Paul was aware of the esoteric teachings. He openly declared, in Romans 2:7, "But we speak the wisdom of God in a mystery, even the hidden wisdom, which God ordained before the world unto our glory." I yearned to understand this wisdom and prayed that God would help me to comprehend it.

I started out meekly, with faith sowed in my heart like a grain of mustard seed, and hoped and prayed God would nurture it until it became a mature tree. I tried to serve God by loving and serving my fellow human beings. The first few years were delightful. I felt like the proverbial born-again Christian–happy, cheerful, optimistic, loving, and loved.

Jesus advised us, "Seek ye first the kingdom of God." I found two important promises in the Bible. One said, "Seek and ye shall *find*," and the other said, "And ye shall *find* me when ye shall search for me with all your heart." I took his words at face value, started my search, and expected with all my heart to find something, though I knew not what.

My Church had told me that the kingdom of God, or heaven, was a place the righteous went to after death—located somewhere in the great beyond. However, Christ taught that the kingdom was *within.* I valued his words above the Church's, so I started my search by looking inward. I devoted much time to prayer. Soon I found I was going into a much deeper, or higher, part of myself than I had expected. I began to feel immense love for God, my family, my friends, and even my enemies. I felt very happy in this prayerful state. I noticed that the deeper I plunged into meditative prayer, with my mind focused on God, the more I was aware of what I can only describe as a sensual feeling. I had read of the mystics' encounters with God—Divine Love—but I knew I wasn't experiencing anything that marvelous. I simply concluded that true prayer should be loving, as we made our petitions known unto God with praise and thanksgiving. I felt I was approaching a "peace which passeth understanding," and during this calm but alert feeling of tranquillity, I often blessed others and wished I could share my joy with them. Sometimes I felt as though I were sharing it with them. I did not know then, as I know now—thanks to the advances being made in psychology, parapsychology, and biology—that I was moving into an altered state of consciousness.

My normal consciousness had expanded and I was feeling transpersonal love, and coming close to transcendental love. Neither did I know that I was, ever so slightly, stirring kundalini. I began to notice unusual activities in other areas of my life. There was an increase in occurrences of mental telepathy, and I felt very intuitional. My dreams became more spiritual, and I had several out-of-the-body experiences. Concomitantly, I began to have problems relating to the world around me. I had shifts in consciousness during my nonmeditative hours—daydreaming and absent-mindedness—as I was absorbed in the inner world. Though I had not required psychiatric care for many years, I was again bothered with alternating periods of euphoria, anxiety, depression, and, sometimes, despair. I was surprised to find that my peaceful prayer life was often counterbalanced with thoughts of suicide. I could not understand these strange moods. Christ had said, "Come unto me . . . and I will give you rest." He said, "My yoke is easy, and my burden is light." I had expected my life to be filled with constant joy. I had overlooked that one of the fruits of the spirit is long-suffering. I had ignored the suffering of the early Christians after they had taken up their crosses.

In retrospect, I now realize that I had incorporated some simple yogic techniques of concentration and breathing into my meditations. This activity, added to long periods of prayer, was causing *changes,* painful ones, in my mind and body. The physical, mental, and emotional problems that surfaced were so dramatic that I had to quit working. I withdrew from society and had to rely upon my family to care for and support me.

Although I could not then connect my prayer life to the ordeals I was subjected to, I was aware of one thing: I knew I was on a spiritual journey. I knew I could no longer ask for psychiatric help. I had begun a long "dark night of the soul," and it lasted for ten years. My peaceful prayers changed to frantic spiritual cries for help. Not even my family knew I was leading an interior life. Several times my family physician recommended I seek psychiatric assistance, but I refused, and the task of caring for me fell upon his shoulders. Finally, in 1975, when I was thirty-seven years old, I was hospitalized three times in the psychiatric ward of the local hospital under his care. After the third incident, he insisted that I obtain psychiatric aid. For two weeks I balked, but finally relented, knowing I could no longer cope with my agitated mind. I was besieged with migraine headaches and no longer had any control over my life.

Reluctantly, I endured eight months of therapy with a well-meaning psychologist, but one who could not understand, or approve of, my approach to religion. The counseling seemed painful and fruitless. As I look back on it now, the *stress* brought on by the therapy sent me back into the depths of my being, calling upon God to hear me in my times of distress.

During this therapy, I underwent the most terrifying, yet enlightening, experience of my life. In February and March of 1976, I had a slight, fairly constant fever. The first week of April I was bothered by a feeling of internal heat. My lungs felt dried out, my eyes were dry and burning, and I developed several fever blisters on my upper lip. I was unable to sleep well. I ate little, having an aversion to food.

On April 6, 1976, I was very deep in prayer, expressing a strong need for God's intervention in the affairs of my life. Unexpectedly, I was jarred out of my prayer by what felt like a current of energy that seemed to enter my body through my left foot. Subjectively, it seemed like an electrical charge of nervous energy, moving with extreme rapidity up the inside of my left leg, passing through my genitals, and then dispersing in my upper back. This current was constant for four days and nights. With it there was an increased feeling of great body heat. I felt as though I were burning up from the inside out. Relatives could feel heat emanating from the front and back of my head while their hands were an inch away from me. It was a frightening experience. I knew, intuitively, that I had somehow triggered this current through intense prayer, but I had no knowledge of how to stop it.

The first three nights, unable to sleep, I read in the Bible, diligently searching for guidance. I kept rereading the Psalms, and despite my fear, I was comforted by the feeling of empathy I shared with the psalmist. It seemed to be exactly as he had written: I was keeping the night watches, my reins were instructing me in the night seasons, and God was writing his laws in my inward parts. I knew I was "fearfully and wonderfully made." The psalmist also said, "This is my comfort in my affliction: for thy word hath quickened me." I had no doubt I had been quickened. I felt as though my basal metabolism rate had skyrocketed. My mind was *hyper*hyperactive as I tried to understand what was taking place. Physically, I went through a variety of symptoms, including anorexia, headaches, trembling, fever with concurrent chills, nausea, and dizziness. Emotionally, I went up and down the keyboard of euphoria, joy, bewilderment, anxiety, depression, and the familiar despair. I was, at times, deluded and often disoriented. On one occasion, I actually believed I had died. Such peace! I was almost disappointed to realize I hadn't. I was afraid to leave my apartment for fear someone would notice my schizophrenic-like behavior. I gazed into a mirror and observed a "wild" look—the same strange look I had noticed in 1973 after I took a week of biofeedback training.

In 1973 I had also read Gopi Krishna's autobiography. I knew there was something to what he was saying, but I couldn't understand it. So I stashed the book away in the attic. However, on April 9, the fourth day of this incessant activity, I retrieved his book, and Gopi Krishna's words took on new meaning for me. This time, I did understand—in part! He was describing in minute detail some of the things I was experiencing. His experiences were far more enlightening, and fearsome, than my own. I never saw the inner light I so fervently prayed for. Yet I recognized the physical, mental, and emotional characteristics of kundalini—aroused, but not fully risen.

There was one thing Gopi Krishna wrote that convinced me he knew about the things that were happening to me. He wrote of the involuntary, increased genital activity. This factor is what prevented me from seeking medical treatment. From the immense reading I had done in the areas of mysticism, metaphysics, and the hidden wisdom, plus my understanding of the Scriptures, I suspected that I may have brought into greater circulation "the water of life." Again the psalmist had said it: "There is a river, the streams whereof shall make glad the city of God. . . ." And so had Jesus: "He that believeth on me, as the Scripture hath said, out of his belly shall flow rivers of living water" (John 7:38). Gopi Krishna, I now saw, was writing from a yogi's point of view about things I had learned from a Christian perspective. I knew the Hindu writings predated the Bible. I also knew, as a seeker after truth, that I had to reconcile Gopi Krishna's experiences with my own Christian philosophy.

I wanted, immediately, to do more research. However, the physical, mental, emotional, and sometimes spiritual distress I felt made it impossible for me to do much of anything except pray. Despite my discomfort, I believed that what was happening to me was *good,* regardless of contrary appearances. I believed, "All things work together for good to them that love God." Yet, while trying to adjust to this marvelous energy that was coursing through my mind and body, now intermittently, I exhibited so many psychiatric symptoms that the psychologist could no longer work with me. Unfairly, I felt that he had abandoned me, and it sent me back to deep prayer, asking God to deliver me from my afflictions. I asked for help in trying to regain control of my life. The bioenergy was still confusing me, and I was unable to concentrate my efforts in a constructive way to help myself. I couldn't pull my life together. I needed assistance.

Finally, in December 1976, by the grace of God, I was led to an open-minded, tolerant, compassionate, caring Christian psychiatrist, Bill Grimmer—an extraordinary man. He was not *afraid* of the occult. He was not *afraid* of kundalini. He was willing to try to help me sort out the complexities of my life. Primarily, his *interest* in my well-being was the deciding factor in the therapy. In his efforts to help me, he read Stanley Dean's *Psychiatry and Mysticism,* Gopi Krishna's *Kundalini, The Evolutionary Energy in Man,* Lee Sannella's *Kundalini—Psychosis or Transcendence?,* Edgar Mitchell's *Psychic Exploration,* and miscellaneous articles about kundalini. Added to that burden, he read eight voluminous notebooks I wrote for him, filled with the flotsam and jetsam of my life, as I tried to explain to him *how* and *why* I had been led into the mystical life.

Gopi Krishna's book inspired me to "let go" of the secret I had nourished for so many years. It is possible that decision kept me from degenerating into schizophrenia, from which there might not have been a return. Sannella's book helped me to realize that my experiences tallied closely with the "physio-kundalini" model he has observed in the Western world, and which he distinguishes from genuine psychosis. My psychiatrist helped me to remember that I am still a Christian, not a yogi. He encouraged me to continue in my search—to reread the Scriptures and the writings of the mystics—to find the common denominator. He helped me by "accepting" me and allowing me to grow. (Incidentally, Sannella, in his book, makes an excellent point about acceptance: Psychiatrists should listen, and possibly learn, from the patient undergoing the kundalini process. All the patient needs is a genuine concern and a willingness to understand on the part of the physician. The process, per se, is self-directing and self-healing, and, unmolested, will go in the direction of health.)

Rereading Gopi Krishna's life story, I realized that I was indebted to him for having the courage to write of his experiences and his philosophy. His life, somehow, touched my own. I knew that he was a forerunner, that the time was coming when the hidden wisdom would be revealed to the public—to be researched, studied, understood, and applied. My own experiences with kundalini, small in comparison, taught me that my soul is metaphysically linked with all others. It also taught me that there are divine ways of overcoming the doctrinal differences that seem to separate people, cultures, and nations. Most of all, it taught me that the Christian Bible presents this central fact: There is a Living God—a vibrant, active, creative Being who is the silent mover of all things.

As I reread the Scriptures and the writings of the mystics, I was amazed at the new insights I gained. It was as though old familiar passages had changed into new gems of wisdom. I was understanding things from a higher perspective. I was learning to recognize (re-cognize, know again) the basic truth in the words of the mystics, which they all hinted at but could not openly reveal. The mystics of all religions have expressed their knowledge in terms of their own faith. The accomplished yogis explained their attainments in terms of kundalini. The Christian mystics, unaware of the Hindu term, described the same phenomenon, but named the animating, motivating spiritual force at work within them as the Holy Spirit. They were aware of Divine Love. The kundalini experience is often accompanied by burning sensations in the body. The Christian experience is described as the "baptism" of the Holy Spirit. In Matthew 3:11, John the Baptist says, "I indeed baptize you with water unto repentance; but he that cometh after me is mightier than I, whose shoes I am not worthy to bear: He shall baptize you with the Holy Ghost and with *fire*." Despite the example of Pentecost, the Church teaches the baptism of water and leaves the baptism of fire to some unknown future time. The Church seems to be ignoring the reports of the mystics. The mystics testify with the writer of Hebrews 12:29, "For our God is a consuming fire." Other examples abound.

Brother Lawrence: "Sustain me by thy power lest the *fire* of thy love consume me."

St. Anselm: "Pierce with the arrows of thy love the secret chambers of the inner man. Let the entrance of thy healthful flames set the sluggish heart alight; and the burning *fire* of thy sacred inspiration enlighten it."

St. Hildegard: "Omnipotent Father, out of thee flows a fountain in *fiery* heat; lead thy sons by a favorable wind through the mystic waters."

St. Simion:

> What is this new mystery, Master of the Universe,
> That You have manifested in my regard, the debauched and impure?
> What is this great marvel that I consider in my own interior
> And which I do not understand, and which remains hidden to me?
> . . . its ray rises small and then makes itself be seen as a flame
> in the center of my heart and of my bowels, turning without stopping and illuminating all the interior of my entrails and rendering them light. . . .
> You who are proclaimed invisible to All?
> How do You become and make Yourself seen by me as a flame?
> And how do You burn matter, You who are immaterial by essence?

Jacob Boehme, in his *Confessions,* describes his own spirit as "the living, running fire." Likewise, Richard Rolle, the "father of English mysticism," reported his mystic experiences in a book whose title has obvious meaning here: *The Fire of Love.*

Reading St. John of the Cross, having some familiarity with the concepts of kundalini and the belief in the possibility of the baptism of fire, one may find that he was trying to explain what was happening in his mind and body—as well as his soul—as he communed with God. From one of his poems, *Songs of the Soul in Intimate Communication and Union with the Love of God,* come these thoughts:

> Oh flame of love so living,
> How tenderly you force
> To my soul's inmost core your fiery probe. . . .
>
> Oh lamps of fiery blaze
> To whose refulgent fuel
> The deepest caverns of my soul grow bright,
> Late bloom with gloom and haze,
> But in this strange renewal
> Giving to the belov'd both heat and light. . . .

Coming out of one of his dark nights of the soul, he was tenderly caressed in a strange renewal that sounds exactly like the enlightenment process of kundalini. Note that he claims the "flame of love" is *living!* He encountered the *living* God through love.

The major goal of the Christian mystic has always been to enter into the ultimate consummation of divine communion with God, through Christ, devotion to Mary, other saints, and sometimes even archangels. The goal had behind it the desire to *feel* divine love. The available literature attests that many of the mystics actually felt as though they were having a genuine, authentic love affair with God. The sexual connotations —usually veiled, sometimes overt—lead one to believe the mystics did, indeed, know and understand that divine healing love was flowing through their bodies. That this love was accompanied by heat, fire, the burning passion of fever, and the other symptoms of kundalini was obviously made known to them by their reported discomforts. It is conceivable to believe that the mystics who searched the Scriptures for instruction, guidance, and the way to live the holy life may have understood them in a far more intelligent way than we do.

Gopi Krishna suggests that the food the body uses to feed the transforming process is supplied by the sexual organs. Although he does not favor complete celibacy, he suggests there is a critical period, possibly as long as a year or two, in which the sexual fluids should be retained. What did the mystics think when they read, in Matthew 25:1–13, of the ten virgins, five of whom could not go to the wedding ceremony because they took no oil with them, whereas the five virgins with oil were permitted to go with the bridegroom? Is it possible they understood this to mean that the five virgins who were admitted to the marriage of the soul were admitted *because,* for a crucial period, they had retained their sexual fluid, their life energy, as part of their preparation to receive the groom, the Holy Spirit?

The spiritual groom, it is worth noting, did not present himself exclusively to the female mystics. St. John of the Cross thought of his soul as being feminine, and he believed he was the bride of Christ, despite his masculinity. St. Bernard, a twelfth-century mystic, alternately believed he was not only Christ's bride, but also Mary's spouse.

St. Paul wrote in the seventh chapter of I Corinthians that it would be better for a man if he did not marry. He went on to say that if a man did marry, he and his wife, by mutual consent, should refrain from coming together for a season—and that the season should be devoted to prayer. Was St. Paul suggesting that there was a sexual element involved in the efficacy of prayer? He added that the married are more apt to try to please their spouses, whereas the unmarried are more apt to try to please God. Surely, the mystics pondered deeply on these things. In the King James Version of the Bible there is a statement that has been retranslated out of the newer versions. It declares, in I John 3:8, "Whosoever is born of God doth not commit sin; for his seed remaineth in him; and he cannot sin, because he is born of God." Consider the mystics thinking deeply on this verse. Doesn't it seem likely the mystics would understand that there is a connection between the sexual activity and the holy life? Not an imaginary one, as so many psychotherapists believe, but a divine link with God?

The mystics may not have understood the Hindu concept of kundalini, but they certainly were aware of the process they were going through. Perhaps they understood it as the purging process they had prayed for when they asked God to *transform* them by the renewing of their minds and the cleansing of their hearts. The Christian mystics may have known much more than we are giving them credit for, but may have been hampered in *explaining* what they knew. Perhaps this was because their tradition had no extensive psychophysiological terminology such as we have today. Perhaps the mystics could have been more precisely expressive of their experiences if they had lived in an age of free expression, open investigation, and honest evaluation of their most sacred secrets.

If this were so, they could have admitted that their relationship with God was a decidedly sexual one at times. They could have complemented such terms as rapture, bliss, ecstasy, and divine union with words like sensual, sexual, erotic, and orgasmic. There was no shame in the minds and hearts of the mystics. The mystic who was admitted to the divine marriage was, undoubtedly, cognizant of the fact that it was in part a sexual marriage. Something happened to him in his periods of meditation, his prayers, and his intense devotional efforts to love God and be loved by God. That something, so it seems, was the awakening of kundalini. To the Christian mystic, this phenomenon was viewed from a radically different frame of reference than the yogic tradition. According to his background, his beliefs, and the knowledge he had, it was the flowing forth of the waters of life. "But whosoever drinketh of the water that I shall give him shall never thirst; but the water that I shall give him shall be in him a well of water springing up into everlasting life" (John 4:14).

The mystic knew experientially what that water was and where it came from, even if he lacked the metaphysical vocabulary to adequately articulate it. He *knew.* That is precisely why he was considered a mystic. He had uncovered one of the mysteries of God's relationship with man. Can anyone doubt that St. John of the Cross, one of the more eloquent mystics, was aware of this truth? In his poem *Song of the Soul That Is Glad to Know God by Faith,* he wrote:

How well I know that fountain's rushing flow
Although by night
Its deathless spring is hidden. Even so
Full well I guess from whence its sources flow. . . .
Its clarity unclouded still shall be:
Out of it comes the light by which we see. . . .
The current that is nourished by this source
I know to be omnipotent in force. . . .
An eternal source hides in the Living Bread
That we with life eternal might be fed. . . .
Here to all creatures it is crying, Hark!
That they should drink their fill though in the dark. . . .
This living fount which is to me so dear
Within the bread of life I see it clear
Though it be night.

"This living fount" is the "well of water springing up into everlasting life," and St. John of the Cross discovered it "within the bread of life," which he knew was his own body. In Romans 12:1, St. Paul beseeches us to present our bodies "a living sacrifice, holy, acceptable unto God. . . ."

The mystics are often considered as neurotic, love-starved, sexually frustrated individuals (and some may well have been), escaping into a nonexistent world of sexual fantasy. However, conventional psychology has overlooked the fact that because the mystics' needs were not satisfied in the exterior world, they withdrew into the interior world, the realm of Spirit, where their needs were met in a very realistic way—a way not understood by those who try to analyze such things without having first experienced them. The mystics had learned to sublimate their sexual drives, and as a result, were fulfilled in a manner that science is only beginning to investigate. Some mystics were married, while others remained single. Of the latter, some had previous sexual relationships, while, apparently, some had no such prior relationships. Yet they all reported that their spiritual love life far surpassed the fulfillment of any earthly love, and was accompanied by a sense of at-one-ment with God and all their fellow human beings. Dag Hammarskjöld, a mystic, wrote in his *Markings*, "How easy psychology has made it for us to dismiss the perplexing mystery with a label which assigns it a place in the list of common aberrations." The time has come for psychology to *understand* the mystery it has been dismissing.

The writings of the mystics and the yogis give credit to the theory that there is a spiritual force, working within and through the biology of man, expressing itself via the medium of the mind. Their writings show that they were trying to describe the transcendental insights they were privileged to enjoy. Yet we must ask: Aside from a limited technical vocabulary, why have the mystics been so confined in describing the physical aspects of enlightenment?

The answer is guilt. Not their guilt–they became as little children in their innocence as the life force flowed through their bodies–but world guilt. The sexual guilt that lies covered over in the person with a more "normal" sex life would certainly not give acceptance or approval to those claiming to have a sexual relationship with God. Unfortunately, as the mystic realized his own guiltlessness, there was no common knowledge about this life energy. He knew no one could understand him except another mystic, so his sacred life became a secret one, written about in prose and poetry that inspires many but is understood by the few.

From all the literature I have read about kundalini–religious, philosophical, scientific, and particularly medical–it seems to agree with the literature concerning mysticism. Yet the literature in both fields seems to express frequently that the mystic was not sure just what was "going on" in his life. From my reading of the Christian mystics, and my understanding of the Scriptures, I think the mystic was more than a bystander watching the proceedings take place in his body and mind. If the mystics had awakened kundalini, and if it is a self-regulating, self-directing, and enlightening experience, why do so many writers think the mystic was not enlightened enough to realize his own situation?

In Psalms 119:93, the psalmist says, "I will never forsake thy precepts: for with them thou hast quickened me." Is it too difficult to imagine the mystic crying out to the Lord, "Quicken thou me according to thy word," and eventually being quickened, and feeling the increased activity in the mind and body? Perhaps the mystic knew what God meant when he said in Jeremiah 31:33–34, "I will put my law in their inward parts, and write it in their hearts; and I will be their God, and they shall be my people." Perhaps they understood the psalmist, who wrote in Psalms 51:6, "Behold, thou desirest truth in the inward parts: and in the hidden part thou shalt make me to know wisdom."

There is no doubt that many of the mystics were self-realized. They had awakened kundalini. The pranic Holy Spirit had descended upon them. They became *aware* that they did, in fact, live and move and have their being in God. It was no longer a belief. It became knowledge to them. Their consciousness had expanded to a new level of perception with the opening of the inner eye. "If thine eye be single, thy whole body shall be full of light" (Matthew 6:22).

At times, St. Paul reports, he came to his followers in weakness and fear, with much trembling, speaking not in "enticing words of man's wisdom, but in demonstrations of the Spirit and of power." What kind of power is this that makes a man weak, fearful, and trembling, yet demonstrates the Spirit? His symptoms sound very much like certain signs of kundalini. Can anyone doubt he was aware of the power within him? The Holy Spirit was moving St. Paul, preparing him for the work he had to do—that of spreading the message: "Now to him that is of power to stablish you according to my gospel, and the preaching of Jesus Christ, according to the revelation of the *mystery,* which was *kept secret* since the world began, but is now made manifest, and by the Scriptures of the prophets, according to the commandment of the everlasting God, made known to *all* nations for the obedience of faith" (Romans 16:25–26).

St. Paul says the mystery is now made known to *all* nations. Is this the same mystery that, once understood, made the mystic into a mystic? Is this the same mystery that Gopi Krishna and others calling for kundalini research are trying to unveil? How long can the Western world ignore the findings of psychic and spiritual researchers in other countries—findings that are in agreement with recent discoveries of our own scientists? We cannot continue to look at the Christian mystics apart from the mystics and yogis of other cultures. Neither can we disregard the insights of psychology, parapsychology, biology, and metapsychiatry, as research reveals the truth. Clearly, the Christian mystics experienced a tremendous force—which they termed the Holy Spirit—that has striking parallels with the traditional descriptions of kundalini. Can we not presume then that there is a common origin for the experiences of higher consciousness that happened to all the mystics and yogis? The true mystic is just as much aware of that source as is the true yogi.

Christianity is being faced with a gigantic challenge—to understand its origins and teachings in the light of scientific knowledge. Perhaps, the Church—grown proud and rigid in its doctrines—may have to humble itself, following the example of Jesus. We may have to admit that we have been "teaching for doctrines the commandments of men" (Matthew 15:9). Walt Whitman, who was recognized by R. M. Bucke in his book *Cosmic Consciousness* as a true mystic, wrote in the Preface to his first edition of *Leaves of Grass*, ". . . re-examine all you have been told at school or church or in any book, dismiss whatever insults your own soul, and your very flesh shall be a great poem and have the richest fluency not only in its words, but in the silent lines of its lips and face and between the lashes of your eyes and in every motion and joint of your body." Whitman may have understood what Christ meant when he said in John 10:34, "Is it not written in your law, I said, Ye are gods?" If we are gods, as Christ says we are, why are we so unaware of our true nature? Is it because we do not understand our own Bible? Christ tells us plainly, in Luke 17:21, "Neither shall they say, Lo here! or lo there! for, behold, the kingdom of God is *within* you." How can we continue to think of the kingdom as a place reserved for us in the future, when we are told it is within us?

It is time for Christianity to re-examine the Bible—to understand all those seemingly unintelligible parts we have thus far skipped over, dismissing as incomprehensible. God does not expect us to remain ignorant forever. The entire Bible is filled with "hidden wisdom," and science and religion together can find that knowledge if they will only search for it. We must not be afraid of the "occult." The Bible itself is one of the greatest occult books ever written, in the sense that it is filled with concealed, secret, esoteric wisdom, hidden in symbols, allegories, parables, and similes. The Book of Revelation is yet to be deciphered.† There is a time for all things, and it is time to investigate Revelation with the insights gleaned from the study of parapsychology and kundalini. The answers are there if we will look for them with an open mind.

To Christians who may oppose such an investigation, I can only repeat Christ's words: "But woe unto you, scribes and Pharisees, hypocrites! for ye shut up the kingdom of heaven against men: for ye neither go in yourselves, neither suffer ye them that are entering to go in" (Matthew 23:13). When Christ repeatedly said, "Woe unto you," he was never personally condemning those he addressed. Christ was a man of love—not condemnation. He was, in effect, telling his listeners that there are certain cosmic laws that require people to reap that which they have sown. He was *warning* the reigning hierarchy that if they not only refused to seek the kingdom themselves, but also closed it to those who were searching for it, they were then *condemning themselves*—to the inevitable karmic results of spiritual darkness—rather than awakening

† See "The Restored New Testament" by J. M. Pryse, which follows. *Editor.*

themselves to the spiritual light that could be found within.

Rather than opposing a joint investigation of cosmic laws and an understanding of all Scriptures, Christians, having been taught by Christ the value of wisdom, love, kindness, and compassion, should give forth a loving invitation to all seekers to join together in harmony–in the common cause of trying to understand the principles that underlie spiritual evolution.

Speaking for myself, as a baptized Christian, I welcome the contributions of the members of all religions, all sciences, and the humanities, as we try to comprehend our unity as human beings in the mystical body of Christ. We are all children of one God–one Creator–and are bound together as one family on the planet Earth in a vast universe. Our family should be able to live and learn in true fellowship. "Come now, and let us reason together" to expand our spiritual awareness.

FROM
THE RESTORED NEW TESTAMENT

J. M. Pryse

In the following introductory analysis it will be shown that the Apocalypse [Book of Revelation] is a coherent whole, symmetrical, and having every detail fitted into its appropriate place with studied care. In its orderly arrangement and concise statement the book is a model of precise literary workmanship. But it contains a series of elaborate puzzles, some of which are based upon the numerical values of certain Greek words, thereby serving to verify the correct interpretation of the more important symbols; and as the detailed explanation of these in the analysis would interrupt the interpretation of the book as a whole, for the sake of clearness the solution of these puzzles will here be given in advance.

In the Apocalypse four animal-symbols or beasts (*thēria*) are conspicuous *dramatis personæ:* (1) a lamb (or "little Ram," *arnion*), having seven horns and seven eyes, and who is identified as Iēsous, who becomes "the Conqueror"; (2) a beast resembling a leopard, with a bear's feet and a lion's mouth, and having seven heads and ten horns; (3) a red dragon, having seven heads and ten horns, and who is "the Devil and Satan"; and (4) a beast having two horns like a lamb but speaking like a dragon, and who is called the pseudo-seer, or false teacher (*pseudo-prophētēs*). Of these four the leopard is particularly referred to as "the Beast"; and concerning him the Apocalyptist [St. John] says:

"Here is cleverness (*sophia*): he who has the Nous, let him count the number of the Beast; for it is the number of a man, and his number is 666."

1. The Conqueror (*ho nikōn*)

ὁ	70
ν	50
ι	10
κ	20
ω	800
ν	50
	1,000

2. Intuitively Wise (*epistēmōn*)

ἐ	5
π	80
ι	10
στ	6
η	8
μ	40
ω	800
ν	50
	999

3. The Higher Mind (*Iēsous*)

Ἰ	10
η	8
σ	200
ο	70
υ	400
ς	200
	888

4. The Cross (*stauros*)

στ	6
α	1
υ	400
ρ	100
ο	70
ς	200
	777

5. The Lower Mind (*hē phrēn*)

ἡ	8
φ	500
ρ	100
η	8
ν	50
	666

6. Desire (*epithumia*)

ἐ	5
π	80
ι	10
θ	9
υ	400
μ	40
ι	10
α	1
	555

7. The Serpent-coil (*speirēma*)

σ	200
π	80
ε	5
ι	10
ρ	100
η	8
μ	40
α	1
	444

8. Incontinence (*akrasia*)

ἀ	1
κ	20
ρ	100
α	1
σ	200
ι	10
α	1
	333

(8.) Licentiousness (*akolasia*)

ἀ	1
κ	20
ο	70
λ	30
α	1
σ	200
ι	10
α	1
	333

The Numbers of the Names

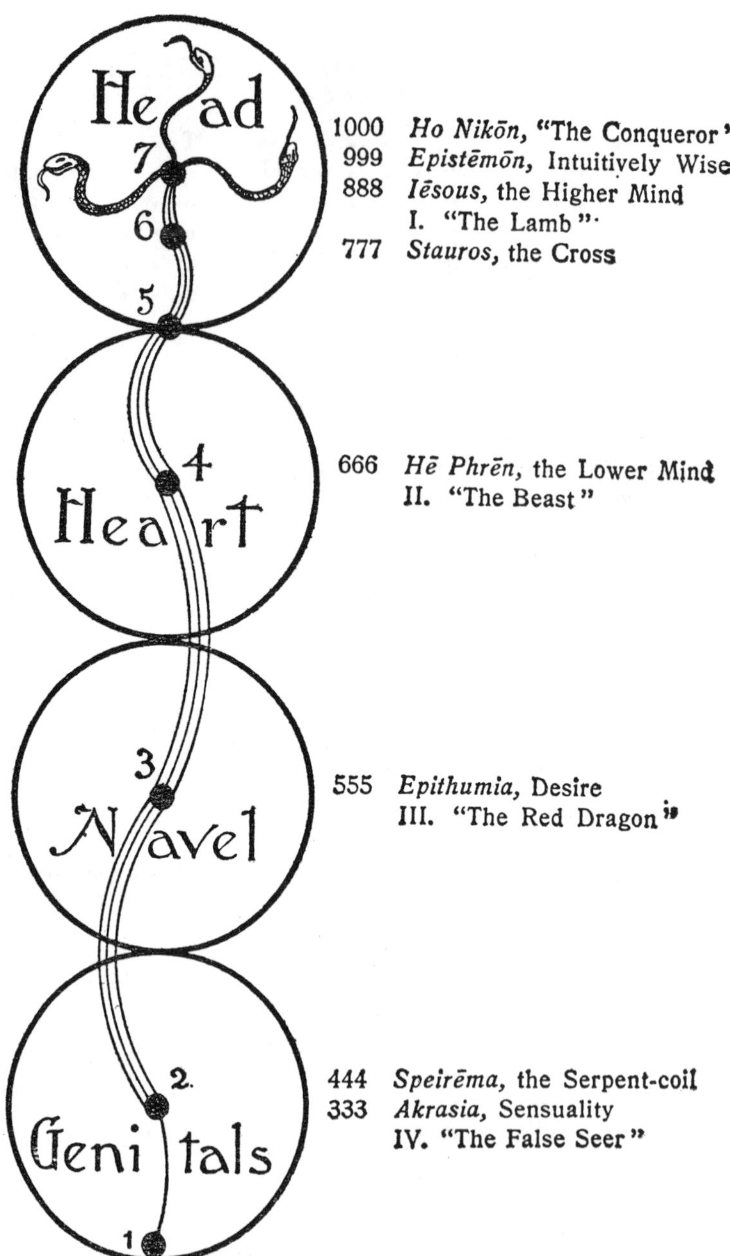

The Gnostic Chart Concealed in the Apocalypse

The "cleverness" of this puzzle lies in its very simplicity; for the words "the Nous" (ὁ νοῦς), the familiar term in Greek philosophy for the higher mind or man, naturally suggest the correct answer, the Phrēn (ἡ φρήν), the cognate term for the lower mind or man. As numbers are expressed in Greek by the letters of the alphabet, and not by arithmetical figures, the number of a name is simply the sum of the numerical values of the letters composing it. Thus the numerical value of *hē phrēn* is 666. If this were the whole of the puzzle, it would be almost puerile; but it is, in fact, only a part of, and the clue to, an elaborate puzzle, which in its entirety is remarkably ingenious. It will be noticed that the Beast, the phrenic mind, is the faculty ruling over one of the four somatic divisions, from which the natural inference is drawn that the three other beasts likewise are the regents of the three other somatic divisions. The Lamb, Iēsous, would therefore stand for the highest of these, the Nous. Now, the word *Iēsous* gives the sum 888. The red Dragon, "the archaic serpent, who is the Devil and Satan," fits neatly into place as the ruler of the third somatic division, *epithumia,* which word yields the number 555. The fourth beast, the "false prophet," takes his place in the fourth division as the generative principle, *akrasia,* "sensuality," the number of his name being 333. Plato applies to this principle the word *akolasia,* which has the same meaning and the same numerical value.

Placing these four names, with their numbers, in the form of a diagram of the four somatic divisions, it becomes apparent that the puzzle is still only partly solved, for evidently a complete series of numbers is intended. A space is left where the diagram, to fill out the meaning, requires the cross, and another space for the "good serpent," the regenerative force; the "bad serpent," the Devil, the lust for life which leads to generation, being already included. The number of the cross, *stauros,* is 777 (the letters στ being taken, of course, as ϛ = 6). The spiraling electric force, "the coil of the serpent," is the *speirēma,* which word gives the number 444. Now, the action of this force upon the brain, where its triple current forms the cross, gives the noetic perception, direct cognition (the *epistēmē,* or highest degree of knowledge, so beautifully defined by Plato), and to express this in the diagram it becomes necessary to insert the word *epistēmōn,* the philosophic equivalent for the word *christos;* its numerical value is 999. Further, he who has attained to this higher knowledge forthwith becomes the conqueror, and as "the Conqueror" is the hero, so to say, of the Apocalyptic Drama, his name must be placed at the head of the list, as *ho nikōn,* with its number, 1,000.

The diagram thus completed makes clear the basic teaching of the Apocalypse, which treats of the *speirēma* and its energizing through the vital centers as the Conqueror gains mastery over them and builds up for himself, out of that primordial substance, his immortal vehicle, the monogenetic or solar body. This deathless solar vesture is symbolized as a city which comes down out of the sky, enveloped in the radiance (*doxa*) of the God, and it is portrayed with poetic imagery of exquisite beauty. The description, with its wealth of detail, should be enough to show very clearly what the city really is; but Iōannēs [St. John] has supplied conclusive proof of the true meaning by inserting in the description a puzzle which reads as follows:

"The divinity who was talking with me had for a measure a golden reed, to measure the city, its gateways, and its wall. The city lies foursquare, and its length is as great as the width. He measured the city with the reed, by *stadia,* twelve thousand; its length, width and height are equal. And he measured its wall, one hundred and forty-four cubits, [including] the measure of a man, that is, of a divinity."

As the expression "by *stadia*" (ἐπὶ σταδίων) shows that the measurement should not be taken in *stadia,* it naturally follows that it should be reduced to miles. Therefore, dividing 12,000 by 7½, the number of *stadia* to the Jewish mile, the quotient is 1,600, and this is the numerical value of the words *to hēliakon sōma,* "the solar body." (The number 1,600 is found also in Chapter 14:20, where it has the same significance.) In the authorized version the preposition *epi,* "by," is not translated, being omitted as redundant—which merely shows the untrustworthiness of an empirical translation. That version also reads, "a hundred and forty and four cubits, [according to] the measure of a man, that is, of an angel," the inserted words making the passage meaningless. The "wall" of the solar body is its aura, or "radiance," *hē doxa;* but the letters of that name amount to only 143. As a puzzle, that number would be too transparent, nor would it harmonize with the other numbers given in relation to the city, as the twelve thousand *stadia,* twelve gateways, twelve foundations, etc., all of which have a real or an apparent reference to the zodiac. Therefore Iōannēs increased it to 144, the square of twelve, by adding another *alpha,* which he calls "the measure of a man, that is, of a Divinity." In the formula, "I am the *Alpha* and the *Ō* [*mega*], the first and the last," *alpha* is the symbol of the divine man, or Divinity, before his fall into matter; and *ō mega* is the symbol of the perfected man, who has passed through the cycle of reincarnation and regained the spiritual consciousness.

The city is described as having the form of a cube. To solve this element of the puzzle it is only necessary to *unfold* the cube, thereby disclosing a cross, which represents the human form–a man with outstretched arms.

Although Iōannēs speaks of measuring "the city, its gateways, and its wall," he does not give the measure of the gateways, for the very obvious reason that it is wholly unnecessary, since the word "gateway" (*pylōn,* from *pylē,* "an orifice") sufficiently indicates their nature: they are the twelve orifices of the body. In the Upanishads the human body is often called poetically the twelve-gate city of God's abode.

In literary construction the Apocalypse follows to some extent the conventional model of the Greek drama: although in narrative form, it divides naturally into acts, or scenes, in each of which the scenic setting is vividly pictured; and interspersed with the action are monologues, dialogues, and choruses. As a mere literary device, these scenes are represented in a series of visions; and in this Iōannēs has adopted the style of the Hebrew seers, from whom he obtained much

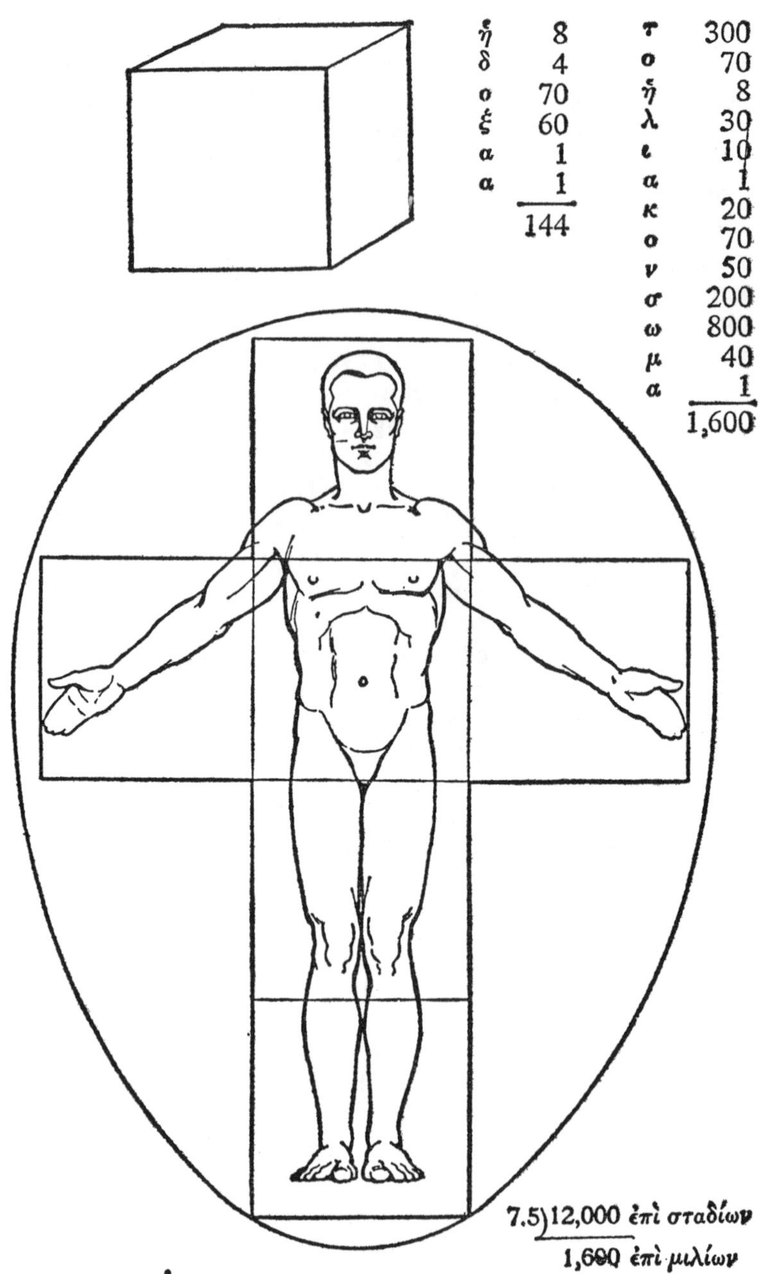

The Cubical City Unfolded

of the quaint symbolism, ornate imagery, and mystifying phraseology he artfully employs. But with the material obtained from this source Iōannēs has skillfully combined symbols drawn from the pagan Greek and other arcana, weaving these materials into a harmonious whole, wonderfully systematic and complete, and having all the details worked out with painstaking exactness. Then, having thus darkly veiled his teachings by this symbolism, utterly baffling to the conventional symbologist, he has ingeniously supplied means for verifying the import of each of the principal symbols, and this he accomplished by word-numbers and other puzzles.

By sentimental literalists the Apocalypse is generally accepted as a record of visions actually seen by "the Seer of Patmos," although it requires but little discrimination to perceive that the visionary style is merely an artifice of the Apocalyptist, adopted for the purpose of introducing the fabulous characters of his drama and mystifying his readers. It is only the psychics, the *mystai* or "veiled ones," who see symbolical visions. The true seer, the *epoptēs,* beholds the things of nature and of supranature as they really *are,* and not as they *seem:* perceiving that all the forms and processes of external nature are themselves but the shadowy symbols of the eternal Ideas of the intelligible world, he passes beyond this fabric of material and psychic glamor, this veil by which the True is covered and concealed, and penetrates to the first principles of things, the archetypal, spiritual realities.

A few of the technical words employed by the New Testament writers are fraudulent substitutes for terms used in older Greek. Thus *angelos,* "messenger," takes the place of the word *daimōn,* Deity in manifestation, including the hosts of lesser deities, powers, and essences. Philōn Judaios says (*De Gigant.,* i. 253) that the beings called angels in the Mosaic writings are simply the *daimōnes.* As the anglicized word "angel" summons to the mind only the theological and popular conception of a celestial being whose function in the universe is undetermined and dubious, *angelos* will in this work be rendered "Divinity," a word which covers in range of meanings the various significations of the Greek word. Similarly, *apokalypsis,* literally, "uncovering," "unveiling," is a substitute for *epopteia,* "beholding," a word technically denoting initiation into the greater mysteries. The Apocalypse is, as its title implies, an account of the initiation of Iōannēs himself. In the subtitle he calls it "the Initiation of Anointed Iēsous," that is, of his own illumined Nous, the "witness" for the universal Logos, as Iōannēs in the material world, the "slave" (*doulos*) of the true Self, is the "witness" for the individual Logos.

Many actors, apparently, play their parts in the drama of the Apocalypse; yet in reality there is but one performer—the neophyte himself, the sacrificial "Lamb," who awakens all the slumbering forces of his inner nature, passes through the terrible ordeals of the purificatory discipline and the telestic labors, and finally emerges as the Conqueror, the self-perfected Man who has regained his standing among the deathless Gods. He is the hero of, and the sole actor in, the drama; all the other dramatis personæ are only personifications of the principles, faculties, forces, and elements of Man, that minor world so vast and mysterious, whose ultimate destiny it is to become coextensive with the divine and illimitable universe.

In the brief prologue to the drama, the Anointed Iēsous, the illuminated Mind, is depicted as the first-born from the dead (the moribund inner faculties), the ruler of the lower powers, yet having been crucified by them on the cross of matter, the physical body. Now, at his coming, they who wounded him shall weep and wail over him. In the New Testament allegory there are two crucifixions: one relating to the soul's descent into matter, the generation of the physical form, and the other to its ascent to spirit, or regeneration in the solar body.

Then, "in the Breath," that is, in samādhi, the sacred trance, Iōannēs has a vision of the Logos, his own spiritual Self, in the self-luminous pneumatic body, of which he gives a magnificent description, partly literal and partly symbolical. He sees him walking to and fro among seven little lampstands, and holding in his right hand seven stars; announcing himself to be the ever-living Self, who became "dead" (incarnated), but is now alive throughout the eons, the Logos explains that the lampstands are the "seven Societies in Asia," and the seven stars their Divinities. That is, they represent respectively the seven Rays of the Light of the Logos (his seven forces), and the seven centers or chakras in the body, through which they energize. Asia is the native land of Iōannēs, therefore typifying the body, the homeland of the soul; and the seven Societies (groups or ganglia) are designated by the names of Asian cities, each of which, by some well-known characteristic or something for which it was noted, calls to mind the somatic center it represents. These cities are given in the same order in the Apocalypse as are the chakras in the Upanishads, thus: (1) Mūlādhāra, sacral ganglion; Ephesos, a city celebrated for its great temple of Diana, the "many-breasted mother," who appears in the Apocalypse as the "Woman clothed with the Sun, the moon underneath her feet," the lunar goddess and the Apocalyptic heroine alike personifying the regenerative force, the sushumnā, mystically called the "World-Mother." (2) Adhishthāna, prostatic ganglion; Smyrna, noted for the fig industry; the fig is preëminently a phallic symbol. (3) Manipuraka, epigastric ganglion; Pergamos, celebrated for its temple of Æsculapius; the epigastric, or solar plexus, is the controlling center of the vital processes of the body, and of the forces utilized in all systems of psychic healing. (4) Anāhata, cardiac ganglion; Thyateira, a city noted for the manufacture of scarlet dyes; the name being thus a covert reference to the blood and the circulatory system. (5) Vishuddhi, laryngeal ganglion; Sardeis, a name which suggests the *sardion,* sardine or carnelian, a flesh-colored stone, thus alluding to the laryngeal protuberance vulgarly termed "Adam's apple." (6) Ājñā, cavernous ganglion; Philadelphia, a city which was repeatedly destroyed by earthquakes; the manifestation of the kundalinī at this sixth center is especially violent, and so Iōannēs describes the opening of the sixth seal (mūlādhāra, which brings the īdā and pingala to their culmination at this center) as being accompanied by a "great earthquake." (7) Sahasrāra, conarium, or pineal body, the "third eye"; Laodikeia, noted for the manufacture of the so-called "Phrygian powder," which was esteemed a sovereign remedy for sore and weak eyes, presumably the "eye-salve" mentioned by Iōannēs in the message to this seventh Society.

To each of these Societies the Logos sends a message; and in these communications, which he dictates to Iōannēs, the nature and function of each center are indicated: a particular aspect of the Logos is presented to each one, a good and a bad quality being ascribed to each center, and a reward or prize is promised, specifying the spiritual results accruing to "the Conqueror" from the conquest of each chakra.

In the next vision is shown the Logos enthroned in the sky, with his four septenary powers. Here Iōannēs has constructed a simple little puzzle by employing redundant symbols and by inverting the order of the forces, enumerating the lesser ones first and the greater ones last. He places twenty-four Ancients ("elders") circling the throne, before which also are seven Breaths ("spirits") and a crystalline sea; after which he describes four *Zōa* ("living creatures"), each of whom has six wings. Yet he makes it clearly apparent, later, that the Zōa are superior to the Ancients and next in rank to the Logos. In fact, the four Zōa are the four manifested Powers of the Logos, the archetypes of the four "Beasts," whose nature, as the regents of the four somatic divisions, has already been explained. As these Zōa are septenates, they are said to have six wings each. These wings are identical with the twenty-four Ancients; and the seven Breaths before the throne are likewise identical with the highest septenate, the noetic *Zōon.* The seemingly complicated assemblage thus resolves itself simply into the Nous centered in the brain, with its four septenary powers; and the "glassy sea" is the ether pulsating in the mystic "eye" of the seer. For the "sky" in the Apocalypse is not the "heaven" of the profane, the celestial world supposed by them to be somewhere in the far depths of space.

The four Zōa are the Lion, the Bull, the Man, and the Eagle. These symbols represent the four cardinal signs of the zodiac, constituting the so-called cross of the zodiac: Leo,

Taurus, Aquarius (Waterman), and Scorpio. The constellation Aquila, the Eagle, though extrazodiacal, rising at the same time as Scorpio, is frequently substituted for it. The word zodiac (*zōdiakos*) is derived from *zōdion,* "a little animal," a diminutive form of *zōon,* "an animal." Hence, the zodiacal signs being called zōdia, the four principal ones are the Zōa.

A scroll ("book") is the next symbol introduced. It is simply the human body, esoterically considered: it is "written *inside* and *at the back,*" referring to the sympathetic and the cerebrospinal systems, and "close sealed with seven seals," which seals are the seven major chakras. The sacrificial Lamb, the neophyte who has attained to the intuitive, noetic consciousness–which is symbolized by his having seven horns and seven eyes, that is, mental powers of action and perception–opens the seals (arouses the chakras) successively. As they are opened, however, they change to zodiacal signs, the zodiac being applied to the microcosm, man, as shown in the diagram here presented, the man being depicted as lying in a circle, and not standing upright as in the exoteric zodiac. The seven planets are assigned to the twelve signs of the zodiac in the order followed by Porphyrios, and, in fact, by all ancient and modern authorities. In Sanskrit works the planets are made to correspond also to the seven chakras in the following order, beginning with mūlādhāra: Saturn, Jupiter, Mars, Venus, Mercury, Moon, and Sun. According to this zodiacal scheme, therefore, seven signs, with their planets, extend along the cerebrospinal region, and correspond to the seven chakras, which are the focal centers of the *tattvas,* and have the same planets; while the remaining signs pertain to the five pranas. This arrangement is shown more in detail in the table on page 431.

When the Lamb opens one of the seals, one of the four Zōa thunders, "Come!" A white horse appears, its rider having a bow. This is Sagittarius, the Bowman or Archer. Iōannēs thus starts the kundalinī current at the second chakra, and correctly so, for the sushumnā does not energize until īdā and pingala have reached the forehead, and then it starts from the

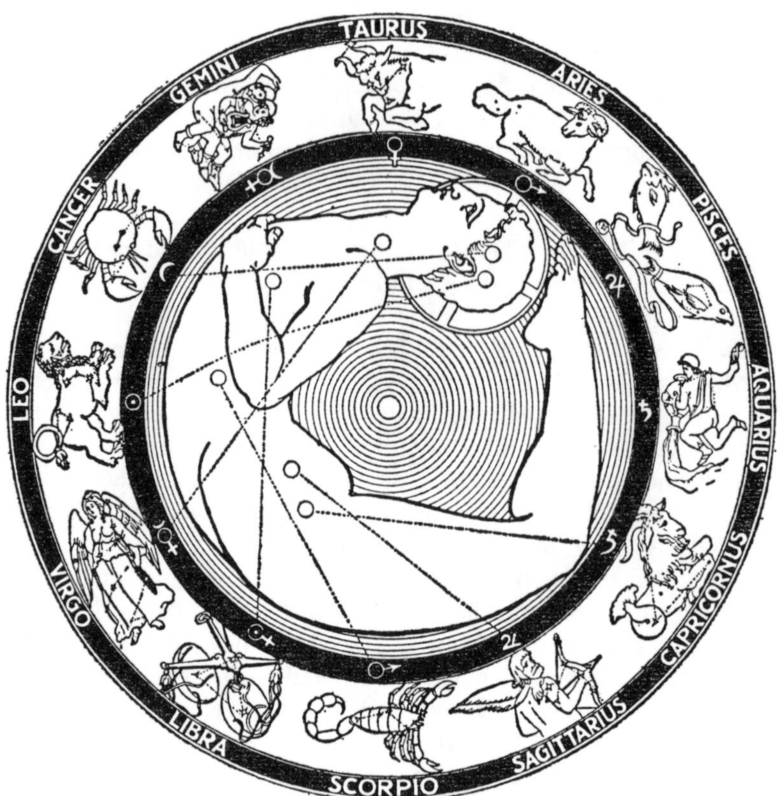

The Apocalyptic Zodiac

first center, corresponding to the terminus of the spinal cord. He therefore avoids calling this the first seal, but says, "one of the seals," and then numbers the others merely in the order in which they are opened.

The second seal being opened, the second Zōon says, "Come!" A red horse comes forth; to its rider is given a great sword, and power to take away peace from the earth. This is Scorpio, the house of Mars, the War-God.

Upon the opening of the third seal, the third Zōon says, "Come!" A black horse appears, its rider having a balance in his hand. This is Libra, the Balance.

When the fourth seal is opened, the fourth Zōon says, "Come!" A "pale" (*chlōros,* "yellowish") horse comes forth, and its rider is Death, accompanied by Hadēs; they are given power over one quarter of the earth, to kill with sword, famine and death, and by the wild beasts of the earth. This is Virgo, the astrological sign of the womb. In the New Testament, as in the Upanishads and other mystical literature, "Death" is the name very frequently applied to the physical, generative world, in which birth, decay, and death hold sway. In her character of the bad virgin, "a queen and not a widow," Virgo appears later in the Apocalyptic drama in the rôle of the Woman in scarlet, who is seated on the red Dragon, the epithumetic nature. But here she is associated with a higher center which has to do with the psychic consciousness, and therefore Hadēs, the psychic realm, is said to ride with Death; and the evil thoughts, desires, and passions of the psychophysical consciousness devastate the earth to the extent that they dominate.

The four horses, corresponding to the four Zōa, as also to the four beasts, are the four somatic divisions.

The fifth seal opened is the cavernous ganglion, to which corresponds the sign Cancer. Although Leo precedes Cancer in the zodiac, its corresponding chakra, the conarium, is the last of the centers to be aroused; for īdā and pingala branch out to right and left at the forehead, and it is only the sushumnā starting at the sacral ganglion, that reaches the conarium. Yet the influence of the two currents, at this stage, causes a partial awakening of the lower centers in the brain; and this is stated by Iōannēs in an ingenious little allegory about the uneasy ghosts ("souls") of those who had been sacrificed (atrophied, that is) because of the evidence they held. For it is by the atrophy of these noetic centers that man has lost the evidence of spiritual realities.

The sixth seal opened is the sacral plexus, to which corresponds the sign Capricornus. When this chakra is awakened, the sushumnā passes along the spinal cord and impinges upon the brain. Words cannot adequately describe the sensations of the neophyte upon his first experience of the effects

The Seven Powers, *Δυνάμεις* or *Shaktis*, and Their Correspondences

The Five Noetic Faculties, or Prānas	Plexi, or Chakras	Elements (Tattvas), or Occult Fires		The Seven Powers, or Shaktis	Colors and Metals
Occult Wisdom (Memory). Vyāna. (Gemini.)	Sacral. Mūlādhāra. (Capricornus.)	Earth. Prithivī. Sushumnā	Triple Fire of Most Sacred Earth.	Serpentine Power, Regenerative. Kundalinī Shakti.*	Yellow and Silvery White. Lead.† ♄
Reason (Power of Consecutive Thought). Apāna. (Aquarius.)	Prostatic. Adhishthāna. (Sagittarius.)	Water. Pingala Apas. Idā Lunar Fire.		Creative Power of Thought. Kriyā Shakti.	Pale Blue. Tin. ♃
Will (Power Stimulating the Mind to Act). Samāna. (Taurus.)	Epigastric. Manipuraka. (Scorpio.)	Fire. Tejas. Creative Fire.		Power of Will. Ichchhā Shakti.	Red. Iron. ♂
Cognition (Power of Apprehending). Prāna. (Pisces.)	Cardiac. Anāhata. (Leo.)	Air. Vāyu. [Sun-Fire. Solar "Breath," or		Power of Knowledge. Jñāna Shakti.	Green. Gold.‡ ☉
Direct Cognition (Power of Spiritual Intuition). Udāna. (Aries.)	Pharyngeal. Vishuddhi. (Libra.)	Æther. Ākāsha.	Triple Divine Fire.	Supreme Power. Parā Shakti. Bliss (Ānanda).	Dark Blue (Indigo). Copper. ♀
	Cavernous. Ajñā. (Virgo.)	Undifferentiated. Avyakta.		Occult Power of Speech. Mantrikā Shakti. Consciousness (Chit).	Orange-yellow (Golden). Mercury.§ ☿
	Conarium. Sahasrāra. (Cancer.)	Primordial. Brahmā.		Divine Substance. Daivaprakriti. Being (Sat).	Violet and Silvery Opalescent. Silver.‖ ☽

* Sanskrit works usually give the navel (epigastric plexus) as the seat of *kundalinī shakti*, and divide *ichchhā shakti* between the sacral and the prostatic; this may fit the notion of those who are devoted to the contemplation of the navel, but it is nevertheless incorrect. In thus dislocating the *kundalinī*, *apāna* is erroneously made to correspond with *prithivī*, and *vyāna* with *apas*. In later Sanskrit works the *prānas* are spoken of merely as the five vital airs, *vāyus*, and to them are added five subairs, these ten forces being said to govern the functions of the physical body.

† Alchemically, lead is regarded as debased silver. In the native state it is almost always found combined with sulphur.

‡ Thin gold leaf appears green by transmitted light.

§ Alchemically, mercury is regarded as "living gold," and gold as "killed mercury." The one symbolizes pure fluidic intuition; and the other, formulated thought, which has lost its living force by becoming concrete.

‖ Light transmitted through a very thin plate of silver appears violet.

produced by this mighty power: it is as if the earth crumbled instantly to nothingness, and sun, moon, and stars were swept from the sky, so that he suddenly found himself to be but an unbodied soul alone in the black abyss of empty space, struggling against dread and terror unutterable. Thus Iōannēs vividly pictures it, in terms of cosmic phenomena, as a seismic cataclysm, seemingly the end of the world. To the neophyte unprepared for this ordeal, failure may mean merely a short period of blank unconsciousness, or it may mean instant death—for this vital electricity has all the destructiveness, when misdirected, of the thunderbolt. The sixth center, ājñā, is the great "lunar" chakra, where the currents bifurcate; and at this point the resurgent "solar" forces, the prānas, form a cross in the brain. These solar forces Iōannēs pictures as five Divinities, of whom four stand at the corners of the earth, presiding over the four winds, and a dominant Divinity, the fifth, bearing the signet ring of the living God, ascends from the fifth direction of space, "the birthplace of the sun"—quite naturally, since he is in fact an aspect of that "Sun," the Nous. With his signet ring he seals 144,000 out of the tribes of the children of Israel. The twelve tribes are simply the twelve zodiacal signs, symbolizing the twelve forces of the Logos, which differentiate into countless minor forces. These, in the microcosm, are the nādīs of the Upanishads, which enumerate variously the nādīs centering in the brain, but usually place the number at 72,000. Iōannēs, however, holds to the zodiacal scheme: as each of the signs of the zodiac is subdivided into twelve minor signs, he multiplies these by 1,000—a number often used in mystical writings to express an indefinite term—and so arrives at a total of 144,000, or double the 72,000 of the Upanishads; but according to the latter the nādīs are innumerable in their ramifications.

After this is seen a great multitude, from all nations and peoples of all languages, white-robed and pure, who wave palm branches and sing a pæan before the throne; they are said to be those "coming out of the great ordeal." This "great ordeal" is reincarnation, the vast misery of being bound for ages to the wheel of birth. But this concourse of the "redeemed" who sing the chorus in this scene are the liberated elements in the aspirant's own nature; they are not a throng of people exterior to him. By evoking the marvelous potencies of his spiritual selfhood the Conqueror thereby regerminates all that was good, beautiful, and true in each of his past incarnations.

The seventh seal is the conarium, its zodiacal correspondence being Leo, which is the house of the Sun. Here reigns the Silence from which issue the seven spiritual "voices," or sounds. These mystic sounds Iōannēs describes figuratively as trumpet calls given successively by seven Divinities. They become audible when the chakras in the brain are awakened. The first four have a relation to the four somatic divisions, and react upon them; hence Iōannēs ascribes to the trumpet calls an obscuring or destructive effect upon the earth, the sea, the rivers and springs, and the sky, which correspond to the somatic divisions. At this stage of the telestic meditation the physical body is already in a state of trance, and it is now the lower psychic consciousness that is to be temporarily paralyzed or placed in abeyance; so, leaving the physical consciousness out of the reckoning, Iōannēs terms the psychic the "third" as applied to each of the four planes, to which correspond the first four trumpet calls. The results produced by the three remaining trumpet calls he terms "woes," since they entail very trying ordeals, the issue of which is certain failure to the unpurified neophyte, of whom it has been said: "His vices will take shape and drag him down. His sins will raise their voices like as the jackals laugh and sob after the sun goes down; his thoughts become an army and bear him off a captive slave." Thus, at the fifth trumpet call appears "a star fallen from the sky to the earth," who is the "Divinity of the abyss" and has the key to its crater, or opening, and whose name is Apollyōn, "he who utterly destroys," the "Murderer"; he opens the crater of the abyss, and from it emerges a locust-swarm of centaurs, who with their scorpionlike tails inflict torments on men. This "star" is Lucifer, the fallen "son of the morning," the *debased psychic mind of man,* which is indeed the ruler over the abysmal depths of desire, the bottomless pit of the passional nature, and the "murderer" truly of all that is pure, beautiful, and true. This fifth trumpet call refers to the carnal mind energizing in the sympathetic nervous system, the seat of the epithumetic consciousness, "the throne of the Beast"; and the next trumpet call, the sixth, bears relation to the cerebrospinal axis, the Apocalyptic "river Euphratēs," and to what may be termed the psychoreligious consciousness, which manifests itself in the emotional worship of the unreal mental images of Deity–the lower phase of religion that indulges in irrational theologies, superstition, sorcery, fanaticism, and persecution. The neophyte who has not thoroughly freed his mind from these pseudoreligious illusions will inevitably fail in the mystic meditation, which requires that all thought-images and preconceptions must be erased from the mind, so as to present it as a clean tablet for the inscription of truth. After this sixth trumpet call, the four Divinities fettered at the river Euphratēs are loosed: they are the four manifested prānas, the solar regents of the seasons, ruling the quaternary divisions of the year, month, day, and hour. The liberation of these forces is followed by the appearance upon the scene of an army of warriors mounted on lion-headed, serpent-tailed horses, who represent the countless powers of the Nous. A "strong" Divinity, the fifth, then descends from the sky, enveloped in a cloud, with a rainbow about his head; his face is luminous like the sun, and his feet resemble pillars of fire. This description of him is very similar to that of the Logos; he is *udāna,* the unmanifested divine power that is the revealer of secret truths. The strong Divinity cries out with a lionlike roar, and seven thunders utter their voices. Concerning the utterances of these seven thunders Iōannēs is very reticent. However, as the Greek language has but the one word (*phōnē*) for both "voice" and "vowel," the meaning obviously is that the "great voice" of the Logos, who is the seven vowels in one, is echoed by the seven vowels, the sounds by which the higher forces are evoked; and these the seer is forbidden to write down. Aι this stage of the sacred trance the neophyte, having attained to the noetic consciousness, begins to receive the mystery-teachings, the "sacred, unspeakable words" (ἄῤῥητα ῥήματα) which, as Paulos says, it is not lawful for a man to disclose. When he shall have mastered the next noetic center, the "third eye" of the seer, he shall pass beyond the illusions of time; "time shall be no more," and "the God-mystery shall be perfected." The Divinity gives a little scroll (booklet) to Iōannēs, who eats it; and though honey-sweet in his mouth, it makes his belly bitter. The scroll symbolizes the esoteric instructions he has received, which are indeed bitter to the lower man, for they inculcate the utter extirpation of the epithumetic nature. He is then told that he must become a teacher, opposing the exoteric beliefs of the masses.

By a side scene, a parenthetical explanation is given of the adytum, or shrine of the God, and the "two witnesses" of the "strong" Divinity, the Nous. The adytum–the temple cell or fane in which the God is enthroned–is the seventh of the noetic centers; and the two witnesses are īdā and pingala, the sushumnā being the third witness, "the believable and true."

When the seventh trumpet call is sounded, there is a choral announcement that the God, the true Self, has come to his own and will reign throughout the eons. The adytum is opened, disclosing the ark, the mystic receptacle in which were placed the "tablets" whereon was inscribed the contract of the God with man. Thereupon appears the Woman clothed with the Sun, star-crowned and standing on the moon; travailing, she gives birth to a man-child. She symbolizes the Light of the Logos, the World-Mother, that is, the pristine force-substance from which is molded the solar body–her "man-child." The red Dragon, the epithumetic nature, seeks to devour her child; but it is caught up to the God's throne, and the Woman flees to the desert, where she is nourished three and a half years. This means that after the formation of the solar body has begun, any strong passion or emotion may disintegrate and destroy it; and that during the first half of the cycle of initiation (here placed at seven years) the nascent body remains in the spiritual world, as it were, while the sushumnā force abides in its "place" in the material form, or "desert." For, strictly speaking, the solar body is not really born at this stage, but only has its inception. In the allegory, however, Iōannēs could hardly employ the more accurate but less delicate mystery-representation of the Eleusinia.

Here the sacred trance ends for the present; and next follows a battle in the sky. The Dragon and his Divinities are hurled down from the sky by Michaēl and his hosts; that is, the *mind* is now purified from the taint of impure thoughts. Michaēl and his fellow Chief-Divinities (*archangeloi*), Uriēl, Raphaēl, Gabriēl, etc., of whom he alone is named in the Apocalypse, are the Regents of the seven sacred planets, he himself being Hermēs, the Guide of Souls and Initiator in the Mysteries. But the Dragon, though ejected from the intellectual nature, continues his persecutions on the lower plane.

The Beast, the phrēnic nature, is described next. One of his seven heads (the seven dominant desires) has been slain, but comes to life; it represents the desire for sentient existence, the principle which causes the soul to reincarnate. This *will* to live, this passionate clinging to sensuous life, is expatiated on by Plato. Although the aspirant has apparently extirpated this longing, so far as the grosser affairs of the material world are concerned, it revives when he enters into the subtler planes of consciousness and perceives the psychic realms of existence. In Buddhistic literature it is termed *tanha* (the *trishna* of Sanskrit philosophical works); and in one ritual it is said: "Kill love of life; but if thou slayest *tanha,* take heed lest from the dead it rise again." Because this principle keeps man under the sway of reincarnation, Iōannēs says significantly: "If any one leads into captivity, into captivity he goes; if any one shall kill with the sword, with the sword must he be killed."

Another beast appears, who is the symbol of the generative principle. He participates in the nature of each of the other beasts, for he has two horns like the Lamb, talks like the Dragon, and has the magical powers of the Beast. He is called the Pseudo-Seer. His false seership is a certain very low form of psychism which, though not necessarily sensual, is due to the generative nervous ether. From this source come most of the "visions" of religious ecstatics, and the material manifestations produced by some spiritist mediums; and, in a more general way, it is the source of the emotional element in exoteric religion, or so-called religious fervor, which is in reality but a subtle sort of eroticism. As a blind emotional impulse to worship, it stimulates the lower mind, the *phrēn,* or Beast, to project an image of itself upon the mental screen and to worship that illusionary concept; and this—the "image of the Beast"—is the anthropomorphic God of exoteric religion.

Next appears again the Lamb, who by strict classification is one of the four beasts, though really too exalted to have that title applied to him, since he is the Nous, the regent of the highest of the four somatic divisions. With him are his many virginal attendants, who, as a prelude to the next act of the drama, chant a new pæan, to the accompaniment of many lyres. The neophyte has now become, as it were, like a lyre, with all the loose strings of his psychic nature tightened and tuned, tense and vibrant to the touch of his true Self. . . .

After this long but necessary digression, the action of the drama is resumed: the Conqueror appears, mounted on a white horse; "he treads the wine-vat of the ardor of the God's fecundating energy"; his mantle is blood-hued, and upon it and upon his thigh is inscribed his title of supreme ruler. The word "thigh" (*mēros*) is euphemistic; the *phallos, membrum virile,* is intended. This particular euphemism is common in the Old Testament (Genesis 24:2, *et passim*). Moreover, it will be noticed that here the Conqueror has the sword of Mars, and is riding the white horse of the Archer who, at the opening of the first seal, the adhishthāna chakra, "came forth conquering and to keep on conquering." Thus the incarnated Logos is shown to bear a direct relation to the lowest centers. Now, it would be utterly impossible to elucidate the Apocalypse and ignore this delicate but perfectly pure subject, concerning which even the most communicative expositors of the esoteric philosophy have been extremely reticent; and so the present writer, being opposed to all undue secrecy, and believing that in this matter harm has resulted from the suppression of the truth, feels justified in dealing with the subject frankly and without constraint, though with necessary brevity. As every practical "pyrotechnist" knows, the human brain contains certain centers or components, including the pituitary body and the conarium, the higher functions of which are almost completely dormant in the normal individuals of the present races of mankind, who are therefore termed in the New Testament and other esoteric writings "the dead"; yet it is only through these organs of the brain that the spiritual Self of man, his overshadowing God, can act upon the consciousness of the psycho-intellectual self. This corpse-like condition of the finer organs of the brain does not preclude very high development of the ordinary intellectual faculties, apart from the epistemonic power; indeed, there are and always have been men who are lamentable examples of brilliant intellectuality combined with the densest spiritual stupidity. In the case of the true genius, the poet, artist, intuitive philosopher, and religious mystic of saintly purity, there is a partial awakening of these centers; while in the case of the seer (excluding from that class the mere psychic clairvoyant) the higher faculties are so quickened that he becomes cognizant of the interior worlds, the planes of true Being. But when the brain is fully restored to its true functions by the energizing of the *speirēma,* the *paraklētos* of the New Testament, that "Light of the Logos" which is literally the *creative force of the Logos,* then it, the brain, becomes an androgynous organ, wherein takes place the immaculate conception and gestation of the self-born spiritual man, the *monogenēs,* who is in very truth "born from above." This is the process of regeneration and redemption which is expressed by myth and symbol in all the great world religions of antiquity. There being a direct and intimate relationship and correspondence between the sacred centers in the brain and the lower procreative centers, it follows that true spirituality can be attained only when a pure and virtuous life is led; while for the neophyte who would enter upon the telestic labor, the task of giving birth to oneself, perfect celibacy is the first and absolute prerequisite. Unless he is inspired by the loftiest aspiration, guided by the noblest philosophy, and restrained by the most rigid moral discipline, his possibility of success is extremely remote; and the mere dabbler in the pseudo-occult will only degrade his intellect with the puerilities of psychism, become the prey of the evil influences of the phantasmal world, or ruin his soul by the foul practices of phallic sorcery —as thousands of misguided people are doing even in this age. To follow the mystic "path" the aspirant must keep himself pure physically, mentally, and psychically.

V

Sage Advice to the Seeker

If the latent power of kundalini slumbering at the base of the spine, awaiting release, is the atom bomb of the human body, as has been claimed, its potentials for benefiting or destroying the individual—and hence society—are profound. Its elucidation and control may be as essential as is the control of the energy of the atom. What is it? Where does its power come from? What do we do about it?

If the sages of the ages are correct that the release of kundalini power can be cataclysmic for a body which is physically, emotionally and—most important—spiritually unprepared by sustained spiritual discipline, then we are indeed "playing with fire"!

Can science, concerned with physical facts and physical phenomena, expand its paradigm to include the spiritual warnings so that experiments with kundalini's physical effects do not create havoc?

Will the growing popular enchantment with vaunted kundalini values—from sexual excitement to spiritual bliss—become a siren song luring the unwary and unprepared to destruction?

Or will we with care and caution discover safe paths to individual and social regeneration through correct understanding and release of this unprecedented potential power?

These thoughtful and socially-responsible questions raised by Jeanne Rindge, president of the Human Dimensions Institute, in a special issue of *Human Dimensions* (see Appendix), should be pondered by everyone concerned with kundalini. Its potential for harm and destruction to bodies and minds is great. We have seen evidence that kundalini, if improperly aroused, without right guidance and preparation in the student, can be horribly painful and destructive—even fatal. The "white light" experience of the mystics can become the "ugly glaring light" of a schizophrenic; the "signs and wonders" performed by saints can turn into psychic phenomena and paranormal experiences that terrify people who naïvely venture beyond the limits of their understanding and preparation. In those who are not sustained by a sensible, healthy manner of living—one that is regulated, balanced, and ethical, not ascetic or orgiastic—kundalini can turn malignant and bring about deteriorating health, terrible bodily heat and chills, pain, many forms of physical and mental illness, and even sudden death.

Gopi Krishna points out in his books that there is another condition, too, even worse for humanity. Kundalini gone astray, he says, has created the evil geniuses in history. In such cases the kundalini energy was active since birth, as in all geniuses. However, their lives were so filled with difficulties that the kundalini energy became malignant because the finer qualities of mind necessary for psychological stability had not been made a part of their upbringing. The absence of those finer traits constitutes nature's safeguard barring access to the highest levels of consciousness. Short of enlightenment, though, the serpent energy can indeed turn venomous and from someone born with high intelligence produce a Rasputin, a Hitler.

This section is intended as a final word of warning. As people seek in various ways to know and to grow, some naïvely think that higher consciousness can result from forcefully practicing certain disciplines in mechanical fashion. This sort of sophisticated "power trip" is warned against by spiritual masters in the kundalini tradition. *Don't* meditate to awaken kundalini, they say, because you will probably harm yourself. Forcing it prematurely is possible but extremely dangerous. Rather, seek to grow in love and understanding. Seek to refine your character and cultivate your mind through selfless service, discriminating studies, and dedicated spiritual training. Do that, and kundalini will awaken gently, automatically, and without the unhealthy effects that are being seen more and more frequently. *Desiring* something—even such a noble goal as the awakening of kundalini—is misguided.

Nor is awakening kundalini in itself a magical key to samadhi. Swami Kripalvananda, in his *Science of Meditation* (see Appendix), cautions against what he terms "the menace of kundalini" during advanced stages of spiritual practice.

> The seeker who dares to awaken the kundalini power without the grace and guidance of a guru might become insane, succumb to diseases, or even die. This is because he does not possess the necessary knowledge, steadiness of mind, or patience required for this difficult undertaking.
>
> Many seekers are found wandering here and there in search of a guru who will awaken their kundalini. . . . Although thousands may claim that they know kundalini and that their kundalini is awakened, it is doubtful if even one of them really has such knowledge or experience.
>
> To awaken the kundalini power is one thing, but to make it move upward into the passage of the sushumna is something else. In the beginning, as the kundalini is awakened, the seeker feels a lot of enthusiasm. But as he advances in [meditation], he begins to encounter various menaces of kundalini. Only one with great courage can cope with these menaces; it is simply not possible for all to do so.

The brief articles assembled in this section call attention to various difficulties and dangers that may be encountered on the path of spiritual development. They are presented without further comment.

In closing, the words of American-born yogi Ram Dass, formerly Dr. Richard Alpert, professor of psychology at Harvard, seem appropriate. Ram Dass describes his spiritual awakening in several engaging books, notably *The Only Dance There Is* and *Grist for the Mill.* He reports the following insightful experience with his guru, Maharaj-ji, which is offered here as sage advice to the student: "When I asked Maharaj-ji, 'How do you raise kundalini?' he said, 'Serve people.' Which is like a real *schlock* answer. And I've worked with that, and it's so far out, and I see as I orient myself to seeing this whole thing as a process with everyone I meet, I keep getting into these spaces of incredible love and connectedness and that's the kundalini. . . . It's like . . . don't just sit there doing breathing exercises–serve people."

THE DANGER OF AROUSING KUNDALINI

Alice A. Bailey

How this fire at the base of the spine can be aroused, the form its progression should take (dependent upon the Ray), the blending of the fire with pranic fire and their subsequent united progression, are things of the past with many, and fortunately for the race, the work was achieved without conscious effort. The second blending with the fire of manas (mind) has to be effected. Scarcely as yet have men succeeded in directing the fire up more than one channel of the threefold column; hence two-thirds of its effect in the majority is yet confined to the stimulation of the organs of race propagation.

Only when the fire has circled unimpeded up another channel is the complete merging with the fire of the manas effected, and only when it progresses geometrically up all the three—with simultaneous action and at uniform vibration—is the true kundalini fire fully aroused, and therefore able to perform its work of cleansing through the burning of the confining web and of the separating particles. When this is accomplished the threefold channel becomes one channel. Hence the danger.

He who directs his efforts to the control of the fires of matter, is (with a dangerous certainty) playing with a fire that may literally destroy him. He should not cast his eyes backward, but should lift them to the plane where dwells his immortal Spirit, and then by self-discipline, and control of the mind and a definite refining of his material bodies, whether subtle or physical, fit himself to be a vehicle for the divine birth, and participate in the first Initiation. When the Christ-child (as the Christian so beautifully expresses it) has been born in the cave of the heart, then that divine guest can consciously control the lower material bodies by means of consecrated mind.

I do not in any way intend to take up the subject from such an angle as to convey rules and information that will enable a man to vivify these centers and bring them into play. I sound here a solemn word of warning. Let a man apply himself to a life of high altruism, to a discipline that will refine and bring his lower vehicles into subjection, and to a strenuous endeavor to purify and control his sheaths. When he has done this and has both raised and stabilized his vibration, he will find that the development and functioning of the centers has pursued a parallel course, and that (apart from his active participation) the work has proceeded along the desired lines.

Much danger and dire calamity attend the man who arouses these centers by unlawful methods; and who experiments with the fires of his body without the needed technical knowledge. He may, by his efforts, succeed in arousing the fires and in intensifying the action of the centers, but he will pay the price of ignorance in the destruction of matter, in the burning of bodily or brain tissue, in the development of insanity, and in opening the door to currents and forces, undesirable and destructive. It is not the part of a coward, in these matters concerning the subjective life, to move with caution and with care; it is the part of discretion. The aspirant, therefore, has three things to do:

1. Purify, discipline and transmute his threefold lower nature.
2. Develop knowledge of himself, and equip his mental body; build the causal body (soul) by good deeds and thoughts.
3. Serve his race in utter self-abnegation.

KUNDALINI IS NOT THE SOLE TRUTH

M. P. Pandit

Gopi Krishna writes from direct experience, in addition to his vast knowledge of ancient Sanskrit treatises and his considerable research in the tantric tradition. Thus his work should provide the much-needed corrective to the lack of understanding that is present in the West regarding tantra yoga and kundalini.

There is one point, however, on which it is not possible to agree with Gopi Krishna. He says in *The Awakening of Kundalini*, "An enlightened consciousness is never possible without a biological transformation" and asserts that the brain mechanism has to undergo a radical change before a more divine consciousness can be embodied. Yogic experience indicates that the process is just the reverse: A change of consciousness is anterior, alterations in the physiological system are a consequence. It is the consciousness that builds the form and shapes it to its needs. Further, the changes in consciousness effected by the direct descent of the higher consciousness through the head center–rather than the ascent of the kundalini from below–must be accounted for. There are lines of yogic discipline–Sahaja Marga, for example–in which it is expressly forbidden to go below the center at the chest level because they do not want to touch the kundalini; and yet they do register changes in consciousness, mental illumination, and spiritual transformation. Kundalini is a great truth, but not the sole or main truth.

In fact, from the point of view of Sri Aurobindo's integral

yoga, kundalini disciplines don't have much relevance. What is being laboriously attempted, dangerously pursued, and problematically achieved in kundalini yoga can be assured in a yoga like Sri Aurobindo's in a very natural way. And without one's mind deciding, "This is to be my way of progress"; but rather by throwing oneself open to a divine consciousness and grace, letting it descend into oneself, and letting it decide which centers of consciousness are going to be operated upon, which one is most open and ready. It is more in the natural way of evolution to let things develop in this manner rather than having a systematized procedure.

Even if one has a capable guru who works with the kundalini, it is not sufficient for reaching transformation as understood from Sri Aurobindo's point of view. Kundalini yoga practiced under a capable guru can lead to the realization of a certain overhead consciousness [awareness of some higher planes associated with the overhead chakras], but one who does this may nevertheless continue to experience anger, desire, etc. And, generally speaking, in such people these emotions are *more* intensified. Nevertheless, that continuous joy, happiness, delight is there. For some people there is more knowledge; for some there are more powers such as writing, painting, psychic abilities.

Still, you cannot say that such a person will have a spiritual consciousness. It is left to him to use his state for further development. If a person takes advantage of that state to transform himself or to divinize himself, then we may say he has true spiritual consciousness. But usually people remain at that level, saying that they have attained the ultimate, that Shiva and Shakti have joined–the power and the Self have joined –and that the purpose of the manifestation of kundalini is fulfilled. Thus the possibility of genuine transformation in the tradition of Sri Aurobindo is forsaken through ignorance and a subtle addiction to bliss.

THE TWO PATHS TO KUNDALINI

Sri Chinmoy

Blessed is he who practices kundalini yoga as part of his self-discovery and not in order to acquire power in hypnotism, black magic, or other low forms of occultism which operate in and from the vital world. A genuine student of kundalini yoga is he who tries to unite the vital power and the spiritual knowledge in perfect harmony with the evolving spirit of life. A genuine seeker never considers the hidden powers or occult powers as his goal. He cares only for God. He longs only for God's loving presence in his life.

The kundalini power is the dynamic power in us. When the dynamic power and spiritual knowledge go hand in hand, the perfect harmony of the universal consciousness dawns and the conscious evolution of the human soul reaches the transcendental self.

There are two ways for one to enter into kundalini yoga: through the tantric process and through the vedantic process. The tantric approach is systematic and elaborate but, at the same time, quite dangerous. The vedantic process is simple and mystical, but it is safe and in no way less convincing or less fulfilling.

The tantric method is dangerous because it deals first with the lower vital and emotional life. The approach is dynamic and courageous. Either one will purify himself by entering bravely into the vital world and coming out triumphant, or one will be totally lost in the ignorance of the vital world if he is not strong enough inwardly to conquer the vital forces there.

The vedantic way is safe because the seeker concentrates and meditates to raise, purify, and illumine his consciousness before he tries to deal with the obscure, impure lower vital forces that want to bind him. When the seeker enters into the lower vital world with the light of illumination, to his wide surprise he sees that the lower vital world is illumined, purified, and divinized.

The tantric process demands from the seeker constant and conscious awareness of the inner and upward movement from the muladhara chakra to the sahasrara chakra. The vedantic process demands from the seeker conscious and constant awareness of the evolving and liberating consciousness.

If anybody here would like to practice kundalini yoga, I advise that seeker to follow the vedantic method, which is safe and, at the same time, sure. If you follow the vedantic method, you are destined to reach the goal certainly and safely.

* * * * *

Q: Is the awakening of the kundalini a sign that God-realization is imminent? At what stage of the soul's evolution does the kundalini rise?

A: There is no hard and fast rule. There are many people who have realized God without ever having developed kundalini power. It is not at all necessary to open up the centers in order to realize God. They have seen the gradual development, revelation, and manifestation of the soul's potentialities and possibilities but have not developed their kundalini power. Here, the soul's manifestation means the soul's evolution. Again, there are those who have developed kundalini power who will not realize God for another two or three incarnations. So there is no direct connection between the kundalini power and the soul's development.

The opening of the centers need not be an indication of God-realization. But when there is intense meditation, very powerful meditation of the highest type, then automatically the centers open up. Also, when one realizes God, everything comes. At that time the centers automatically open, whether the seeker wants to utilize them or not.

Q: So the awakening of the kundalini does not mean that one is realizing God?

A: When one's kundalini is awakened, one becomes conscious of his inner psychic power, but this does not mean he is realizing God. God-realization is infinitely superior to the awakening of the kundalini and infinitely more fulfilling. When one's kundalini is awakened, one feels the inner vibration and inner power at his command. But this inner power does not mean the infinite peace, light, and bliss of the Supreme.

When the kundalini is awakened, it is like having a penknife with which one can do various things. But when one realizes God, one feels that he has the capacity to use the atom bomb. When one realizes God, his divine consciousness bursts into the earth's atmosphere and spreads over all the length and breadth of the world. But when the kundalini is awakened, one has only limited power. After the awakening of the kundalini, one sees the limitation of kundalini power. Then one wants to go high, higher, highest and naturally one will march on until the infinite goal is realized. . . .

Q: Does sexual indulgence prevent one from acquiring occult power through kundalini yoga?

A: Kundalini yoga is the yoga of absolute purity. It is one of the most sacred yogas and physical, vital, mental, and psychic purity are of paramount importance. The three major nerves–ida, pingala, and sushumna–will suffer immensely and immediately if there is any sexual indulgence. And it is not only physical relations that are bad. If somebody enjoys lower vital thoughts, impure thoughts, in the mind, that is also harmful. There are many who have concentrated on the centers and who were about to open them when unfortunately they entered into the lower vital world.

There are many Indian spiritual seekers who have said that when the kundalini is awakened, the vital heat, dynamic heat inside the subtle body very often causes them great discomfort. This energy comes from the subtle body, but it is felt in the physical body. Very often seekers who are about to develop spiritual powers find that the intense inner power is too difficult to bear. So they enter into the ordinary lower vital world and lose the kundalini experience.

To have the kundalini experience for a minute or two or for a few days is not difficult. The most difficult thing is to open up the centers. But this is not the end of our journey. Opening up the centers will give us psychic power or occult power or spiritual power. But the most important thing is to live in the divine consciousness. . . .

ORDERED MEDITATION AND LOVING SERVICE

Alice A. Bailey

This process of ordered meditation, when carried forward over a period of years and supplemented by meditative living and one-pointed service, will successfully arouse the entire system, and bring the lower man under the influence and control of the spiritual man; it will awaken also the centers of force in the etheric body and stimulate into activity that mysterious stream of energy which sleeps at the base of the spinal column.

When this process is carried forward with care and due safeguards, and under direction, and when the process is spread over a long period of time there is little risk of danger, and the awakening will take place normally and under the law of being itself. If, however, the tuning up and awakening is forced, or is brought about by exercises of various kinds before the student is ready and before the bodies are coordinated and developed, then the aspirant is headed toward disaster.

Breathing exercises or pranayama training should never be undertaken without expert guidance and only after years of spiritual application, devotion, and service: concentration upon the centers in the force body (with a view to their awakening) is ever to be avoided; it will cause overstimulation and the opening of doors on to the astral plane which the student may have difficulty in closing. I cannot impress too strongly upon aspirants in all occult schools that the yoga for this transition period is the yoga of one-pointed intent, of directed purpose, of a constant practice of the Presence of God, and of ordered regular meditation carried forward systematically and steadily over years of effort.

When this is done with detachment and is paralleled by a life of loving service, the awakening of the centers and the raising of the sleeping fire of kundalini will go forward with safety and sanity and the whole system will be brought to the requisite stage of "aliveness."

I cannot too strongly advise students against the following of intensive meditation practices for hours at a time, or against practices which have for their objective the arousing of the fires of the body, the awakening of a particular center and the moving of the serpent fire. The general world stimulation is so great at this time and the average aspirant is so sensitive and finely organized that excessive meditation, a fanatical diet, curtailing the hours of sleep or undue interest in and emphasis upon psychic experience will upset the mental balance and often do irretrievable harm.

Let the students in esoteric schools settle down to steady, quiet, unemotional work. Let them refrain from prolonged hours of study and of meditation. Their bodies are as yet incapable of the requisite tension, and they only damage themselves. Let them lead normal busy lives, remembering in the press of daily duties and service who they are essentially and what are their goal and objectives. Let them meditate regularly every morning, beginning with a period of fifteen minutes and never exceeding forty minutes. Let them forget themselves in service, and let them not concentrate their interest upon their own psychic development. Let them train their minds with a normal measure of study and learn to think intelligently, so that their minds can balance their emotions and enable them to interpret correctly that which they contact as their measure of awareness increases and their consciousness expands.

Students need to remember that devotion to the path or to the master is not enough. The Great Ones are looking for *intelligent* cooperators and workers more than they are looking for devotion to their personalities, and a student who is walking independently in the light of his own soul is regarded by them as a more dependable instrument than a devoted fanatic.

THE HIGH PURPOSE OF KUNDALINI

G. S. Arundale

It is sometimes thought that the development of kundalini leads to clairvoyance and continuous interplane consciousness, or to the linking of the various levels of consciousness, so that other states of consciousness may be connected with waking consciousness. This does take place in due course, but of far greater importance is a very real transubstantiation, in which the higher consciousness becomes jewels in the setting of the lower, the higher taking up its abode in the lower, that is to say in the waking consciousness itself. The lower knows itself to be a setting, and offers its substance for the jewels of the higher. This is in fact a setting up of continuous consciousness. Whether in fact clairvoyance, etc., arises or not, though in course of time it will, is of far less importance than the definite establishment of the higher consciousness–buddhic and later nirvanic–in the waking consciousness, this being the high purpose of the arousing of kundalini. This means . . . an extraordinary vivification of intuition–pure knowledge untainted, undistorted, by the personal equation; for into awakened buddhic and nirvanic consciousness no un-universalized personal equation can ever enter. The personal equation is transcended, the desires of the lower self begin to be transmuted into the will of the One Great Self. . . .

The burning sensation, so often associated with kundalini, and by no means confined within the channels of its passage through the body, is not necessarily inevitable. There may be a sensation of cold, of pressure, of a bursting, the latter generally within the head. Some students have experienced an uncomfortable warmth throughout the trunk of the body, with extension into the head, so that the whole of the upper part of the body seems intensely hot, streaming forth heat in all directions.

But always, and this is an acid test of the rightness of the experience, the whole body becomes comparatively universalized as to its sensitiveness. The whole body becomes, as it were, a gauge of the Real, so that discrimination . . . is alive from the feet to the very top of the head itself. This is a reflection on the physical plane of the absence in the inner bodies of the localization of faculties which is so apparent in the physical body itself. There arises, with the vivification of kundalini, a blending of the lower with the higher bodies, so that there begins to be one vehicle–receptive and active in every part of its being.

KUNDALINI IN ACTION

Roy Eugene Davis

. . . Over the years students may have been informed, as a result of their reading, of the dangers which lie in wait for one who awakens kundalini prematurely. The two main fears seem to be that increased activity of energy through the lower chakras will create an insatiable sexual urge or that increased flow of currents through the system will add to mental confusion and cause emotional instability.

As to whether or not one who awakens this heretofore dormant energy will experience an increase in sexual desire depends upon the person. Some will note this to be true and will be able to handle the matter appropriately: either by learning to express more fully and completely with the husband or wife or, if this is not desired or not possible, the energy can be directed into the upper chakras and the emphasis placed on creative work and meditation. Total aliveness is a characteristic of one who is truly awakened. We can do what we will with the energy at our disposal.

As to the possibility of psychological disturbance; a person who is not mentally and emotionally stable has no business working with subtle forces anyway. This is why, in the *Yoga Sutras of Patanjali,* the first two steps leading to meditation practice are concerned with attitude, behavior, and, in general, living in harmony with the environment. One who has serious psychological problems should not try to find a cure through meditation or by working with subtle forces. Many who are not yet ripe for spiritual awakening dabble on the fringes of the occult sciences and become mediums, sorcerers, and pseudospiritual leaders. One who is looking for thrills, phenomena, power over others, or magical abilities is not yet ready for this path which has enlightenment as the goal.

Some powers may be realized but they will only be utilized by a serious student of the truth to clear the mind and consciousness and bring him into a greater realization of Life. Even in the East magicians, mediums, workers of spells, and misguided users of occult power are not unknown. I have met swamis who claimed to have been trained in the ashrams of the Himalayas who were taken in this country, by those of superficial perception, as true spiritual leaders. Some of these men could demonstrate mastery (through autosuggestion) over blood circulation, suspend breathing for an hour or more while entranced (not samadhi), manufacture scents through the chanting of mantras, prophesy as a result of observing the flow of breath in their body at the time of being presented a question (a method known to some) and remain impervious to pain. Still, upon careful questioning they proved to be ignorant of the truths revealed in their own sacred scriptures and were lacking in genuine God-realization.

Many of these "wonder-workers" find, as do others who build a following through the display of special gifts, that there is always the temptation to "fake it" when they temporarily lose the power to perform. Also, the lure of money and fame causes them to prostitute their abilities and deny what principles they may have had at the beginning of their career.

One may ask, "What about Jesus and other enlightened men and women who performed miracles?" My only answer can be: when a person is self-realized he will do what he is led to do and, whatever expression this takes, he will neither be motivated by ego nor bound by his actions. . . .

Not all masters impart a specific method for working with kundalini. Some give the impulse, the awakening of the energy, and then instruct the student to meditate and let happen what will happen at the right time. In this manner kundalini moves from chakra to chakra according to the readiness of the disciple and brings about whatever changes are needed.

No attempt is made to force the circulation of currents; things are allowed to work naturally. In due time, after some years in most instances, the chakras are activated by the ascending flow of kundalini and spiritual consciousness is realized.

Once awakened, whether by personal initiation or not, this force will continue to be active. Sometimes, one becomes aware of the activity of kundalini during calm moments, meditation and whenever relaxed. Over a period of years the organism will be transformed and purified. This is a little-understood point; when a person is able to *bring through* this powerful force, then other people, usually family members and close associates are, unknown to themselves, uplifted and benefited. As a focal point through which kundalini can express, we silently bless our fellow man. Some people have, as their goal, final liberation with the idea of not returning once they leave this plane of expression. However, they and others who plan to return, can assist in the regeneration of man by living in the consciousness of Spirit on this planet. . . .

It is not really necessary for one on the path to become overly fascinated by the subject of kundalini and the workings of the chakras. As we rest more and more in the awareness of our true nature, whatever reorganization of physiological and psychic processes which is necessary will automatically take place. The practice of the presence, meditation, and remembrance of the nature of the soul will assure any serious person of success on the spiritual path.

Appendix

Suggestions for Further Exploration

BOOKS

Arundale, G. S. *Kundalini: An Occult Experience.* Wheaton, Ill.: Theosophical Publishing House, 1970.

Bentov, Itzhak. *Stalking the Wild Pendulum.* New York: E. P. Dutton, 1977.

Chinmoy, Sri. *Kundalini: The Mother Power.* New York: Chinmoy Lighthouse Publishing, 1974.

Davis, Roy Eugene. *Darshan: The Vision of Light.* Lakemont, Ga.: CSA Press, 1971.

Desai, Yogi Amrit. *God Is Energy: Five Articles on Kundalini Yoga.* Kripalu Yoga Ashram, Sumneytown, Pa.: privately printed, 1977.

Dychtwald, Ken. *Bodymind.* New York: Pantheon, 1977.

Eliade, Mircea. *Yoga, Immortality and Freedom.* Princeton, N.J.: Princeton University Press, 1970.

Grewal, Rishi Singh. *Kundalini.* Santa Barbara, Calif.: privately printed, 1930. Available through the Bear Tribe, P.O. Box 9167, Spokane, Wash. 99209.

Hills, Christopher. *Nuclear Evolution.* Boulder Creek, Calif: University of the Trees Press, 1977.

——. *Supersensonics.* Boulder Creek, Calif.: University of the Trees Press, 1976.

Karanjia, R. K. *Kundalini Yoga.* New York: Kundalini Research Foundation, 1977.

Kripalvananda, Swami. *Science of Meditation.* Gujurat, India: Sri Dahyabha Hirabhai Patel, 1977. Available through the Kripalu Yoga Ashram, Sumneytown, Pa. 18084.

Krishna, Gopi. *The Awakening of Kundalini.* New York: E. P. Dutton, 1975.

——. *The Biological Basis of Religion and Genius.* New York: Harper & Row, 1972.

——. *The Dawn of a New Science.* Kundalini Research Foundation (475 Fifth Avenue, New York, N.Y. 10016), 1978.

——. *Higher Consciousness.* New York: Julian Press, 1974.

——. *Kundalini, The Evolutionary Energy in Man.* Berkeley, Calif.: Shambhala, 1970.

——. *Panchastavi.* Kundalini Research Foundation (475 Fifth Avenue, New York, N.Y. 10016), 1978.

——. *The Riddle of Consciousness.* New York: Kundalini Research Foundation, 1976.

——. *The Secret of Yoga.* New York: Harper & Row, 1972.

Kundalini Research Institute, *Kundalini Yoga/Sadhana Guidelines.* Kundalini Research Institute (778 William St., Pomona, Calif. 91768), 1976.

——. *Kundalini Meditation Manual.* Kundalini Research Institute (778 William St., Pomona, Calif. 91768), 1976.

Lansky, Philip. *Consciousness and the Ergotrophic and Trophotropic Systems of Arousal.* Privately printed, 1975.

Available in Xerox copy for $15 from the author at P.O. Box 13056, Philadelphia, Pa. 19101.

Maharaj, Dhyananyogi Mahant Madhusudandasji. *Light on Meditation: A Definitive Work on Kundalini and Raja Yoga.* Scotts Valley, Calif.: Keshavdas Carl Kuntz, 1976.

Motoyama, Hiroshi. *Science and the Evolution of Consciousness.* Brookline, Mass.: Autumn Press, 1978.

Muktananda, Swami. *Guru.* New York: Harper & Row, 1971. Reprinted in expanded edition as *Play of Consciousness.* Oakland, Calif.: SYDA Foundation, 1974.

Mumford, John. *Sexual Occultism.* St. Paul, Minn.: Llewellyn, 1975.

Narayanananda, Swami. *The Primal Power in Man or the Kundalini Shakti.* Rishikesh, India: Narayanananda Universal Yoga Trust, 1970.

Pandit, M. P. *Kundalini Yoga: A Brief Study of Sir John Woodroffe's "The Serpent Power."* Madras, India: Ganesh & Co., 1968.

Peck, Robert L. *American Meditation.* Box 251, Windham Center, Conn. 06280, privately printed, 1976.

Radha, Swami Sivananda. *Kundalini: Yoga for the West.* Timeless Books: 1215 Washington Mutual Bldg., West 601 Main Avenue, Spokane, Wash. 99201, 1978.

Rajneesh, Bhagwan Shree. *Dynamics of Meditation.* Bombay, India: Life Awakening Center, 1973.

Rele, Vasant G. *The Mysterious Kundalini.* Bombay, India: D. B. Taraporevala Sons, 1970.

Sannella, Lee. *Kundalini: Psychosis or Transcendence?* San Francisco, Calif.: H. S. Dakin, 1976.

Saraswati, Paramahans Satyananda. *Tantra of Kundalini Yoga.* Monghyr, India: Bihar School of Yoga, 1973.

Sharma, Y. Subbaraya. *Sri Kundalini Sakthi–Serpent Power.* Bangalore, India: privately printed, 1971.

Sivananda, Swami. *Kundalini Yoga.* Sivanangagar, U.P., India: Divine Life Society, 1971.

Thompson, William Irwin. *Passages Around Earth.* New York: Harper & Row, 1974.

Tirtha, Swami Vishnu. *Devatman Shakti (Kundalini) Divine*

Power. Delhi, India: Swami Shivom Tirth, 1974.

Wolfe, W. Thomas. *And the Sun Is Up: Kundalini Rises in the West*. Academy Hill Press (292 Academy Hill Road, Red Hook, N.Y. 12571), 1978.

Woodroffe, Sir John. *The Serpent Power*. Madras, India: Ganesh & Co., 1974.

PERIODICALS

Beads of Truth
3HO Foundation
1620 Preuss Road
Los Angeles, Calif. 90035

Official voice of Yogi Bhajan's organization and approach to kundalini yoga.

Human Dimensions
Human Dimensions Institute
4620 West Lake Road
Canandaigua, N.Y. 14424

Vol. 5, No. 3, 1976 is a special issue on kundalini containing some of the articles included here.

Kundalini Quarterly
Kundalini Research Institute
P.O. Box 1020
Claremont, Calif. 91711

Official voice of the research arm of Yogi Bhajan's 3HO Foundation. Publishes research data and kundalini-related articles.

Spiritual India and Kundalini
"Shanti Villa"
1615 Madarsa Road
Kashmere Gate
Delhi 110006, India

Official voice of Gopi Krishna's research organization, and also an outlet for the views of others interested in the pursuit of kundalini research. Published quarterly. Available through the Kundalini Research Foundation

Ltd., Bio-Energy Research Foundation, and Kundalini Research Institute of Canada (see addresses listed below), and can be purchased directly by subscription.

SPECIAL ARTICLES

Campbell, Joseph. "Kundalini Yoga: Seven Levels of Consciousness," *Psychology Today,* Vol. 9, No. 7, Dec. 1975.

Jung, Carl. "Psychological Commentary on Kundalini Yoga," *Spring* 1975 (Part I) and 1976 (Part II). Transcript of a seminar given in 1932. Available from Spring Publications, 28 East 39th Street, New York, N.Y. 10016.

Krishna, Gopi. "Beyond the Higher States of Consciousness," New York *Times,* Oct. 6, 1973.

White, John. "Kundalini Research," *Psychic,* Vol. 7, No. 6, Jan.–Feb. 1977.

——. "Sex and Sublime Awareness," *Human Behavior,* Vol. 6, No. 8, Aug. 1977.

ORGANIZATIONS

Allahabad Institute for Kundalini Research
28 Hamilton Road
Georgetown, Allahabad 2110002
U. P., India
Dr. Jamuna Prasad, Director

Collects documentary case histories of people who claim to have an awakened kundalini, and investigates such cases within northern India. Submission of cases is requested.

Bio-Energy Research Foundation
P.O. Box 1846
Rancho Santa Fe, Calif. 92067
George Tompkins, Director

Supports the work of Gopi Krishna and promotes the

concept of kundalini research. Offers books and tapes (audio and video cassettes) of Gopi Krishna's discourses for sale. Organizes discussion groups in Southern California on the scientific and spiritual implications of kundalini research. Distributes *Spiritual India and Kundalini* magazine.

Center for Spiritual Awareness
P.O. Box 7
Lakemont, Ga. 30552
Roy Eugene Davis, Spiritual Director

Offers literature, books, and instruction in meditation and yoga from the lineage of Paramahansa Yogananda. Publishes *Truth Journal.*

Central Institute for Kundalini Research
14 Karan Nagar
Srinagar, Kashmir
India
Gopi Krishna, Director

Sponsors kundalini research, both scientific and scholarly, which it disseminates through books, tapes, conference proceedings and a journal, *Spiritual India and Kundalini.* North American affiliates: Bio-Energy Research Foundation, Kundalini Research Foundation Ltd., and Kundalini Research Institute of Canada.

Himalayan International Institute
R.D. 1
Honesdale, Pa. 18431
Swami Rama, Spiritual Director

Offers literature, books, instruction, and therapy based on yoga in combination with Western psychophysical and medical practices.

Kripalu Ashram
2970 Russell Street
Berkeley, Calif. 94705
Yogeshwar Muni, Spiritual Director

Offers literature and instruction in shaktipat kundalini yoga as taught by Yogeshwar Muni in the lineage of Swami Kripalvananda.

Kripalu Yoga Ashram
7 Walters Road
Sumneytown, Pa. 18084
Yogi Amrit Desai, Spiritual Director

Offers literature and instruction in shaktipat kundalini yoga as taught by Yogi Amrit Desai in the lineage of Swami Kripalvananda.

The Kundalini Clinic
5532 Fremont Street
Oakland, Calif. 94608
Lee Sannella, M.D., Director of Research

Offers a five-member staff of psychiatrists, psychologists, and therapists who work with imbalanced individuals undergoing the kundalini process. Services include differential diagnosis, short-term therapy, and a referral to other resources as needed. The clinic operates a residence center nearby for a small number of persons needing special attention.

Kundalini Research Foundation Ltd.
475 Fifth Avenue
New York, N.Y. 10016
Gene Kieffer, President

Dedicated to the dissemination of information on kundalini, based on documentary and scientific research. Affiliated with the Central Institute for Kundalini Research, the Foundation cooperates with similar organizations and individuals to support research and publish findings. Offers literature, books, and tapes (audio and video cassettes) of Gopi Krishna's discourses, as well as the quarterly magazine, *Spiritual India and Kundalini.*

Kundalini Research Institute
P.O. Box 1020
Claremont, Calif. 91711
and
Kundalini Research Institute/East
411 Marlborough Street
Boston, Mass. 02115
M. S. S. Gurucharan Singh Khalsa, Director of Research
The research arms of Yogi Bhajan's 3HO Foundation. Publishes *Kundalini Quarterly* journal.

Kundalini Research Institute of Canada
9 Richmond Street, East
Suite 403
Toronto, Ont. M5C 1NE
Canada
Joseph Dippong, President
Supports the work of Gopi Krishna and promotes the concept of kundalini research. Offers literature, books, and tapes (audio and video cassettes) of Gopi Krishna's discourses for sale. Distributes *Spiritual India and Kundalini* magazine.

Personal Development Center
P.O. Box 251
Windham Center, Conn. 06280
Robert L. Peck, President
Offers courses in meditation and yoga.

Queens Siddha Yoga Meditation Center
68-20 Selfridge Street
Forest Hills, N.Y. 11375
Don. R. Butler, Spiritual Director
Offers a correspondence course in siddha yoga from the lineage of Swami Muktananda.

Sanatana Dharma Foundation
3100 White Sulphur Springs Road
St. Helena, Calif. 94574
Yogeshwar Muni, Spiritual Director

Offers literature, counseling, and instruction in shaktipat kundalini yoga as taught by Yogeshwar Muni in the lineage of Swami Kripalvananda.

Siddha Yoga Dham
324 West 86th Street
New York, N.Y. 10024

Primary center in the eastern United States for literature and instruction in siddha yoga as taught by Swami Muktananda.

SYDA Foundation
1107 Stanford Avenue
P.O. Box 11071
Oakland, Calif. 94611
Swami Muktananda, Spiritual Director

National headquarters for Swami Muktananda's U.S. mission. Provides literature and a listing of more than two hundred centers/ashrams throughout the United States where instruction in Swami Muktananda's approach to kundalini, called siddha yoga, may be obtained.

3HO Drug Program
1050 North Cherry Avenue
Tucson, Ariz. 85719

Offers residential drug detoxification and drug/alcohol rehabilitation programs and research data based on kundalini yoga as taught by Yogi Bhajan. Also offers workshops and training courses in these techniques throughout the United States.

3HO Foundation
1620 Preuss Road
Los Angeles, Calif. 90035
Yogi Bhajan, Spiritual Director

Offers literature and instruction in kundalini yoga and tantra as taught by Yogi Bhajan. Publishes *Beads of*

Truth journal. Has more than one hundred centers and ashrams affiliated with it throughout the United States.

University of the Trees
P.O. Box 644
Boulder Creek, Calif. 95006
Christopher Hills, Spiritual Director

Offers literature, books, spiritual instruments, tapes, and instruction (through correspondence and residence courses) in meditation and Nuclear Evolution as developed by Christopher Hills.

Yasodhara Ashram
P.O. Box 9
Kootenay Bay, B.C. VOB 1XO
Canada
Swami Sivananda Radha, Spiritual Director

Offers literature, records, tapes, books, and instruction in meditation and yoga. Holds annual seminars and workshops, including kundalini yoga, to explore topics of relevance to spiritual living and modern life.

About the Authors

Swami Ajaya (Allan Weinstock), Ph.D., was trained in clinical psychology and has been a consultant to several mental health centers. He was ordained a monk in the order of Shankaracharya by his guru, Swami Rama. The author of *Yoga Psychology, Levels of Consciousness* and co-author (with Swami Rama and Rudolph Ballentine) of *Yoga and Psychotherapy*, Swami Ajaya has traveled widely, studying with various sages of India. He lives in Madison, Wisconsin.

George S. Arundale was the third international president of the Theosophical Society, succeeding Annie Besant in 1934. A native of England, he went to India at the turn of the century, where he held a series of teaching positions, among them that of professor of history at Central Hindu College in Benares. He is the author of *Kundalini: An Occult Experience* and *Nirvana*.

ALICE A. BAILEY was founder of the Lucis Trust and author/ channel of many books on esoteric wisdom. The Lucis Trust, located in New York City, conducts activities dedicated to the establishment of right human relations by promoting the education and the expansion of the human mind toward practice of spiritual disciplines and values.

ITZHAK BENTOV, author of *Stalking the Wild Pendulum*, was a biomedical inventor.

YOGI BHAJAN, formally known as Siri Singh Sahib Bhai Sahib Harbhajan Singh Khalsa Yogiji, is the chief religious and administrative authority for the Sikh Dharma in the Western Hemisphere. He teaches kundalini yoga at UCLA and is founder-director of the 3HO Foundation in Los Angeles. Many of his discourses are collected in *The Teachings of Yogi Bhajan*.

D. R. BUTLER is an American yogi who devotes full time to students of his correspondence course in siddha yoga. He is a disciple of Swami Muktananda and lives in Forest Hills, New York, where he directs the Queens Siddha Yoga Meditation Center.

HARIDIS CHAUDHURI, Ph.D., was founder and (until his death in 1975) president of the California Institute of Asian Studies in San Francisco. A disciple of Sri Aurobindo, he wrote more than a dozen books and fifty articles, including *The Evolution of Integral Consciousness, The Philosophy of Meditation, Integral Yoga,* and *Being, Evolution and Immortality*.

SRI CHINMOY teaches the path of love, devotion, and surrender to God. Born in 1931, he came to the West in 1964 to establish centers for self-realization. He has written more than three hundred books. Presently located in New York, with centers in sixty cities around the world, Sri Chinmoy serves as director of the United Nations Meditation Group, conducting meditations twice a week for UN delegates and staff.

Roy Eugene Davis is a spiritual teacher in the tradition of his guru, Paramahansa Yogananda. Ordained by Yogananda in 1951, he founded and resides at the Center for Spiritual Awareness. His many books, including *Yoga Darsana* and *God Has Given Us Many Good Things*, extend his teaching to the public. He also travels widely to lecture and teach yoga meditation.

Yogi Amrit Desai is founder and spiritual leader of the Kripalu Health Center in Lenox, Massachusetts. He was initiated into Yoga at age sixteen by his guru, Swami Kripalvananda, who was widely regarded in India as a master of kundalini yoga. Yogi Desai has a B.F.A. degree from Philadelphia College of Art and has lived in the United States since 1960.

Marilyn Ferguson is editor-publisher of *Brain/Mind Bulletin* and author of *The Brain Revolution* and *The Aquarian Conspiracy*.

Erik Floor, Ph.D., is a biochemist. He has done research in neurochemistry, psychophysiology, and genetics at Harvard University, Harvard Medical School, and Massachusetts Institute of Technology.

John R. M. Goyeche, Ph.D., is a psychologist who has experiential knowledge of yoga. He is a member of the Department of Psychiatry at Kurume University in Japan.

Kenneth Grant is author of *Cults of the Shadow, Aleister Crowley and the Hidden God*, and *The Magical Revival*. He lives in England.

Christopher Hills is a British-born scientist-yogi who founded the University of the Trees in Boulder Creek, California. He studied yoga under his guru, Swami Shantananda, in India in the 1960s. In 1970 Hills was elected president of the first World Conference on Scientific Yoga, which was attended by eight hundred yogis and fifty scientists. Hills is the author of many books, including *Nuclear Evolution* and *Supersensonics*.

TONTYN HOPMAN was born in Holland and studied Jungian psychology in Zurich. In 1952 he contacted Gopi Krishna in Kashmir, and later induced him to write his autobiography, *Kundalini*. Hopman published the first edition himself. He worked with Gopi Krishna as secretary of the Central Institute for Kundalini Research.

M.S.S. GURUCHARAN SINGH KHALSA, Ph.D. is a psychotherapist, Director of the Yoga Center in Wellesley, Massachusetts, and a current researcher for and a member of the Board of Directors of the International Kundalini Research Institute, affiliated with the 3HO Foundation, founded by Yogi Bhajan.

SADHU SINGH KHALSA is a researcher at the Kundalini research Institute in Claremont, California, where he specializes in clinical and psychological studies. He earned a master's degree in clinical psychology at Pepperdine University.

GENE KIEFFER is president of the Kundalini Research Institute, which he founded in 1970 to promote the work of Gopi Krishna.

GOPI KRISHNA was founder-director of the Central Institute for Kundalini Research in Srinagar, Kashmir. He was author of many books and articles, including the autobiographical *Kundalini, The Secret of Yoga, Higher Consciousness, The Awakening of Kundalini*, and *The Dawn of a New Science*. He died in 1984.

PHILIP LANSKY holds a B.A. in psychophysiology and an M.D. degree from the University of Pennsylvania. He has lectured on the physiology of consciousness at Tufts University and the East West foundation.

MINEDA J. MCCLEAVE describes herself as 'a friend of God and a friend of Christ.' She lives in Davenport, Iowa where she continues her research and shares her findings with people via correspondence.

Vasant V. Merchant, Ph.D., is an educational consultant and associate professor of Humanities at Northern Arizona University in Flagstaff. She has published a number of articles and lectured extensively around the world on the philosophy and teaching of Sri Aurobino and The Mother.

Swami Muktananda taught the path of siddha yoga. His principle ashram is in Ganeshpuri, India, but he has other ashrams and meditation centers in the United States. He granted shaktipat (the direct transmission of energy) to the readied aspirant, which awakens the kundalini energy. His spiritual teachings are published in many books, the primary one being the autobiographical *Guru (Play of Consciousness)*. He died in 1983.

Geoffrey Nicoletti, formerly a graduate student of theology at Villanova University, was a National Collegiate Poetry winner in 1968. His poetry and religious articles have been published in Europe and India.

M. P. Pandit is editor of *World Union* magazine, published by the Sri Aurobindo Ashram in Pondicherry, India. A disciple of Sri Aurobino for more than forty years, Pandit published dozens of books on yoga, spiritual psychology and higher consciousness.

Robert L. Peck is a physicist and teacher in meditation and yoga. He founded the Personal Development Center in Windham, Connecticut, which he directs. He is also developing advanced technology for New Age living.

James Morgan Pryse was a Theosophist who worked with its founder H. P. Blavatsky, as a staff member at the London Theosophical Society headquarters at the turn of the century. Among his books are *Reincarnation in the New Testament* and *The Apocalypse Unsealed*.

Swami Sivananda Radha is founder and spiritual leader of the Yasodhara Ashram in Kootenay Bay, British Columbia (see Appendix). She received her yogic training at the ashram of her guru,

Swami Sivananda, in Rishikesh, India, in the mid-1950s. Her books include *Kundalini: Yoga for the West and Hatha Yoga: The Hidden Language*. She travels widely, lecturing and teaching yoga and meditation.

SWAMI RAMA was ordained a monk in his early childhood and lived in Himalayan International Institute in Honesdale, Pennsylvania. As a subject for psychophysiology studies, he has been tested extensively in many laboratory situations. He is author or co-author of nearly a dozen books, including *Yoga and Psychotherapy, Lectures on Yoga*, and *Superconscious Meditation*. His spiritual adventures are recorded in his autobiographical *Living with the Himalayan Masters*.

LEE SANNELLA, M.D., a psychiatirst and ophthalmologist in Middletown, California, founded the Kundalini Clinic in Oakland, California, which was designed to help people undergoing kundalini experiences balance themselves holistically.

JOHN SCUDDER may be contacted at P.O. Box 142, Homewood, Illinois 60430.

SWAMI VISHNU TIRTHA lives in Bombay and holds M.A. and LL.B. degrees.

BRIAN VAN DER HORST was formerly a staff writer for the Village Voice newspaper and a columnist for *Playboy* magazine. He is now manager of the Public Information Office for *est*, an educational corporation.

KEN WILBUR is author of *The Spectrum of Consciousness, No Boundary, The Atman Project* and many other books on transpersonal psychology and consciousness studies. He was editor of *Re-Vision Journal*. He completed course requirements for a Ph.D. degree in biochemistry. He lives in Boulder, Colorado.

PAUL ZWEIG is a writer and poet. He also teaches and is chairman of the Department of Comparative Literature at Queens College, New York City.